AF659890

Second Edition

Kundu's Practical Medicine

An overview of physical examination

As per the latest CBME Guidelines |
Competency based Undergraduate Curriculum for the Indian Medical Graduate

Other Books/Chapters by the Same Author

- *Bedside Clinics in Medicine,* Part I (9th Ed), 2024
- *Bedside Clinics in Medicine,* Part II (9th Ed), 2024
- *Pearls in Medicine* (3rd Ed), 2024
- *MCQs in Internal Medicine* (6th Ed), 2022
- *Memorable Memoirs of a Medico,* 2023 (on Amazon portal)

Chapters in:

- *API Textbook of Medicine,* 8th Ed, 2008
- *Postgraduate Medicine,* 2009
- *Rheumatology: Principles and Practice,* 2010
- *Medicine Update*: 2010-15, 2017, 2018, 2021–2024
- *Progress in Medicine,* 2016, 2019, 2020, 2023, 2024
- *Manual of Rheumatology:* 5th Ed, 2018 & 6th Ed, 2024
- Online Appendix of "Kumar & Clark's" textbook, *Clinical Medicine,* 6–10th Ed

Biography (Author)

- Included in *Marquis Who's Who in the World* 2014, 2015, 2016
- *Who's Who in Science and Engineering* 2016-17, and Wikipedia & WikiVisually
- Gifted Teacher Awardee 2022 (by Central API)

Fellow/Member of

- Fellow, Indian College of Physicians (India)
- Fellow, Royal College of Physicians (Edinburgh)
- Member, New York Academy of Sciences (USA)
- Member, International Advisory Panel of "Kumar & Clark's" textbook, *Clinical Medicine,* 7th–10th Ed (Edinburgh)
- Life-member, Association of Physicians of India (API)
- Life-member, Indian Rheumatology Association (IRA)
- Life-member, Indian Medical Association (IMA)

Second Edition

Kundu's Practical Medicine

An overview of physical examination

Arup Kumar Kundu MD, FRCP, FICP, MNAS
Ex-Visiting Faculty and Consultant Rheumatologist
IQ City Medical College
West Bengal, India

Formerly
Professor of Medicine and
In-charge, Division of Rheumatology
NRS MC, KPC MC, IQ City MC, and
RG Kar Medical College, West Bengal, India

and

Thirty years of teaching experience in Govt and private medical colleges
UG and PG examiner in West Bengal and different Indian universities
Prestigious 'Gifted Teacher' awardee in 2022 by API
Biography included in Marquis Who's Who in the World 2014, 2015, 2016
Member, IAP of "Kumar & Clark's" Textbook, 'Clinical Medicine', 7th–10th Ed
Mentor and Instructional Coach, pan-India for teaching in MBBS, MD, DNB

CBSPD

CBS Publishers & Distributors Pvt Ltd

New Delhi • Bengaluru • Chennai • Kochi • Kolkata • Lucknow • Mumbai
Gujarat • Hyderabad • Jharkhand • Nagpur • Patna • Pune • Uttarakhand

Disclaimer

Science and technology are constantly changing fields. New research and experience broaden the scope of information and knowledge. The author has tried his best in giving information available to him while preparing the material for this book. Although all efforts have been made to ensure optimum accuracy of the material, yet it is quite possible some errors might have been left uncorrected. The publisher, the printer and the author will not be held responsible for any inadvertent errors, omissions or inaccuracies.

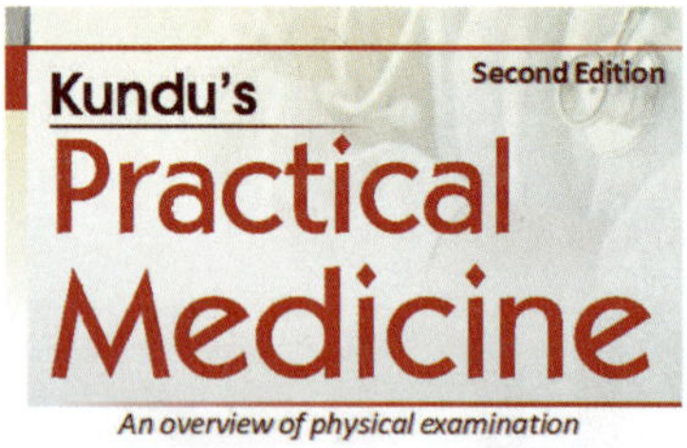

ISBN: 978-93-5466-632-2

Copyright © Author and Publisher

Second Edition 2024
Reprint 2025
First Edition 2023

All rights reserved. No part of this book may be reproduced or transmitted in any form or by any means, electronic or mechanical, including photocopying, recording, or any information storage and retrieval system without permission, in writing, from the author and the publisher.

Published by **Satish Kumar Jain** and produced by **Varun Jain** for

CBS Publishers & Distributors Pvt Ltd
4819/XI Prahlad Street, 24 Ansari Road, Daryaganj, New Delhi 110 002, India.
Ph: 011-23289259, 23266861 Website: www.cbspd.com e-mail: delhi@cbspd.com

Corporate Office: 204 FIE, Industrial Area, Patparganj, Delhi 110 092
Ph: 011-4934 4934 Fax: 011-4934 4935
e-mail: publishing@cbspd.com; publicity@cbspd.com

Branches

- **Bengaluru:** Seema House 2975, 17th Cross, KR Road, Banasankari 2nd Stage, Bengaluru 560 070, Karnataka, India
  Ph: +91-80-26771678/79 Fax: +91-80-26771680 e-mail: bangalore@cbspd.com
- **Chennai:** 7, Subbaraya Street, Shenoy Nagar, Chennai 600 030, Tamil Nadu, India
  Ph: +91-44-26680620, 26681266 Fax: +91-44-42032115 e-mail: chennai@cbspd.com
- **Kochi:** 42/1325, 1326, Power House Road, Opp KSEB, Power House, Ernakulum Kochi 682 018, Kerala, India
  Ph: +91-484-4059061-65,67 Fax: +91-484-4059065 e-mail: kochi@cbspd.com
- **Kolkata:** 147, Hind Ceramics Compound, 1st Floor, Nilgunj Road, Belghoria, Kolkata-700056, West Bengal, India
  Ph: +033-25633055, 033-25633056 e-mail: kolkata@cbspd.com
- **Lucknow:** Basement, Khushnuma Complex, 7 Meerabai Marg (Behind Jawahar Bhawan),Lucknow-226001, UP, India
  Ph: +0522-4000032 e-mail: tiwari.lucknow@cbspd.com
- **Mumbai:** PWD Shed, Gala no 25/26, Ramchandra Bhatt Marg, Next to JJ Hospital Gate no. 2, Opp. Union Bank of India, Noorbaug, Mumbai-400009, Maharashtra, India
  Ph: 022-66661880/89 e-mail: mumbai@cbspd.com

Representatives

- Gujarat 0-9879558667
- Hyderabad 0-9885175004
- Jharkhand 0-9811541605
- Nagpur 0-8692091830
- Patna 0-9334159340
- Pune 0-9664372571
- Uttarakhand 0-9716462459

Printed at: HT Media Ltd, Greater Noida, UP, India

to

My wife Bijoya
for being tolerant, supportive and bearing with my shortcomings all through life, and it is she who always comforts and consoles but never complains or interferes, and

All the students
generations of medical students past, present and future, for their constant inspiration to fulfil my irresistible desire for gaining and sharing knowledge

"Acquire the art of detachment, the virtue of method, and the quality of thoroughness, but above all the grace of humility"

—Sir William Osler (1849–1919)

Canadian physician, Professor of Medicine (Oxford, UK), author, educator, historian and bibliophile who is one of the greatest icons of modern medicine

Preface to the Second Edition

In view of the wide acceptance of the first edition by the medical fraternity, I have ultimately succeeded to bring out the second edition of the book. My intention is to re-orient the students to identify the basic message of the monograph, that is, to depict the real situations and events present in the text, rather than just ideas and theories. The title of the book initiates an impact on the mind of medical students for better understanding of the practical part of medicine. This part of medical science, a simplified approach to practical medicine, is to be practiced by a doctor throughout his/her life.

The intention of writing *Kundu's Practical Medicine* is to groom and prime young medical students from their earlier days in undergraduate curriculum. Teaching a large number of students for more than 30 years made me realise the need for such a kind of book which is lucid, concise, updated and student-friendly. The skill of communication, clinical examination, objective assessment and planning of treatment can only be gained by learning and practice. This book is full of clinical methods and truly exam-oriented. It is a book for quick review and to achieve a basic grip on the practical part of medicine. This book attempts to present all clinical topics required for a modern, clinical curriculum with easy access to major clinical information for medical students.

Though there is a tremendous change in medical practice with a battery of investigations entering into the medical field in every moment, we cannot ignore the importance of face-to-face consultation as well as examination of the patient. One should appreciate that the improved technologies like internet, fax, e-mail, digitalisation, spiral CT scanning, or wireless capsule endoscopy, can never be a substitute for clinically examining a patient which is known as "Practical Medicine".

I expect that the unique narrative style of the book will allay apprehension of the students for the subject of medicine. I presume that this book will help the students to make their eyes 'watchful', ears 'alert', fingers 'tactful', while making the mind 'logical'.

The book contains more than 200 very lively and appealing clinical photographs, multiple tables and charts, line drawings and bulleted lists for quick reference to increase the clinical skills. I think, the present monograph will help the young medical students, dental students, nurses, and a range of other healthcare professionals, while the clinical tutors will find it a helpful source for learning and teaching.

This work would not have been possible without the constant encouragement of my family members, especially to speak of my son Dr Abhishek, wife Bijoya, and my daughter Ushasi, which ultimately made this book a reality. I acknowledge the sincere help extended by Dr Krishnendu Dey who has given some clinical photographs for the book and Mr Ramkrishna Sharma for preparing the colour atlases. I also record my appreciation to Mr Satish Kumar Jain, Chairman and Managing Director, and Mr Varun Jain, Director, CBS Publishers & Distributors for publishing and distributing the book to the students all over India and abroad. Mr YN Arjuna, Senior Vice President (Publishing Editorial and Publicity), CBS Publishers & Distributors, needs special mention for his cooperation to bring out this book in an engrossing look.

Healthy suggestions and constructive criticism from students, teachers, or any thoughtful reader through e-mail to me or the publisher will be received with gratitude.

Dear students, I wish you the very best in your new adventure.

Arup Kumar Kundu
arup2158@gmail.com
arup_kundu@hotmail.com

Contents

Chapter 1

Introduction

It is customary that the 1st year curriculum at the medical school begins with a study of anatomy through laboratory dissection, and its processes at the molecular and cellular level. Along with this embryology, genetics, cellular biology, biochemistry and physiology are also taught concurrently in this time span of 1st year.

In different parts of the world, it is observed that from the 1st year study of *Essentials of Clinical Medicine (with foundation of medicine)* has been included in the curriculum which is an introduction to clinical medicine, including basic patient interview and hypothesis-driven physical examination techniques. In many countries, physician-patient-society-system (P2S2) with clinical skills and doctor–patient relationship are taught. Essentials of Clinical Medicine teaches the art of taking history of medicine, continues the clinical skills development and critical thinking, and explores ethics and professionalism. Thus, it is unequivocal and leaves no doubt that undergraduate students should be well-conversant with basic clinical medicine from the earlier days in their medical school which will help them to build the foundation of medicine in future.

This monograph, which will guide the students extensively to understand a difficult science like medicine, should be completed within first 1 to 2 years in medical school. Students should try to corroborate the clinical link of anatomy, physiology and biochemistry (e.g., the applied anatomy) with the living patient holding the hand of 'clinical medicine'.

PROLOGUE

INSTRUMENTS/TOOLS/APPLIANCES TO CARRY IN THE CLINICAL ROTATION

1. Stethoscope, preferably double-tube
2. Blood pressure machine (aneroid or spring dial type, as it is smaller and lighter)
3. Percussion hammer
4. Pencil torch
5. Tongue depressor (or, spatula)
6. Pins, cotton, measuring tape, skin pencil, clinical thermometer
7. Apron (preferably, half-sleeve).

All the kits should be kept in a small and handy plastic box blended with *intense desire to learn and thirst for knowledge* from the very first day.

KNOW YOUR HOSPITAL

Just try to be acquainted with the 'world of sufferings and illness'. Remember, your hospital is a temple where you are a simple priest; so maintain its sanctity.

KNOW THE CROWD IN YOUR HOSPITAL

They are either the patients or their relatives/accompanying persons/third party. Hospital staffs are always there to extend their help to this crowd who seeks help.

KNOW YOUR TARGET

A great son of India, a Bharat Ratna, Dr Bidhan Chandra Roy (Dr BC Roy), MD, MRCP, FRCS once commented that you doctor may treat your patients by allopathy, homeopathy or naturopathy but you should always keep some 'empathy' for them. Learn the subject and translate it into 'healing touch' for the patients.

KNOW YOUR TEACHER

He/she is an experienced and trusted adviser. He/she is your educator, pedagogue, instructor, tutor, master, and remember he will be your ultimate mentor. In the medical field, a teacher holds the position of a 'parent outside the home'.

KNOW YOUR PATIENT

The patients are the living pages of your book.

They are cured by receiving treatment from team of doctors, while the medical students are being benefitted by the sufferings of the patients (a mutual exploitation!).

KNOW YOUR STETHOSCOPE

It was discovered in the year 1816 by a French physician named RTH Laennec (1781–1826). Worldwide, stethoscope symbolises a doctor. It has four parts like:

1. *Chest piece:* It has two parts, i.e., diaphragm (larger round part) and bell (smaller round part or conical part). The diaphragm helps to hear the different heart sounds, breath sounds, murmurs, etc. The bell is for low-frequency sounds like third or fourth heart sounds, foetal heart sounds, or murmur of mitral stenosis. In the initial days, a student may find difficulty to listen sounds with a bell, and thus they are advised to use the diaphragm more in clinical classes. Stethoscopes from renowned companies like Littman, Sprague or Leatham give better audibility (and, costly too!) in all variety of sounds (Fig. 1.1).
2. *Connecting tube:* A single or double tube connects the head piece with the chest piece.
3. *Head piece:* There are two metal tubes in the head piece which are attached together by a metallic U-connector.
4. *Ear piece:* Two plastic ear pieces are attached in two metal tubes of the head piece. Place the ear pieces in such a way, so that they are in the same line with your external auditory canal (actually needs a little practice for a few days).

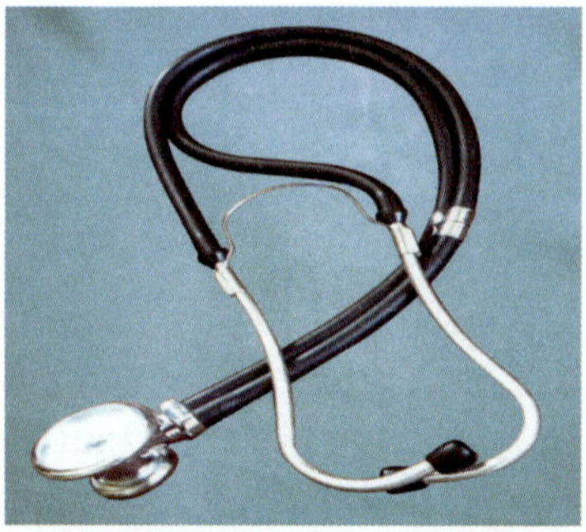

Fig. 1.1: Stethoscope

KNOW YOUR PERCUSSION HAMMER

This medical instrument was first used to examine the knee jerk (tendon reflex) to become a regular part of neurological examination, thus it is also known as patellar hammer (Fig. 1.2). It may be of rounded (plastic shaft with rounded rubber to strike) or conical (metallic shaft with conical rubber to strike) variety. It is basically used in patients of neurology to examine the deep reflexes (i.e., jerks), superficial reflexes (abdominal reflex or plantar response is examined by the blunt tip present at the end of the shaft), or fasciculation.

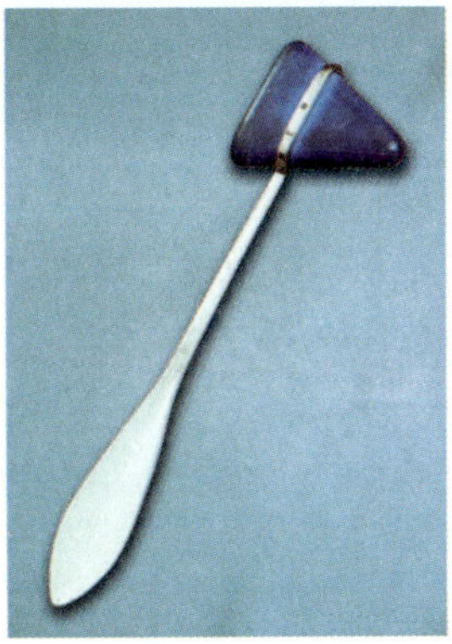

Fig. 1.2: Hammer

KNOW THESE LEGENDS AS WELL AS THE MEDICAL SYMBOLS/TERMS

There are many names/figures in history of medicine like Charaka and Sushruta, Hippocrates, RTH Laennec, WC Roentgen, Robert Koch, Sir William Osler, Willen Einthoven, Edward Jenner (discoverer of smallpox vaccine, the world's first vaccine), Ronald Ross (discovered life-cycle of malaria parasite), Alexander Fleming (discoverer of the world's first antibiotic, penicillin), Godfrey Hounsfield and so on, who have reduced the sufferings of the mankind by their outstanding skills and thereby saved crores of lives (Figs 1.3 to 1.10).

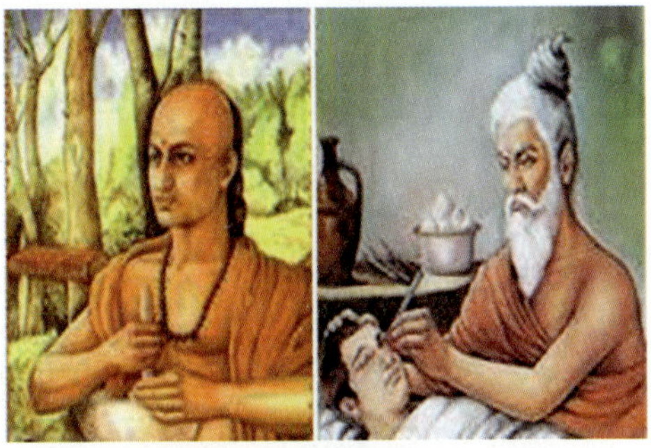

Fig. 1.3: Charaka and Sushruta—the pioneers in developing the medical science in ancient India

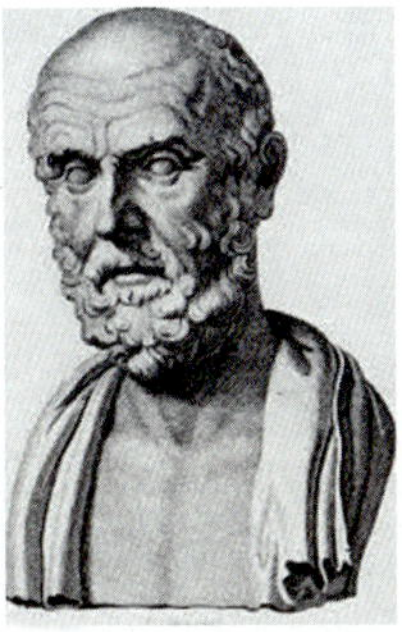

Fig. 1.4: Hippocrates (460-375 BC)—ancient Greek physician, known as 'Father of Medicine'

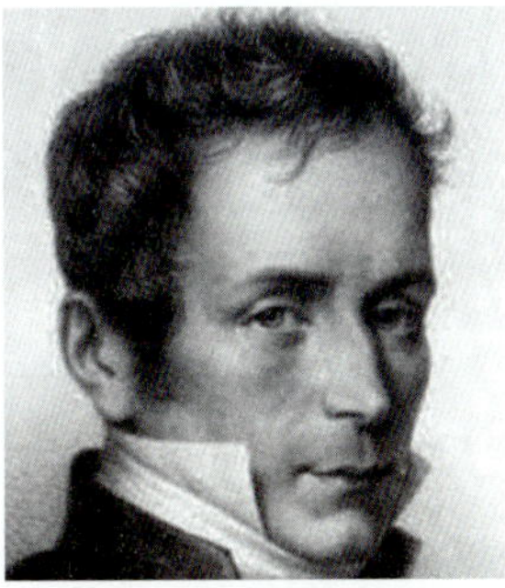

Fig. 1.5: RTH Laennec—the French physician who is the inventor of stethoscope in 1816

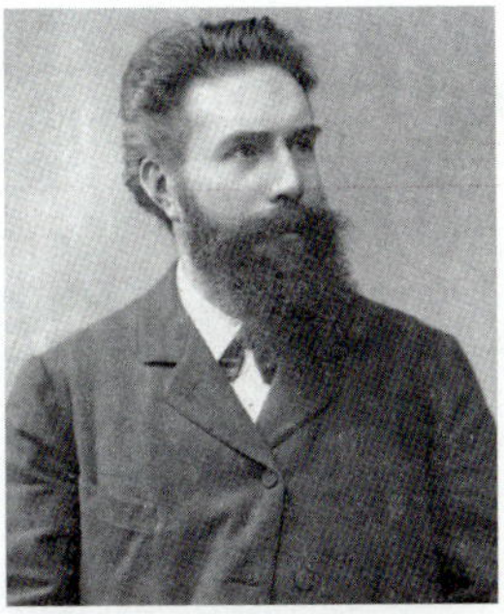

Fig. 1.6: WC Roentgen—the German mechanical engineer and physicist who discovered the X-ray

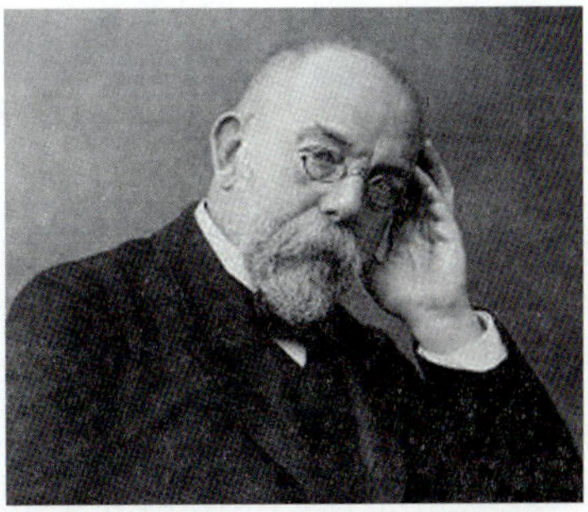

Fig. 1.7: Robert Koch—the German physician who discovered the cause of tuberculosis, the *Mycobacterium tuberculosis*

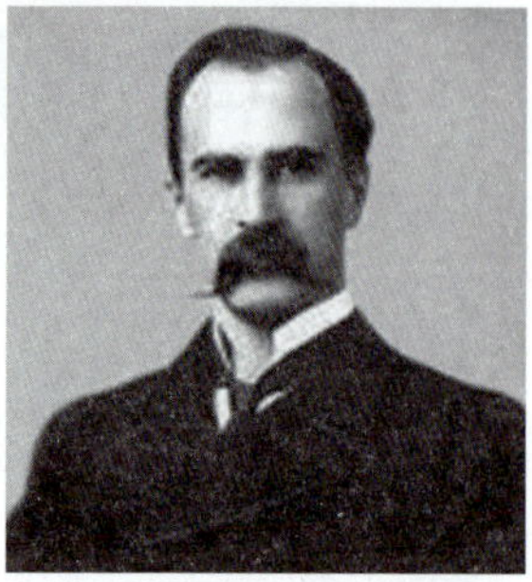

Fig. 1.8: Sir William Osler—the Canadian physician, known as 'Father of Modern Medicine'

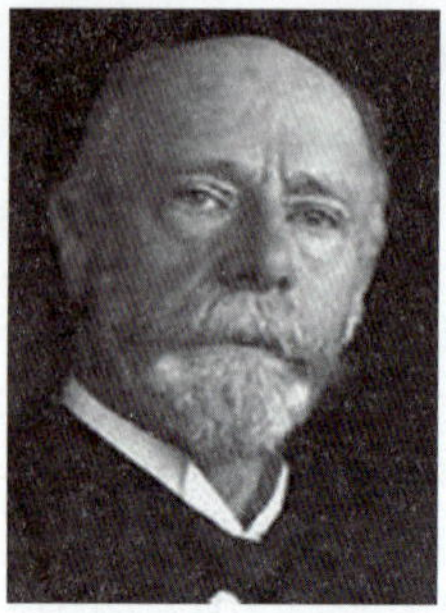

Fig. 1.9: Willem Einthoven—the Dutch doctor who invented the electrocardiography (ECG)

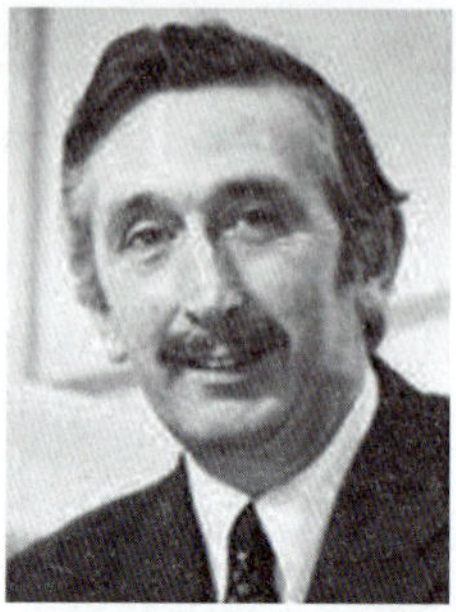

Fig. 1.10: Godfrey Hounsfield—the British electrical engineer who discovered computed tomographic (CT) scan

It is desirable that one student should be acquainted with different 'medical symbols in practice' like Caduceus, Asclepius and the Red Cross (Figs 1.11–1.13).

WHO (World Health Organisation), Geneva, Switzerland is the directing and coordinating authority for health within the United Nations system that is concerned with international public health. The goal of WHO is to build a better and healthier future for people all over the world.

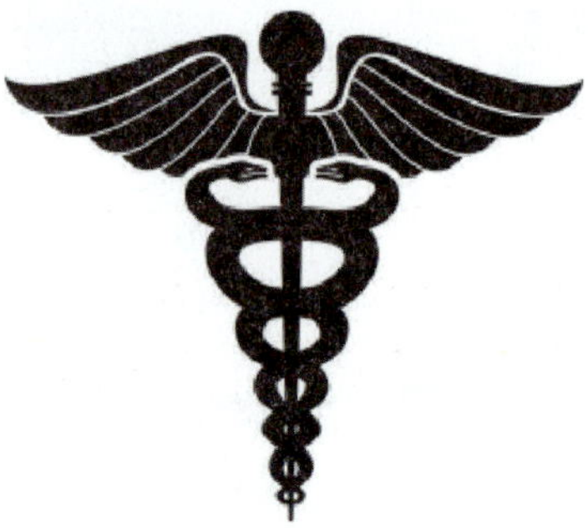

Fig. 1.11: The twin serpent, winged staff—Caduceus is the 'symbol of medicine'

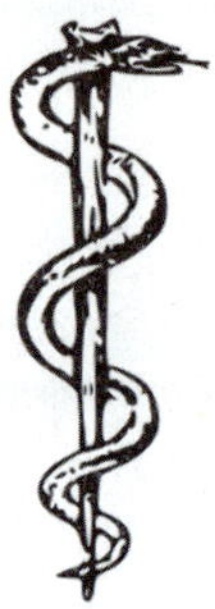

Fig. 1.12: Asclepius—the God of medicine and healing

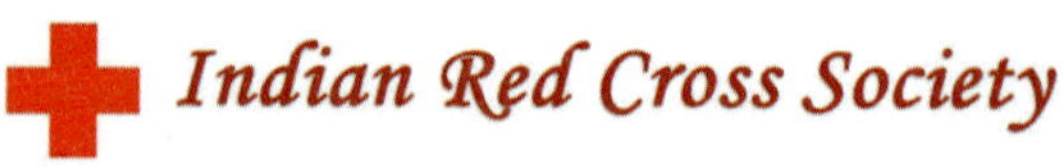

Fig. 1.13: The Red Cross—an international philanthropic organization (Red Cross Society) that cares for the wounded, sick, homeless in wartime, and during and following disasters (according to the Geneva Convention of 1864). The red cross sign should not be used by doctors, hospitals or in first-aid box

INTRODUCTION

In clinical medicine, the patient holds the key position; a 'patient' is one who feels sick physically or mentally, and seeks help of doctor for relief of his/her ailments. Clinical diagnosis is an artistic science, based on three pillars like:

1. History taking (inquiry),
2. Physical examination, and
3. Investigations

Clinical medicine deals with history taking and physical examination, jointly known as clinical examination. Medical events that have already taken place as well as taking place are known as 'history'; *history taking* is an art and is to be learned over years dedicating time at the bedside of the patient keeping patience in mind. In majority of cases, history alone can give clue to diagnosis (approximately, 75%), and builds up the beginning of a doctor–patient relationship. While examining the patients day by day, a doctor develops the keen 'power of observation' and tries to associate different observations and findings to penetrate the diagnosis, which is known as 'clinical eye'. Clinical medicine is otherwise considered as 'approach to the patient at the bedside'. A successful clinician must have sharp 'clinical acumen'.

The clinical state of the patient at the given time is determined by *physical examination*, which is divided customarily by four techniques into inspection (looking), palpation (feeling), percussion (tapping), and auscultation (listening). The physical examination using these four modalities like inspection (minute observations by your eyes), palpation (feeling by your hands), percussion (tapping by fingers or a percussion hammer), and auscultation (hearing different sounds by a stethoscope) are skills acquired by a student over years of sincere training, which also provides the physical contact that communicates a doctor's caring/healing touch to the patient, and helps to build up a doctor–patient relationship. In bedside clinical examination, the physicians use their senses along with traditional tools like stethoscope, sphygmomanometer (i.e., blood pressure measurement machine), thermometer, percussion hammer, measuring tape, etc. to understand and assess the patient, and to find out normal and abnormal signs. Diagnosis of a disease becomes very easy if one bridges basic medicine and clinical medicine.

Appropriate *investigations* assist the clinician to confirm the diagnosis made by clinical examination. Investigations like blood sugar/urea/creatinine, routine examination (R/E) of urine, sputum for AFB (acid-fast bacilli), different radiology (X-ray, ultrasound, CT scan, MRI scan), or even tissue biopsy helps to arrive at a definitive diagnosis. A student must learn to ask for 'rational investigations' related to the patient than to order for 'all investigations'.

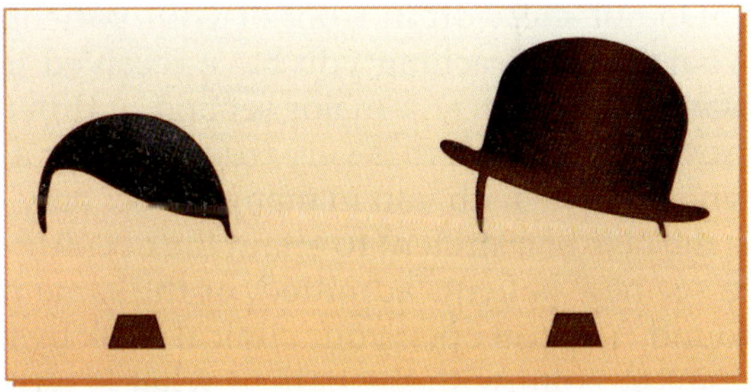

Fig. 1.14: The first picture is of Adolf Hitler and the second one is of Charlie Chaplin, where the hairstyle and the hat-style are sufficient to recognise them though the moustache-style is similar. Clinical medicine is just like this—one has to learn to diagnose diseases by the symbolic expression

It is an old connotation that 'doctors know more but see less'. Thus, remember these lines from the beginning of clinical training: *there is no substitute for watchful eyes, alert ears, and tactful fingers in a logical mind* (Fig. 1.14).

ADVICE TO BEGINNERS STARTING CLINICAL ROTATIONS

Try to learn the vocabulary and grammar of medicine. Clinical medicine cannot be learnt by sitting, reading and cramming in hostel room. If you want to be a driver, you have to sit on the driver's seat for learning with a trainer by your side; ultimately you watch and learn from the trainer driver. Clinical rotations are like this—you have a trainer (i.e., your teacher) who guides you in every aspect and teaches you hand to hand. Remember, you cannot learn the lessons of a driver by seating in the backseat of the car. Sometimes, to learn within a short span of clinical hours, you have to be aggressive and pushy.

Select your 'learning objectives'. Usually there are 1–2 good textbooks on clinical medicine. Ask your teachers, seniors and other students which one they recommend for you. Start with a basic clinical textbook with overview of the clinical topics along with a practical orientation.

Your strategy must be clear. Try to chalk out the major clinical topics and take regular class notes on them. You need not read the chapters in the order mentioned in the book, rather read them as you see patients in clinical classes. Be sure that all the topics are covered during the rotation time; if needed, request your teachers repeatedly from junior to senior ones.

Come early to the hospital, keep moving around in search of patients (so called 'cases'), and stay late if you want to be a professional in future.

Do not miss a single clinical rotation day, whether your teacher is good or bad. Remember, a very bad teacher knows more than you. Come with your apron (half-sleeve), stethoscope, hammer, torch, etc. Be polite, smart, gentle and courteous in your behaviour at the bedside. Be empathetic to your patient while taking history. Do not harass a patient who is in agonising abdominal pain or breathless. Do not hurt your patient physically or mentally; be careful about patient's physical and emotional needs, which enormously help to build-up the doctor–patient relationship. Always remember that you are a trainee and thus it is not wanted that you will divulge the prognosis (i.e., outcome or course of a disease) to the patient or his/her relatives.

Do not show-off in front of your patient. Make it a regular habit to read at home what clinical teaching you have received in the morning wards and just see by this way you can cover a major section of different diseases. 'Two is company, three is a crowd'—the proverb is very true, and thus always try to select 'a friend' or 'a classmate' who is at par with you in many aspect only to accompany you in the clinical wards; it is the task of a student to attain the evening round, either alone or with his/her friend to see new patients admitted, or the same patient which were taught in the morning round. You can open your clinical book by the side of the patient and can corroborate point to point with the patient what is written in the book. Practice 'history writing' repeatedly, and remember rehearsal of final examination starts from very first day of your clinics.

Do not rush to every Tom, Dick and Harry 'cases'. Stick to the 'must know' areas (e.g., details of anaemia) though you may peep through 'desirable to know' areas (e.g., exposure to cold may precipitate Raynaud's phenomenon in a patient suffering from scleroderma) but totally avoid 'nice to know' areas (e.g., pneumonoultramicroscopic-silicovolcanoconiosis is the largest medical word in the Oxford dictionary) in your earlier days of clinics.

Try to observe the black, tarry and offensive stool of melaena (do not hesitate to go to the bathroom with proper permission), coffee-ground vomiting of carcinoma of the stomach, rice-watery stool of cholera, turbid chalky-white urine (present in the urosac) of urinary tract infection, or sputum mixed with blood i.e., haemoptysis (just have a look in the sputum-bowl). Always take the opportunity to observe the procedure of inserting IV drip (Fig. 1.15) (i.e., device used for intravenous fluid infusion), blood transfusion or urinary catheterisation, Ryle's tube introduction, lumbar puncture to collect CSF, paracentesis thoracis (i.e., tapping of pleural fluid) or nebulisation in a patient with respiratory distress in the medical ward. Try to learn these from the very first day of your clinical training as much as you can; that means you should be passionate to learning during your clinical posting days.

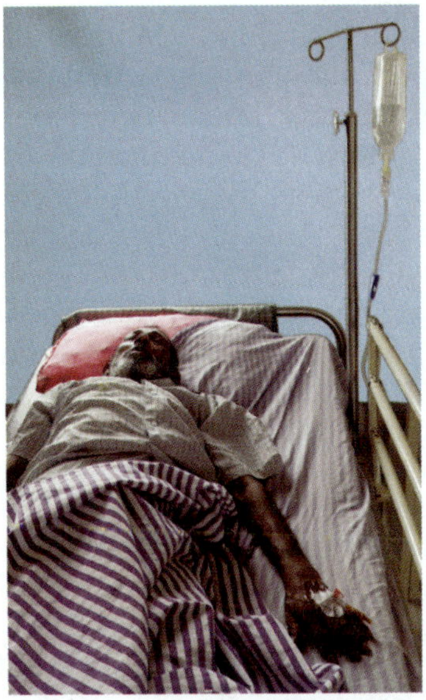

Fig. 1.15: Patient of gastroenteritis receiving IV saline drip in a city hospital—a very common picture in the hospital

Every day, a student will have to learn many new medical terms at the beginning like 'agammaglobulinaemia', which means 'absence of gamma globulin in blood'—where 'a' means absence, 'mia' means 'related to blood'. One student should also be acquainted with the new terminologies in health care system for intensive treatment in medicine like ICU (Fig. 1.16) (intensive care unit), ITU (intensive therapy unit or intensive treatment unit), CCU (critical care unit), NICU (neonatal intensive care unit), PICU (pediatric intensive care unit), SICU (surgical intensive care unit), HDU (high dependency unit), ANCU (acute neuro critical care unit) and MICU (mobile intensive care unit). The common lethal conditions treated in ICU are ARDS (acute respiratory distress syndrome), trauma, head injury, multi-organ failure, and especially sepsis. Every student should know the common gadgets [e.g., pulse oximeter (a spectrophotometric device that measures arterial oxygen saturation i.e., SpO_2), cardiac monitor (a device that shows the electrical and pressure waveforms of the cardiovascular system for measurement and treatment) etc], used in different types of ICUs.

A student should be conversant with three common terms in day-to-day use like 'iatrogenic', 'aetiology' and 'idiopathic'. Iatrogenic means 'doctor-made' or 'treatment-made' i.e., a drug-reaction in a patient is iatrogenic. Aetiology means 'the cause' e.g., one of the aetiology of pleural effusion is tuberculosis. Idiopathic means 'the cause is unknown' i.e., if the cause of a disease is idiopathic or unknown, it is obviously very difficult to treat, and that is why it is told that it is idiotic to the part of the doctor and pathetic for the future of the patient.

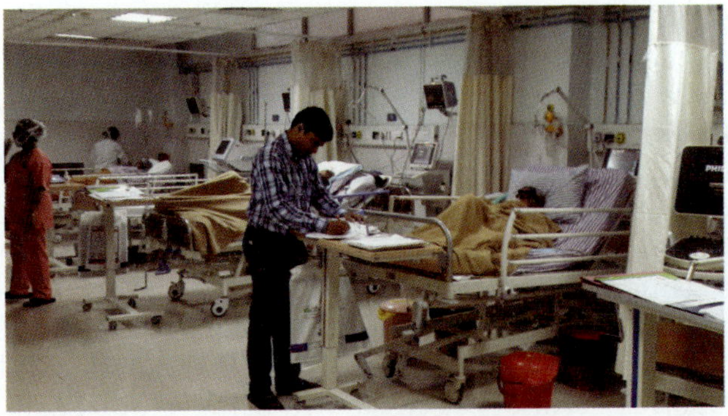

Fig. 1.16: An ICU (intensive care unit) for treatment of severe and life-threatening illness

Two other important terms are 'acute' and 'chronic' in the medical science. For better understanding, a student may consider 'sudden' as acute and 'a condition which is persisting for a long time' as chronic. Progress of a disease may be rapid, or insidious, i.e., proceeding in a gradual or subtle way. 'Placebo' is a term which means a substance containing no medication and prescribed or given to reinforce a patient's expectation to get well by psychological benefit to the patient rather than for any physiological effect (a functional or non-organic pain may sometimes be cured by injecting distilled water by intramuscular route).

The subject of Medicine is full of 'syndrome'. Do not be afraid, it is nothing but 'group of symptoms' or 'symptom complex'.

At the same time, one beginner should know what makes 'informed consent' from a patient; it is a process for getting written permission before conducting a healthcare intervention on a person (e.g., a pleural aspiration in pleural effusion or a splenic puncture in diagnosing chronic kala-azar). One student is expected to learn the skill to 'breaking a bad news' to the patient or their relatives clearly, honestly and sensitively which is one of the most difficult duty of a physician (e.g., to cancer patients about their illness). It is mandatory to remember that a code of ethics binds the doctor to certain modes of conduct in the relationship either with a patient or with colleagues. That is why, some idea should be acquired about the incidences of 'medical negligence' or 'medical malpractice' (i.e., treatment below the accepted standard and/or causes injury or death to the patient), which is a punishable offence by a doctor. Make a habit of keeping patient's records from student life, either in hard copy or in soft copy, which will be enormously helpful in future life.

It is known that practice makes a man perfect. So communicate with your patient repeatedly as you were taught by your teacher at the bedside to write a good and comprehensive 'history'. It is often told by eminent clinicians—'go to the patient, listen to him repeatedly, and see that he will give you the diagnosis'. Everyday, try to learn some 'bedside manners' from your teachers. Now, give a look through the investigations and treatment file to have a complete knowledge about the disease. One must admit that a clinician dedicates minutes after minutes, hours after hours, and days after days at the bedside to become a true professional. It is the positive attitude which helps to attain a good communication skill.

Rapid development in biomedicine and information technology is ushering a new age of medicine; artificial intelligence, genome editing, tissue engineering are just a few of the frontier fields that are changing the practice of medicine. Remember, all are required in the life of a physician but as a physician, first try to learn the art of clinical medicine by going at the bedside and secondly by comforting the patient.

Lastly, one student should have some idea about euthanasia. Euthanasia is also known as assisted suicide, doctor-assisted dying (suicide), or "mercy-killing" of terminally ill patients. There are different euthanasia laws in each country. In India, passive euthanasia is legal under exceptional circumstances (e.g., withdrawal of life support to patients who is in a permanent vegetative state) but active euthanasia (i.e., intentional act of causing the death of a patient experiencing great suffering) is illegal.

You have no holiday during your clinical posting though pauses are vital in life. Remember, 'All work and no play makes Jack a dull boy' that means though hard and laborious work is necessary to achieve our goals in life but concentration on work alone with no recreation tends to make a person dull and unsociable. Thus Osho once told 'life is a balance between rest and movement'.

Remember these points as a newcomer in the field:

1. Set your goals
2. Prepare study notes on a regular basis
3. Do not use too many study resources
4. Clear your queries from your teachers or seniors
5. Regularly attend clinical classes
6. Revision
7. Give some clinical mock test in the presence of your teacher.

According to Bloom's taxonomy, there are three domains of educational activities which should always be remembered by a student:

- *Cognitive (domain of the brain):* Knowledge
- *Psychomotor (domain of the hands):* Skill
- *Affective (domain of mind, feelings, emotion):* Attitude

So, in the summary show some professionalism by maintaining the following facts: Communicate sensitively, maintain patient's dignity, convey thanks to your patient and explain conclusions to the patient, if needed. Try to give your 'human touch' so that a 'case' is converted into a 'patient', and ultimately becomes 'healthy, physically and mentally'.

Be an empathetic listener of your patient. Try to learn the effective communication and interpersonal skills. Have faith and believe in yourself as well as your abilities. With a boundless vision, determination, motivation and dedication anything is achievable by any student.

Before starting your journey to clinical medicine, remember these golden words of Sir William Osler, the father of modern medicine, ".... Medicine is learned by the bedside and not in the classroom. See, and then reason and compare and control. But see first.", and try to take the essence of the comments of the legend told more than 100 years back that "The good physician treats the disease; the great physician treats the patient who has the disease."

Congratulations!

Enjoy being a real doctor and try to serve the community.

A SCHEMATIC HISTORY: GENERAL PRINCIPLES

Interrogation of the patient to gather maximum possible information is the first and foremost part of clinical evaluation. History taking, which is an immensely skilled technique and requires a lot of trial, remains the essence of medical practice. The inquiry (i.e., history) of the patient precedes both clinical examination and treatment. Clinical methods are the skills in clinical practice a doctor achieves during examination of a patient by a combination of study and experience; bedside manners are taught by clinical teachers, and this is how the 'bedside clinical medicine' is learnt (Fig. 1.17). Try to evaluate the patient as soon as he/she enters the consultation room i.e., how the patient walks, interactions during conversations, body language, etc. can give vital clinical clues. Call the patient by name and interrogate by asking "What is your problem?" or 'How can I help you?" Put the patient at ease and encourage him/her to talk freely. Allow the patient to tell their story without interruption because a sympathetic listening instils confidence in the treating doctor and establishes a good doctor–patient relationship. Be polite, humble and respectful in behaviour, and professional in dress. Always maintain the patient's privacy and dignity. The surrounding area and staffs of the hospital/clinic should be sensitive and patient-friendly. In all sense, be an attentive listener and behave friendly. Do not hurt the patient's religious belief. Try to assess the patient's mood, anger, anxiety or frustrations arising out of the disease. Many patients speak either too much (garrulous) or too little but an intelligent doctor knows how to extract the best out of it, and it is achieved only by repeated practice at the bedside.

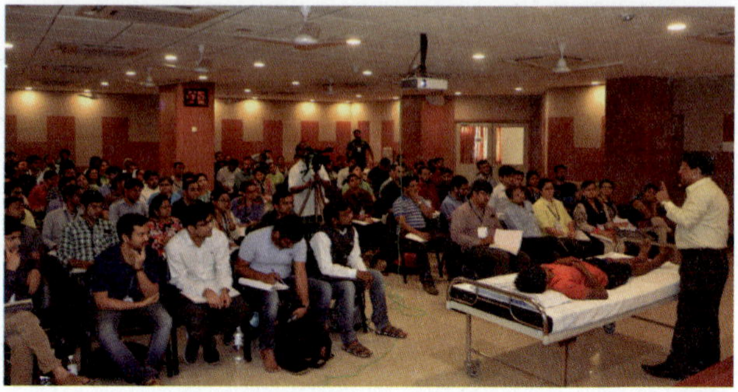

Fig. 1.17: Bedside clinical demonstration of symptoms and signs

If the patient is non-communicable (cannot speak, confused, abusive, emotionally disordered or unconscious), take the help of accompanying persons, or a relative, or a third party to collect information. Negative points are very important in history taking [e.g., absence of history of haematemesis (i.e., blood coming out with vomiting) in a patient of cirrhosis of liver often indicates a good prognosis (i.e., outcome), which points out that oesophageal varices is yet to be formed, or formed but not ruptured yet]. While assessing pain anywhere in the body, give the patient an arbitrary 'pain scale' from 1 to 10, where 1 is very mild pain, while 10 is the severest pain. Try to discourage pseudo-medical terms delivered by the patient like allergy, sciatica, stroke, pleurisy, etc. Highly-sensitive issues like marital disharmony, sexual disorders, substance abuse, and mental derangement should be asked at the last part of history taking. At the first hand, try to avoid 'leading questions', which are very specific and their answer remains between 'yes' and 'no'; but in a patient with central chest pain which is radiating to the left hand may be asked by a leading question like 'is the pain increases with exertion?', while an affirmative answer points towards coronary heart disease and helps in diagnosis.

Do not violate the privacy of the patient for any reason. Maintain the confidentiality which is essential for therapeutic relationship. Never break the 'trust', which is the strongest bondage between treating physician and ailing patient.

In spite of recent boom in investigational facilities, history taking and physical examination remain the essential skills of the attending physician.

SUGGESTED SCHEME FOR HISTORY TAKING SEQUENCE

1. ***Particulars (biodata) of the patient:*** Name, age, sex, race/religion, occupation, address, date and time of admission, date and time of examination
2. ***The history proper***
   - Chief (presenting) complaints
   - History of (H/o) present illness
   - Past history
   - Family history

- Personal and social history
- Treatment history
- Psychiatric history
- Menstrual and obstetric history in women

3. ***Physical examination***
   - *General survey:*
     - Level of consciousness: Whether alert, oriented and co-operative
     - Apparent age
     - Decubitus
     - Build (built)
     - Nutrition (and assessment of body mass index or BMI)
     - Facies
     - Pallor (or anaemia)
     - Cyanosis
     - Jaundice
     - Neck vessels (internal carotid artery and jugular veins)
     - Lymph nodes
     - Thyroid gland
     - Clubbing
     - Koilonychia
     - Pulse
     - Blood pressure (BP)
     - Respiration
     - Temperature
     - Oedema
     - Skin, hairs, nails
     - Skeleton: Height, weight, arm-span, upper segment–lower segment ratio
     - Any obvious deformity (e.g., swelling of abdomen) or outstanding features (e.g., asymmetry in face due to Bell's palsy)
     - General observation: Any acute distress present or not
     - Handedness (right, left, or ambidextrous) with level of intelligence (average, low, high)
     - *Others:* Breasts, hydration, bony tenderness
   - *Systemic examination:*
     - Cardiovascular system (CVS)
     - Respiratory system
     - Gastrointestinal (GI system) and hepatobiliary system
     - Genitourinary system
     - Nervous system
     - Haemopoietic system/lymphoreticular system
     - Musculoskeletal system/locomotor system (optional)

*Always begin with general survey, followed by system review

4. ***Summary of the case:*** Construct two paragraphs encompassing short history with clinical findings in 5–6 sentences

5. ***Provisional diagnosis (P/D):*** Most probable diagnosis considering history and physical examination
6. ***Differential diagnoses (D/D):*** Consider other possibilities in the similar scenario
7. ***Relevant investigations (optional):*** Rational investigations targeting final diagnosis

HISTORY TAKING

1. ***Chief (presenting) complaint:*** Ask the patient directly about his/her problem for which he/she presents to the doctor or hospital. Note down the complaints in patient's own words avoiding medical terminologies ('coughing out of blood' is preferable to 'haemoptysis').
   Record the presenting symptoms with duration (from longest to shortest duration), in chronological order of their appearance in patient's own words.
   Following are the common presentations which result in urgent hospital admission: Chest pain, respiratory distress (breathlessness), fever (pyrexia), pain in the abdomen, loss of consciousness or impaired cognition, weakness of the body (hemiplegia or paraplegia), haematemesis and/or melaena, haemoptysis, severe vomiting and diarrhoea.
2. ***H/o present illness***
   - Chief complains are expanded here in relation to onset (acute, subacute, insidious), progress or course of illness (progressive, static, with remissions and relapses), and duration. The common examples of acute onset within hours is a vascular lesion (i.e., cerebrovascular accidents or CVA)/acute myocardial infarction (AMI) or respiratory distress, subacute onset within days or weeks is infection/inflammation/burning micturtion, while insidious or very slow onset occurs in neurodegenerative disorders, i.e., Parkinson's disease.
   - Positive, plus important negative symptoms (e.g., absence of paralysis in disorders of nervous system, or absence of chest pain in cardiovascular illness) should be recorded.
   - It is better not to use leading questions though it is often required for sensitive history taking. Avoid scientific terms (joint pain is preferable to arthritis).
   - Pain (site, radiation, character, severity, duration, relieving and aggravating factors, associated symptoms) and fever (range, axillary or oral, intermittent/continued/remittent, diurnal variation, chill and rigor, sweating, associated headache/malaise) should be uncovered in details.
   - Record symptoms referable to other systems (e.g., confusion in nervous system occurs in a patient of cirrhosis of liver who develops hepatic encephalopathy) and relevant associated symptoms (e.g., drenching sweat in hypoglycaemic coma).
   - Basic general symptoms (should be recorded in every patient): Appetite, loss of weight, fatigue, sleep, bladder and bowel.
3. ***Past history:*** Ask about previous illness (enlist in chronological order from infancy, if possible), H/o illness recurring in nature (e.g., epilepsy), operations, accidents or admissions to hospital. Note the following points while recording past history:
   - Specific diseases like tuberculosis, rheumatic fever, malaria, kala-azar, jaundice, epilepsy, ischaemic heart disease (IHD), systemic hypertension, diabetes mellitus, STD (sexually transmitted diseases like gonorrhoea, syphilis, AIDS).

- H/o travel abroad (or disease-prone areas), blood transfusion, operations, injury, major psychiatric illness in past.
- Childhood illness like mumps, measles, chickenpox, whooping cough, poliomyelitis; birth history (asphyxiated or not), H/o umbilical sepsis (may lead to portal hypertension in adolescence), immunisation and different vaccinations history taken from the parents.
- *H/o contact* with persons suffering from tuberculosis or any contagious disease.
- *H/o exposure* (sexual) to STD or any H/o promiscuous sex.

4. ***Family history:*** It includes 'first degree relatives' (parents, children and siblings) but in a broader sense all 'blood-relatives' (grandparents, parents, brothers, sisters, uncles, nephew or niece) comes within family history.
   - Does anybody suffer (or suffered) from similar type of heredofamilial diseases like thalassaemia, haemophilia, schizophrenia? Is there any sufferer from diseases of multifactorial inheritance like hypertension, diabetes, IHD, bronchial asthma, epilepsy or migraine?
   - Any sufferer from communicable diseases (e.g., chickenpox, mumps, measles, tuberculosis) at this point of time due to unavoidable H/o contact within the family?
   - Any H/o 'consanguineous marriage' (i.e., marriage among relatives) within the family (may give rise to hereditary autosomal recessive diseases like 'inborn errors of metabolism')?
   - Cause of death of 'first degree relatives' (with age) should be recorded. Try to construct the family tree with 'pedigree chart' (symbolic diagram in construction of a family) reflecting the pattern of inheritance.

   (**NB:** Genetic counselling is the method by which the patients, who are at risk of an inherited disorder, are explained of the outcomes, the probability of transmitting it to the next generations, and the options given to them in management and planning of family.)

5. ***Personal and social history:*** These include H/o the patient, spouse and children only.
   - Personal details e.g., level of education (gives an indirect idea of social status), occupation in various stages of life (e.g., working in coal mines for a long duration may give rise to coal workers' pneumoconiosis, or leptospirosis in paddy field workers), marital status with number of children (ask for health of spouse and children), dietary habit, addiction (e.g., smoking, alcoholism, or drug abuse; or 'substance abuse' like consumption of cocaine, heroin, LSD, 'recreational drugs', tobacco or alcohol'. Try to estimate the amount of consumption of tobacco and/or alcohol), daily lifestyle (hobbies, pets, sedentary or an active life, travelling, sleep, bladder, bowel, marital relationship, sexual history), and ethnic background (e.g., thalassaemia) are considered in personal history.
   - Income and social status should be asked in a decent way. Dietary habit is to be asked to diagnose avitaminosis, malnutrition or obesity; whether a vegetarian, or non-vegetarian, or consumes mixed Indian diet?
   - Record any H/o 'high risk behaviour' i.e., IV drug abuse, multiple unprotected sexual exposure, homosexuality may acquire disease like hepatitis B or C infection,

subacute bacterial endocarditis (SBE) and AIDS. 'Needle sharing' may acquire abscess/cellulitis, thrombophlebitis, hepatitis B or C or HIV infection, or right-sided infective endocarditis.

6. ***Treatment history:*** Following are taken into consideration:
   - Treatment received so far for the present illness; any drug resistance?
   - Regular use of drugs for treatment of diabetes, hypertension, epilepsy, rheumatoid arthritis, or oral contraceptives. Any H/o blood transfusion, anaesthesia or surgery in the past? Ask for total knee replacement, cochlear implant, valve replacement, or pacemaker implantation.
   - Record any H/o allergy or drug reactions (from penicillins, sulphonamides, pollen, metal, etc).
   - Details of use of NSAIDs (non-steroidal anti-inflammatory drugs), which may give rise to acute gastritis, haematemesis or renal toxicity. Corticosteroids used for prolonged period (e.g., for rheumatoid arthritis, bronchial asthma) may be complicated by peptic ulcer, hypertension, diabetes, weight gain, cataract and osteoporosis (Fig. 1.18).
   - Immunisation taken so far for hepatitis B, tetanus, pneumococcal or influenza vaccine; any H/o self medication?

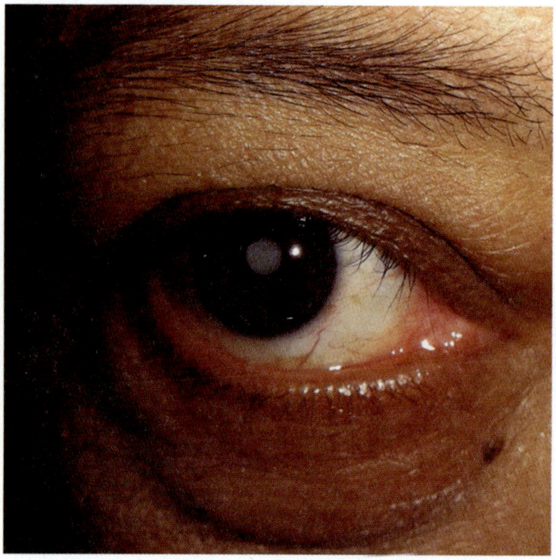

Fig. 1.18: Cataract in right eye after prolonged corticosteroid therapy in bronchial asthma

7. ***Psychiatric history:*** Try to record the 'mood' of the patient i.e., anxiety, depression, phobia, obsession, euphoria or irritability should be noted. Irritable bowel syndrome (IBS), peptic ulcer, bronchial asthma are examples of common psychosomatic disorders. Examples of 'functional disorders' (non-organic diseases, and many a time stress-induced) are chronic fatigue syndrome, irritable bowel syndrome (IBS), fibromyalgia and conversion disorder (previous 'hysteria').
8. ***Menstrual and obstetric history in women:*** Try to include menarche, duration of menstruation, quantity of blood loss (assess indirectly by number of pads used), any dysmenorrhoea or amenorrhoea, date of last menstrual period (LMP), menopause (age at menopause, any post-menopausal bleeding or hormone replacement therapy), and obstetric history (number of pregnancy, outcome i.e., abortion or live birth, complications like toxaemia of pregnancy, mode of delivery i.e., normal or Caesarean section, and last child birth).

Chapter 2

General Examination (History and General Survey)

HISTORY

Q. In history-sheet, what is the importance of 'name'?

Importance of name in history taking lies in:
- It indicates identity of the patient
- Psychological attachment with the patient (if called by name)
- Builds first step to doctor–patient relationship.

Q. Why to mention the age and sex in history-sheet?

Age and sex often help in diagnosing a particular disease like:
- *Age:* Some diseases are common in younger age (e.g., acute rheumatic fever, acute lymphoblastic leukaemia), while some are common in middle age (e.g., gout, rheumatoid arthritis), and old age (e.g., dementia, carcinoma, osteoporosis, parkinsonism, osteoarthritis).
- *Sex:* Systemic lupus erythematosus (SLE) and myxoedema are prevalent in females, while carcinoma of lung is commoner in males. Haemophilia (X-linked disease) virtually affects only the males.

NB: Regarding biodata of the patient, in *obstetrics* (the branch of medical science which deals with childbirth and midwifery) patients, one student should not write/mention 'sex' because all of the patients are female; while in *gynaecology* (the branch of medical science which deals with the diseases specific to women and girls, basically those affecting the reproductive system) as male infertility is being treated in the same department, 'sex' should be mentioned. In *surgery* (the branch of medicine that deals with diagnosis and treatment of disease, injury and deformity by the use of instruments, manipulations or operations) and *paediatrics* (the branch of medicine which deals with children and their diseases), like *medicine*, 'sex' should always be mentioned.

Q. Why race or religion is important in clinical medicine?

Race and religion help in the following way in diagnosing diseases like:
- Spiritual belief, culture and social taboos (Fig. 2.1) are different from religion to religion, which often influence a disease acquired in the society.

- Diet differs from race to race, and religion to religion.
- Consanguinity is a deeply rooted social trend among one-fifth of the world population (i.e., in Middle East, West Asia and North Africa; common in Muslim communities), and is prevalent in some religion and race. Consanguineous marriages (i.e., marriage among relatives, or biologically-related individuals) are associated with increased risk of congenital malformations and autosomal recessive disorders (e.g., mucopolysaccharidosis or phenylketonuria).

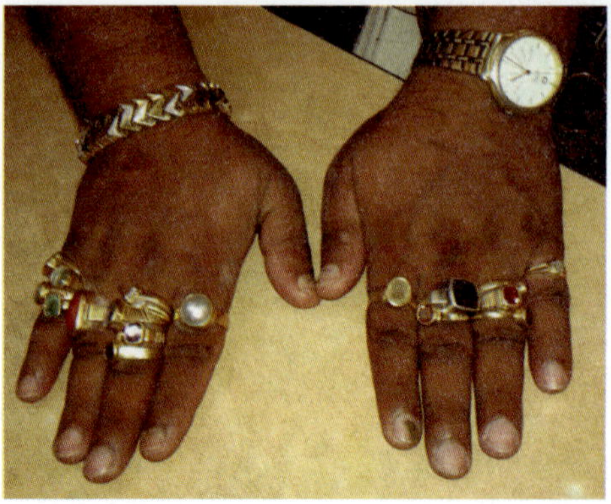

Fig. 2.1: Social taboo—putting on multiple rings in fingers or metallic bracelet in wrist in a false belief to remain happy in life or cure a disease

Q. Role of occupation and address in history-sheet.

Role of occupation and address in history taking are of immense importance like:

- ***Occupation:*** Working place and type of work immensely influence health. Exposure to dust, chemicals or fumes may be complicated by 'occupational respiratory diseases' like pneumoconiosis, asbestosis (from asbestos exposure), nasobronchial allergy or interstitial lung disease; veterinary workers can acquire brucellosis or anthrax; leptospirosis (Weil's disease) is common in paddy field workers. A laborious job may precipitate musculoskeletal pain whereas a sedentary job may initiate weight gain. Unemployment may develop into depression.
- ***Address***
  - Some diseases are common in specific geographical areas like leprosy in Odisha and Andhra Pradesh, and kala-azar in Bihar state of India. Behcet's disease is mostly seen in 'Silk Route' countries around the Mediterranean region and Japan. Chronic arsenic toxicity is common in Taiwan, Thailand, China, Chile, Ghana, Eastern India, and Bangladesh.
  - Hypokalaemic periodic paralysis and sickle-cell disease are common in Odisha, while α-thalassaemia is prevalent in South East Asia, China, Middle East, and thus gives a clue to clinician regarding provisional diagnosis.
  - Often the address reflects the surrounding environment (e.g., environmental pollution in the presence of a factory).
  - Moreover, complete postal address is needed in hospital records to follow-up the patients.

Q. Diabetes and hypertension are mentioned in which part of history?

According to majority of clinicians,

- It is customary to mention them within past history as they have affected the patient in the past and are still continuing (definitely with antidiabetic and antihypertensive medications, respectively).
- A few clinicians prefer to describe them within personal history.

Q. In a patient of mitral stenosis (MS), what past history you have to enquire?

One should enquire in the line of:

- H/o rheumatic fever i.e., polyarthritis, pancarditis, fever, skin rash or subcutaneous nodules should be enquired in a case of MS.

NB: One should be acquainted with selective past history in specific diseases like tuberculosis in pleural effusion, jaundice in cirrhosis of liver, repeated blood transfusions in thalassaemia.

In mentioning past history, never say that 'past history is nothing significant'; it is wise to say in this way: the patient had no history suggestive of malaria, kala-azar, haematemesis or melaena, and so on.

Q. What is your diagnosis/what is your case?

About 'diagnosis': Directly tell the *provisional diagnosis.*

About 'case': Describe the *summary* of the case with salient features; give stress on negative points too (e.g., no H/o haemoptysis in a case of pulmonary tuberculosis). Remember, *summary should be summarised* i.e., first 2–3 sentences for short history, and next 2–3 sentences will encompass clinical examination findings in brief. If some of your friend or the examiner wants to listen detailed history, then you have to be detailed in description of history as well as clinical findings.

Q. 'Your examination hall': prerequisites in observation and description.

Remember, *clinical examination consists of history taking and physical examination.*

A. ***Starter***

- Introduce yourself to the patient and take consent for examination. You may explain briefly what you are going to do.
- Wash your hands before starting clinical examination. You may shake hands with the patient. Wish him/her by good morning.
- Inspect the patient and surroundings for clues (e.g., sputum bowl in a patient with resolving pneumonia).
- Note or mention ongoing oxygen inhalation, IV drip, Ryle's tube, urinary catheter or chest drain, if there is any.
- Always try to stand on the right side of the lying patient during examination as majority of us are right-handed (even during examination in front of examiners).
- Always examine female patients in presence of a female attendant.
- After taking permission, make the position of the patient in bed (e.g., supine or reclining at 45°) with proper exposure of the part to be examined.

B. ***Main course:*** Examine all the systems in *'Long case'* (e.g., in a case of pleural effusion, you have to examine and write CVS, GI system, nervous system, renal system, and so on, over and above the primary respiratory system), and write them in answer script. In *'Short case'*, examine for general survey and specific system asked for (usually nothing to be written). In *spotters (Spot cases)*, just give the provisional diagnosis and its justification (if asked) in front of the examiner.

Set up your mind from the beginning to learn wholeheartedly as well as to face the day of assessment of learning at the end of curriculum.

NB: Some prescription languages one should know at the beginning:
- Rx (recipe)—treat with (take thou)
- bd (bis die)—twice daily (usually in morning and at night)
- tds (ter die sumendus), or tid (ter in die)—thrice daily, usually 8 hourly
- qds (quarter die sumendus), or qid (quarter in die)—four times daily, commonly 6 hourly
- ac (ante cibum)—before food
- pc (post cibum)—after food
- po (per orem)—nothing per mouth
- per os—via the mouth
- mane (om = omni mane)—morning
- nocte (on = omni nocte)—night
- stat—give immediately as initial dose
- sos (si opus sit)—'in an emergency' or ' if needed'(usually given single time)
- prn (pro re nata)—'as needed' (may be given multiple times)
- qs (quantum satis)—sufficient quantity
- q4h—every 4 hours (q means every)
- q6h—every 6 hours
- qd—once a day
- qh—every hour
- hs (hora somni)—at bedtime, hours of sleep.

LEVEL OF CONSCIOUSNESS

Q. Clinical classification of level of consciousness—do you know?

Clinical classification of level of consciousness is:
- *Conscious:* It is a state of awareness of one's self and environment, and relates to the person who is alert, attentive, oriented and co-operative
- *Confusion:* Inability to think with customary speed, clarity and coherence (i.e., disorientation, where the patient is conscious but often talks irrelevantly)
- *Drowsy:* Sleepy but can be aroused easily by external stimulus
- *Stupor:* Appears to be asleep and can be aroused only by painful stimulus
- *Semicoma:* Responds only to internal needs (e.g., shakes body with fullness of urinary bladder) but not to external painful stimulus
- *Coma:* No response either to external stimulus or internal needs.

*As drowsy, stupor, semicoma are ill-defined terms, the level of consciousness is assessed nowadays by Glasgow Coma Scale (GCS) but GCS can never be a substitute of thorough clinical neurological examination. Clinical grading of coma i.e., GCS is assessed by eye opening (4 points), best motor response (6 points) and verbal response (5 points); fully conscious patient scores 15, while deeply comatose gets 3 points.

NB: Always determine whether the patient is fully conscious, alert and cooperative in giving information and permitting examination.

Q. Mention a few other terminologies in relation to higher functions.

They are:

- *Syncope (fainting/black-out):* Sudden and transient loss of consciousness with inability to stand upright due to cerebral ischaemia.
- *Vertigo:* A sense of loss of balance and refers to subjective or objective illusion of rotation.
- *Giddiness:* A swaying type of dizziness.
- *Dizziness:* A sensation of light headedness or faintness.
- *Delirium (or acute confusional state):* Acute confusional state due to acute or subacute brain failure with excitability and hyperactivity e.g., the patient becomes talkative and talks irrelevantly.
- *Illusion:* An instance of a wrong or misinterpreted perception of a sensory stimulus, which later get corrected by proper explanation (e.g., hearing the blowing wind as someone crying).
- *Delusion:* Firm and false belief strongly held and cannot be corrected by any amount of evidences or explanations (e.g., a rope is thought to be a snake).
- *Hallucination:* Perception of visual, auditory, olfactory, gustatory, or tactile experiences in the absence of any external stimulus and with a compelling sense of their reality (e.g., seeing somebody to smoke in a closed room makes the patient thinking that the person is trying to kill him by setting fire in the room).

APPARENT AGE

Q. What is meant by 'apparent age'?

Estimation of apparent age helps the clinician in the following way:

- *Apparent age* means that what is the approximate age of the patient on look-basis. It is the physician's duty to determine how many years the patient looks older or younger than his/her chronological age. Chronological age is known by directly asking the patient.
- Patient's apparent age *may match* his/her chronological age (or more simply, patient looks of his age), or *may not match* (e.g., thalassaemia, Down's syndrome, hypogonadism and pituitary dwarf look younger, while precocious puberty, progeria, chronic sun-exposure make the patient look older—may be helpful in clinical diagnosis).

DECUBITUS

Q. What is 'decubitus'?

It is the posture of the patient in bed assumed by him/her in most of the time of day and night. Many a time, by looking at the decubitus, a pin-point diagnosis can be ascertained.

Q. Describe different types of decubitus in clinical practice.

The common variants of decubitus are:

1. *Of choice:* Comfortable in any position in bed.

2. *Propped-up:* A dyspnoeic patient may adopt propped-up position with the help of a 'back-rest' placed in the head end of the bed. The patient may have mild (adopts 45°), moderate (adopts 60°) or severe (adopts 90°, or orthopnoea where patient sits on bed) dyspnoea.
3. *Squatting:* A patient with Fallot's tetralogy is being relieved of dyspnoea by adopting squatting posture, which increases peripheral resistance and reduces the right-to-left shunting of blood through ventricular septal defect (VSD).
4. *Stooping forward position (in sitting position):* Patients suffering from severe dyspnoea out of pericardial effusion, acute severe asthma, cardiac asthma or chronic obstructive pulmonary disease (COPD) may be seen in Mohammedan's prayer position in bed.
5. *"Stooped posture" (increased thoracic kyphosis):* The patient bends forward in standing condition in parkinsonism, ankylosing spondylitis, and osteoporosis of spine with collapse (widow's stoop). These patients find difficulty while lying in dorsal decubitus position in bed as a result of increased convexity of thoracic spine.
6. *Orthopnoea:* Dyspnoea in lying down position and feels somewhat comfortable in upright position (i.e., in sitting posture), and is commonly seen in acute left ventricular failure (LVF), COPD, cardiac tamponade or severe ascites. Sitting posture helps in reducing venous return to heart and accentuates free diaphragmatic movement by descent of liver.
7. *Trepopnoea:* Dyspnoea in left or right lateral decubitus position only, and is seen most often in heart disease (congestive cardiac failure or CCF). It may be observed in pleural effusion and pneumothorax e.g., a patient of left-sided pleural effusion or pneumothorax feels dyspnoeic when he/she adopts right lateral position in bed.
8. *Platypnoea (orthodeoxia):* Dyspnoea only on adopting sitting posture i.e., just opposite to orthopnoea. It is found in hepato-pulmonary syndrome, massive pulmonary thromboembolism, left atrial myxoma or in selective paralysis of intercostal muscles.
9. *Lateral decubitus:* Patients with pleural effusion and pneumothorax prefer to lie on the affected side as it allows maximum expansion of normal lung; moreover, pleural fluid may compress the mediastinum, if the patient lies on the healthy side.
10. *Prone position:* Colics (renal or biliary), abdominal aortic aneurysm, acute pancreatitis (better relieved by lying down with knees drawn towards the chest).
11. *Curled-up:* Seen in renal and biliary colic.
12. *Restless and tossing:* Colics and acute myocardial infarction (AMI).
13. *Listless attitude (patient lies still in bed):* Found in coma, peritonitis (abdominal movement causes pain), angina pain and hysteria.
14. *Opisthotonus:* Bending the whole body backwards like an arc (hyperextension) is opisthotonus, while bending in forward direction (hyperflexion) is emprosthotonus; seen in tetanus and strychnine poisoning.
15. *Hemiplegic decubitus (posture):* It is due to corticospinal tract or pyramidal tract lesion. The *upper limb* of affected side will be flexed (at elbow, wrist and fingers), adducted, semipronated and lying helplessly; while the *lower limb* of affected side will be extended, adducted, plantiflexed and lying helplessly.

16. *Head end down (by placing bricks or wooden blocks in foot end of bed):* After lumbar puncture (to reduce headache), balanced traction in orthopedics, postural drainage of bronchiectasis and lung abscess, deep venous thrombosis (DVT) in legs and in treatment of bulbar palsy.

NB: 'Decubitus angina' is a variant of angina, and occurs when a patient lies down horizontally. Typical anginal pain in this condition occurs as a complication of heart failure as change in body position results in redistribution of fluids in the body.

'Decubitus ulcer' is the other name for bedsore, which is denuded areas of skin, commonly occurs over bony prominences and is formed as a result of prolonged immobilisation.

BUILD

Q. What is build (or built)?

- *Definition:* 'Skeletal framework' of a person in relation to his/her age and sex as compared to a normal person. It is of two types:
  - Short stature or dwarfism (below 3rd percentile), and
  - Tall stature (above 97th percentile)—less common
- *'Stature'* is the total height measured from crown to heel. *Upper segment* is the distance from 'crown to pubis' and *lower segment* is that of 'pubis to heel'.
- Build and stature are important because short and tall stature may specify some diseases.
- *'Arm-span'* is the distance between fingertips when hands are stretched parallel to the ground.
- While describing build, it may be of *average, short (dwarf), or tall.*
- If the height of an adult is < 4 feet, the same may be called as *'dwarf'*.

**Anthropometry:* Measurement of height and weight, arm-span, and upper segment–lower segment ratio.

Q. Enumerate causes of short and tall stature in clinical practice.

- In *short stature* or dwarfism, the height of a person is much below in relation to chronological age and sex of that person as compared to a normal individual. The causes are:
  - Constitutional (commonest)—delayed growth and puberty
  - Heredofamilial
  - Protein-energy malnutrition (PEM)
  - Cretinism (hypothyroidism—coarse facies, lack of intelligence, normal genitals)
  - Pituitary dwarf (hypopituitarism—'chubby' facies, normal intelligence, sexual infantilism)
  - Rickets
  - Achondroplasia
  - *Others:* Fallot's tetralogy, Down's syndrome, Turner's syndrome, gross kyphoscoliosis, pseudohypoparathyroidism, mucopolysaccharidosis, thalassaemia, progeria.

- Causes of *tall stature* (height is longer in relation to chronological age and sex of that person as compared to a normal individual) are:
  - Constitutional (idiopathic)—commonest cause
  - Racial, or familial
  - Marfan's syndrome
  - Gigantism (cerebral) and acromegaly
  - Hypogonadism (lack of testosterone accentuates uninhibited longitudinal growth)
  - Klinefelter's syndrome
  - Homocystinuria (inherited disorder of amino acid metabolism with 'marfanoid' habitus where dislocation of lens occurs downwards)
  - Supermales (XYY) and superfemales (XXX).

Q. What is the normal body ratio?

At birth, upper segment: Lower segment is 1.8:1; by the age of 10 years, the ratio becomes 1:1, and is approximately 0.9:1 in adults as legs grow more rapidly than trunk.

Q. Differentiation of 'short stature' by body ratio: just give an outline.

- Upper segment = lower segment
  - Constitutional
  - Heredofamilial
  - Pituitary dwarf
- Upper segment > lower segment
  - Cretinism
  - Achondroplasia
  - Juvenile myxoedema
- Upper segment < lower segment
  - Spinal deformity
  - Post-menopausal osteoporosis of spine.

Q. Differentiation of 'tall stature' by body ratio: just give an outline.

- Upper segment = lower segment
  - Constitutional
  - Pituitary causes (gigantism and acromegaly)
- Upper segment > lower segment
  - Precocious puberty
  - Adrenal cortical tumour
- Upper segment < lower segment
  - Marfan's syndrome
  - Klinefelter's syndrome
  - Hypogonadism
  - Homocystinuria.

NB: Arm-span > height is found in conditions with tall stature where lower segment > upper segment.

Q. Describe different diseases in short with alteration of stature (body habitus).

Many a time the first impression of the following conditions with specific body habitus may lead to a pin-point diagnosis:

Turner's syndrome (gonadal dysgenesis): Girls with short stature, receding chin with low set ears, webbed neck (Fig. 2.2), low hair line, 'shield-like' chest (flat breasts), widely-spaced nipples, cubitus valgus (increased carrying angle), primary amenorrhoea, lack of secondary sexual character, streak gonads, short 4th metacarpals, sterility; may have associated coarctation of aorta; karyotype is 45, XO.

Cretinism: Short stature; hypothyroidism since birth due to thyroid agenesis. Dull, idiotic, expressionless face, depressed bridge of nose, broad flat nose, hypertelorism with thick and everted lip, macroglossia, pot-bellied abdomen with umbilical hernia; lethargic with severe mental retardation (Fig. 2.3).

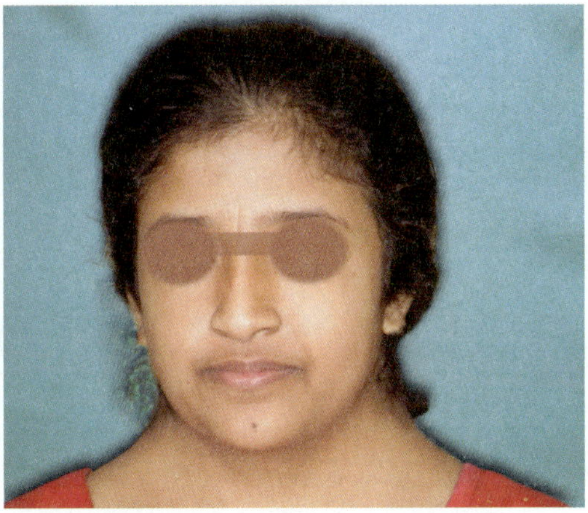

Fig. 2.2: Turner's syndrome with webbed neck (i.e., a fan-like fold of skin extending from shoulders to neck)

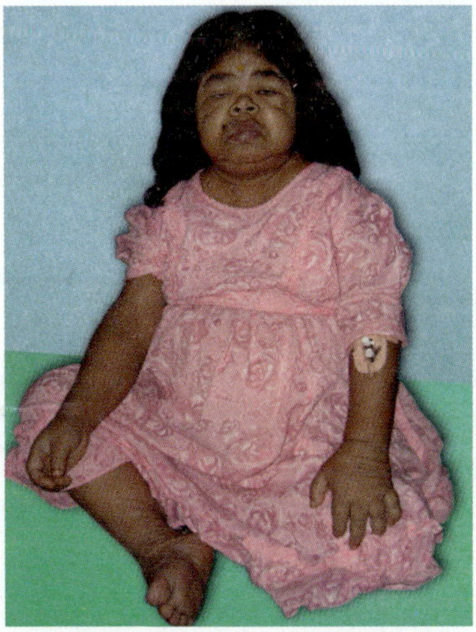

Fig. 2.3: Dwarfism with depressed bridge of the nose, broad and flat nose with big nostrils, thick lips, and an idiotic face—features of cretinism

Marfan's syndrome: Tall stature, long and narrow facies (dolicocephaly), thin built, lower segment > upper segment, arm-span > height, long slender fingers and toes (arachnodactyly), high arched palate, hyperextensible joints, pectus excavatum or carinatum, ectopia lentis (displaced upwards), may have associated aortic regurgitation (AR) or mitral valve prolapsed.

Klinefelter's syndrome: A tall and obese male with eunuchoid body habitus, lower segment > upper segment, bilateral gynaecomastia (Fig. 2.4) with loss of secondary

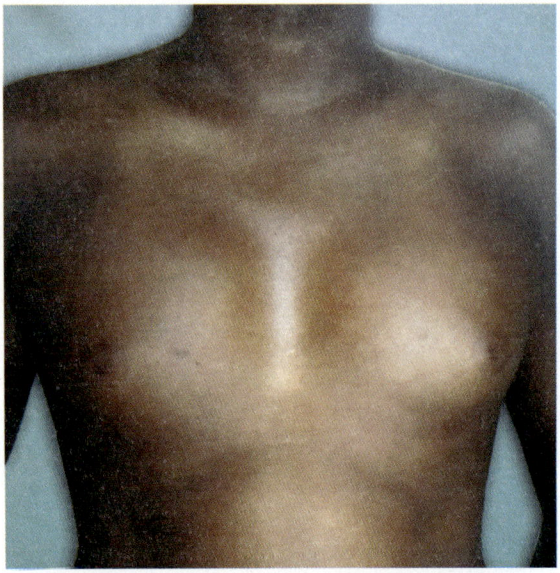

Fig. 2.4: Gynaecomastia in hypogonadism (Klinefelter's syndrome)

sexual characters (lack of beard and scanty pubic hairs), small and firm testes with small penis, feminine voice, infertility, mild mental retardation, chromatin (Barr) body present in buccal smear with chromosomal pattern 47, XXY.

Rickets: Dwarfism, frontal bossing of skull, rickety rosary and Harrison's sulcus over anterior chest wall, pigeon chest, kyphoscoliosis, delayed dentition, bowing of legs.

Achondroplasia: Dwarfism, large head, saddle nose, short limbs, increased lumbar lordosis, kyphoscoliosis; normal trunk size with normal mental and sexual development. These patients are commonly seen as jokers in a circus.

Mucopolysaccharidosis (e.g., Hurler and Hunter syndrome): Dwarfism, characteristic gruesome and extremely unpleasant facies, may be with corneal clouding, kyphoscoliosis with joint stiffness.

Pseudohypoparathyroidism: Short stature, stocky built, round face, short neck, mental retardation, short 4th and 5th metacarpals and metatarsals (Fig. 2.5).

Acromegaly: Enlarged face with prognathism (*see* characteristic 'facies' below), deep and husky voice, 'spade-shaped' hands (broad hands with thick, large, square-tip fingers).

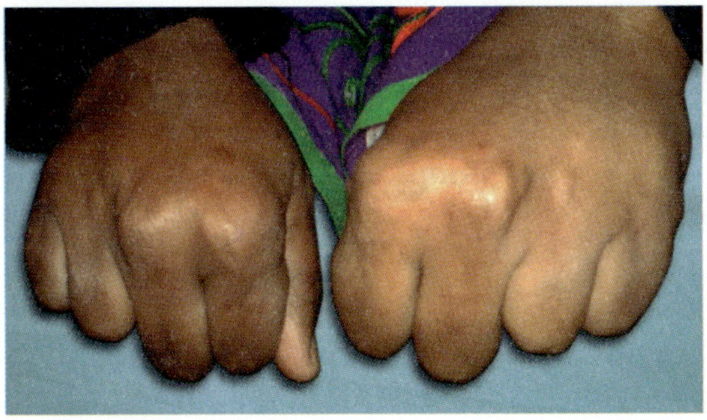

Fig. 2.5: Short 4th and 5th metacarpals in pseudohypoparathyroidism—4th and 5th knuckles are absent bilaterally due to short metacarpals

Gigantism: Large body stature including height, and girth as well; other features are like acromegaly.

Down's syndrome (mongolism): Small, round and flat face, upwards-slanting eyes (*see* characteristic 'facies' below), short and broad hand with single palmar flexion crease (simian crease), clinodactyly in little finger, sandle-gap in feet, hypotonia, pleasant personality with fond of music, short stature with mental retardation (Fig. 2.6).

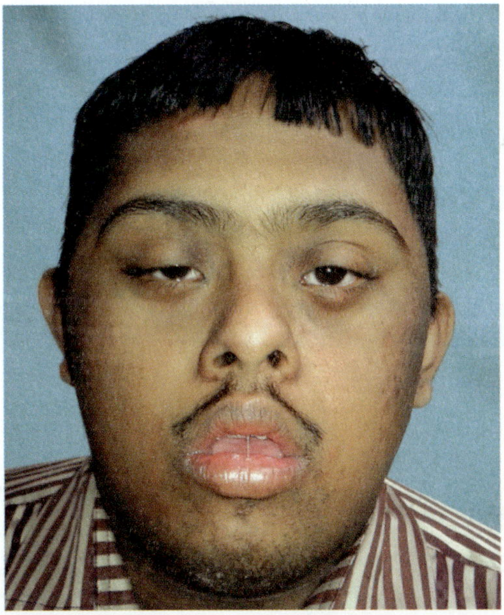

Fig. 2.6: Down's syndrome (mongolism) with mongoloid slant of eyeballs and an idiotic look

Q. What is eunuchoidism?

Hypogonadism, lack of sexual maturation and tall stature with long legs are collectively known as eunuchoidism, and develops as a result of pre-pubertal testicular failure (i.e., androgen loss reflects eunuchoidism).

Q. What is body constitution or somatotypes?

- It is divided into 3 types:
  - *Normosthenic:* Normal body build
  - *Asthenic:* Lean body, narrow shoulders, flat chest with thin limbs
  - *Sthenic:* Short neck, thick trunk, broad shoulders and thick-short limbs

Q. What is progeria?

It is the 'premature ageing', which mimics senile appearance of a person, and is manifested by accelerated atherosclerosis, alopecia, dwarfism, mild mental retardation, angina, AMI, and hypertension; death usually occurs before 20 years.

Q. Mention the common investigations done in short stature.

Short stature is evaluated by:
- *History:* Family and personal history including natal history (i.e., birth history)
- *Clinical examination:* Height, weight, arm-span, secondary sexual characters
- Thyroid function test
- Growth hormone (GH) assay
- *Radiology for bone age:* Skull, and non-dominant hand and wrist
- Chromosomal karyotyping.

Q. Name some autosomal and sex-linked disorders.

Autosomal dominant	*Autosomal recessive*	*X-linked disorders*	*Y-linked manifestations*
1. Huntington's disease 2. Marfan's syndrome 3. Nail-patella syndrome	1. Cystic fibrosis 2. Sickle cell disease 3. Hartnup disease	1. Haemophilia 2. Glucose-6-phosphate dehydrogenase (G6PD) deficiency 3. Colour blindness	1. Hairy ears in males (hyper-trichosis) *There is no Y-linked disorder

NUTRITION

Q. How to assess nutrition at the bedside?

- Nutrition is 'nourishment of the body', and is assessed at the bedside by:
  - Subcutaneous fat—by picking up 'skinfold thickness' between finger and thumb in mid-triceps region (ideally by Harpenden or Schofield's calliper); other sites are biceps, infrascapular and suprailiac regions.
  - Bulk of muscle mass—measure the mid-arm or mid-thigh circumference by a tape from a fixed point i.e., from elbow or knee joint respectively.
  - Signs of vitamins, minerals and nutrient deficiency—assessed by diagnosing glossitis, cheilosis, angular stomatitis, koilonychia, Bitot's spot, etc.

Q. Normal value of skinfold thickness and mid-arm circumference: do you know?

They are as follows:
- *Average adult triceps skinfold thickness:* Males 12.5 mm, females 16.5 mm.
- *Average adult left mid-arm circumference:* Males 25.5 cm, females 23 cm.

Q. Enumerate the division of 'nourishment' of body.

The division goes like this:
- Normal
- Underweight (e.g., malnutrition, emaciation, cachexia)
- Overweight
- Obesity.

Q. Define the undermentioned terms.

- *Malnutrition:* Undernutrtion as a result of vitamin, mineral and essential amino acid deficiency.
- *Emaciation:* Generalised undernutrition (i.e., loss of total body fat and muscle bulk).
- *Cachexia:* Combined anorexia, anaemia and emaciation is known as cachexia (i.e., a profound state of general ill-health), and is seen in tuberculosis, disseminated malignancy and COPD. Actually, cachexia is accelerated loss of lean body mass, caused by decreased intake and increased metabolic rate in the context of a chronic inflammatory response.
  - Sarcopenia—decrease in muscle mass (old age, COPD).
- *Overweight:* Body weight is 10% excess over the limit of standard weight in relation to age and sex of that individual.
- *Obesity:* Body weight is 20% excess over the limit of standard weight in relation to age and sex of that individual.
  - *Morbid obesity:* It is 100% more overweight over the upper limit of standard weight, or body mass index (BMI) ≥40.

Q. Enumerate causes of obesity.

Different causes of obesity are:
- Idiopathic (simple obesity)
- Physical inactivity
- Drugs—prolonged corticosteroid therapy or use of tricyclic antidepressants, cyproheptadine, oestrogen-containing oral contraceptive pill
- Hypothyroidism (i.e., myxoedema)
- Hypogonadism
- Insulinoma
- *Syndromes with obesity*: Cushing's syndrome, Laurence-Moon-Biedl syndrome, Fröhlich's syndrome, Pickwickian syndrome, Prader-Willi syndrome.

*'Diabesity' is a new term when an obese person suffers from diabetes mellitus (DM).

Q. Mention the types of obesity.

Different types of obesity are:
- *Android:* Excess deposition of fat in waist; mainly in men (*apple-shaped obesity*).
- *Gynoid:* Excess deposition of fat at hip or thigh (mainly in women; *pear-shaped obesity*).
- *Truncal:* Excess deposition of fat over face, neck and upper trunk (e.g., seen in Cushing's syndrome).

- *Visceral or abdominal:* Excess deposition of fat in abdominal viscera and omentum. It is also known as *apple-shaped obesity* (central obesity with more fat deposition in abdomen rather than subcutaneous fat around abdomen), which is more dangerous than healthy *pear-shaped obesity* (more fats in hips and thighs, non-harmful). Mesenteric fat is more atherogenic than peripheral fat, and is correlated with insulin resistance. Apple-shaped obesity caries more risk of developing diabetes mellitus (DM), ischaemic heart disease (IHD), hypertension and dyslipidaemia (symptom complex of metabolic syndrome).

NB: BMI >30 is also associated with sleep apnoea syndrome, fatty liver, gout, degenerative joint disease and gallstones.

Q. What is body mass index (BMI)?

- Obesity is assessed by body weight (*see* above) and BMI
- BMI = Weight (kg)/Height $(m)^2$
- WHO classification of body mass index (BMI) is:

Nutritional status	*BMI/Quetelet index*
Underweight	<18.5
Normal	18.5–24.9
Overweight	25–29.9
Moderately obese	30–34.9
Severely obese	35–39.9
Morbidly obese	≥40

- *Waist-hip ratio:* It clinically measures visceral obesity at the bedside, and is equal to waist circumference (cm)/hip circumference (cm). A ratio of >1.0 in males and >0.9 in females indicates obesity, and increases morbidity and mortality.
  - *Waist circumference:* Measured mid-way between superior iliac crest and lower costal margin in the mid-axillary line. A measurement in males >102 cm and in females >88 cm indicate high-risk abdominal obesity associated with metabolic complications. Waist circumference is a strong predictor of abdominal obesity.
  - *Hip circumference:* Measured from greater trochanter of one side to greater trochanter of other.
- Ideal *body weight for an adult* can be arrived approximately by Broca's index, i.e., desired body weight in kilogram (kg) = height in centimetre (cm)–100

Q. Causes of weight gain and weight loss in clinical practice.

- *Gain in weight:*
  - *Causes of obesity (see above)*, overeating, familial.
  - Fluid overload e.g., CCF, nephrotic syndrome, cirrhosis of liver, hypoproteinaemia, pregnancy.
  - *Others:* Hypogonadism (males and perimenopausal women), acromegaly, polycystic ovarian disease (PCOD), depression, bulimia nervosa, cessation of smoking.
- *Loss of weight:*
  - *Causes of emaciation:* Tuberculosis (Fig. 2.7), diabetes mellitus (especially, type 1), thyrotoxicosis, malignancy (disseminated), AIDS (acquired immune deficiency syndrome), anorexia nervosa or severe depression.

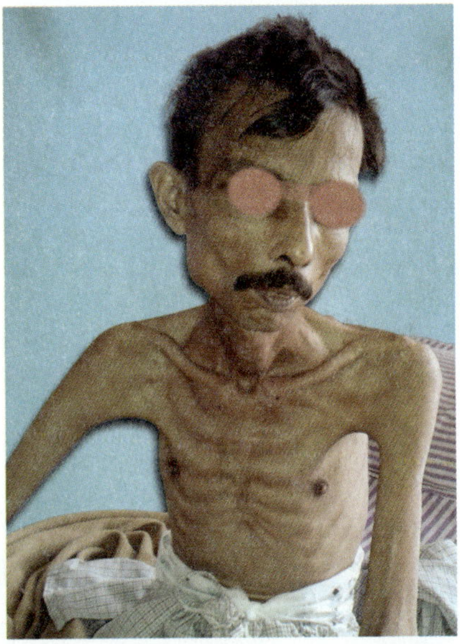

Fig. 2.7: Emaciation—the 'skin and bones' condition in disseminated tuberculosis

- Malabsorption syndrome.
- Chronic malnutrition (e.g., kwashiorkor, marasmas).
- *Others:* Motor neuron disease (MND), COPD, CCF (cardiac cachexia), cirrhosis, Addison's disease, Sheehan's syndrome, pheochromocytoma, chronic infections, emphysema, metformin-induced.

NB: Weight loss in CCF and cirrhosis may be masked by retention of fluid in body. Weight loss is discovered by the patients by loose-fitting clothes or gradually tightening belt notches.

Q. When the weight loss is considered 'significant'?

It is the 'unexplained and unintentional' weight loss of >3 kg in the previous 6 months, and is associated with significant morbidity and mortality. It may terminate in infections (e.g., tuberculosis), lymphoma, carcinoma or diabetes. 'Voluntary' weight loss is not uncommon in models, gymnasts, in treatment of obesity and while on anorexic drugs.

Q. What is the interrelation between appetite and weight loss?

- Weight loss associated with loss of appetite:
  - Malignancy (advanced)
  - Tuberculosis (disseminated)
  - Anorexia nervosa
  - AIDS
  - Addison's disease
- Weight loss associated with normal/increased appetite:
  - Diabetes mellitus (uncontrolled)
  - Thyrotoxicosis

- Kala-azar (chronic)
- Pheochromocytoma
- Malabsorption syndrome.

Q. Vitamins: Fat-soluble and water-soluble with their deficiency features.

Fat-soluble vitamins	*Deficiency symptoms*
Vitamin A	Toad's skin (phrenoderma), night blindness, Bitot's spots, xerophthalmia, keratomalacia
Vitamin D	Rickets (before puberty) and osteomalacia (after puberty)
Vitamin E	Dry hair/loss of hair, muscular weakness, leg cramps, mild haemolytic anaemia, visual scotoma
Vitamin K	Impaired coagulation, bleeding and easy bruising
Water-soluble vitamins	*Deficiency symptoms*
Vitamin B_1 (thiamin)	Dry beriberi (peripheral neuropathy with wrist/foot drop, Korsakoff's psychosis, Wernicke's encephalopathy), and wet beriberi (anasarca due to heart failure)
Vitamin B_2 (riboflavin)	Magenta-coloured tongue, cheilosis, angular stomatitis, corneal opacity, seborrhoeic dermatitis, anaemia, polyneuropathy
Vitamin B_3 (niacin)	Cheilosis, angular stomatitis, raw-beefy tongue, pellagra (dermatitis, dementia, diarrhoea)
Vitamin B_5 (pantothenic acid)	Fatigue, irritability, burning feet, insomnia
Vitamin B_6 (pyridoxine)	Peripheral neuropathy, hypochromic anaemia, cheilosis, glossitis, convulsions
Vitamin B_9 (folate)	Megaloblastic anaemia, peripheral neuropathy, glossitis, cheilosis
Vitamin B_{12} (cobalamin)	Pernicious anaemia (i.e., megaloblastic anaemia), peripheral neuropathy, sore tongue, optic atrophy, subacute combined degeneration of spinal cord
Vitamin H (biotin)	Alopecia, anaemia, muscle pain, paraesthesia, seborrhoeic dermatitis
Vitamin C (ascorbic acid)	Scurvy: Swollen and spongy gum which bleeds easily, perifollicular haemorrhage, ecchymosis, haemarthrosis, anaemia, poor wound healing.

*Fat-soluble vitamins are deficient in obstructive jaundice (those vitamins cannot be absorbed in the absence of bile) and water-soluble vitamins are mostly deficient in malabsorption syndrome.

ANAEMIA/PALLOR

Q. How to define anaemia?

It is the qualitative or quantitative diminution of RBC and/or haemoglobin (Hb) concentration in relation to standard age and sex, and is clinically manifested by pallor.

Q. What are the sites to be looked for anaemia?

- Anaemia is examined in good natural light, and the sites examined are:
  - Lower palpebral conjunctiva—retract the lower eyelids downwards and ask the patient to look upwards (both eyes at a time) (Fig. 2.8).
  - Tongue (especially, the tip and the dorsum).
  - Palate (especially, the soft palate).

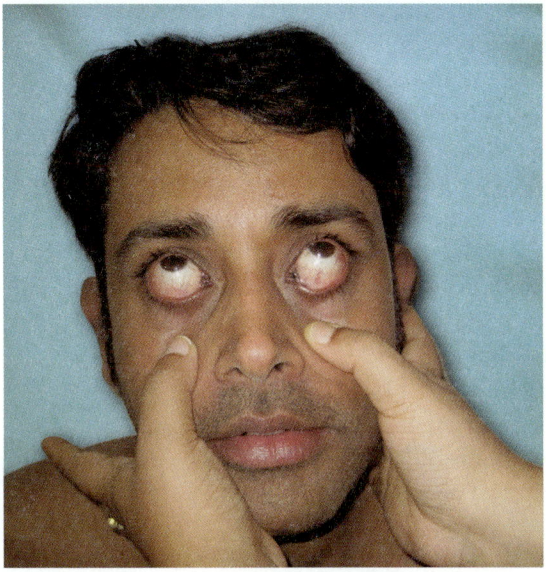

Fig. 2.8: Clinical examination of anaemia (examining lower palpebral conjunctiva)

- Nail-beds (nail-beds are windows of capillary network)—press the base of the nail to observe blanching and flushing, and compare with your own nail-bed.
- Palms, soles and general skin surface.

NB: Anaemia is seen earliest in soft palate.

Q. What is pallor?

Pallor can be described in the following way:

- Pallor (paleness) is the waxy appearance of skin and mucous membrane (normally, they are pink-coloured). It depends on thickness and quality of skin, and quality and amount of blood in the capillaries. A person with low haemoglobin or reduced RBC always looks pale. Anaemia is a pathological condition while pallor is a clinical entity. Pallor and anaemia are not interchangeable terms; there are many causes of pallor, and anaemia is commonest of them.
- For example, a person looking severely pale may not be anaemic (e.g., Sheehan's syndrome).
- Pallor of mucous membrane is commonly due to anaemia. It is very difficult to detect pallor in thick-skinned persons.
- Palmar creases become pale when Hb level goes below 7 g/dL. *'Facial pallor'* is commonly seen in shock and low cardiac output states (e.g., left ventricular failure or LVF).
- Pallor may be:
  - *Temporary:* Fright, shock (due to vasoconstriction), emotional outburst, haemorrhage.
  - *Permanent:* Anaemia due to any aetiology, oedematous part of body or myxoedema.
- False pallor is due to anasarca (generalised oedema) or myxoedema.

- Pallor is a better term than anaemia while doing general survey.
- *The opposite term for pallor is plethora (ruddy 'weather-beaten' appearance).*

Q. How will you grade anaemia clinically?

- Remember, the normal haemoglobin concentration in males and females are: *Males:* 14.6 to 15.5 g/dL, and *Females:* 13.3 to 14.6 g/dL. *Haemoglobin concentration varies* substantially according to age, sex, *race, ethnicity*, and by altitude. *Anaemia is clinically classified as mild, moderate and severe types,* and the clinical assessment is highly subjective (may not correspond laboratory values). The clinical grading goes like this:
  - *Mild anaemia:* 60–80% of Hb (9–12 g/dL)
  - *Moderate anaemia:* 40–60% of Hb (6–9 g/dL)
  - *Severe anaemia:* Less than 40% of Hb (<6 g/dL).
- According to WHO, haemoglobin level of <13 g/dL in adult male, and <12 g/dL in adult female are known as anaemia.

Q. What are the differential diagnoses (D/D) of anaemia?

These are the causes of 'pallor without anaemia', and are enlisted below:

1. Peripheral circulatory failure, shock (ashen-grey pallor), exposure to cold
2. Acute myocardial infarction
3. Myxoedema
4. Nephrotic syndrome
5. Tight aortic stenosis (AS) or mitral stenosis (MS)
6. *Others:* Vasovagal attack, thick skin (e.g., scleroderma), Sheehan's syndrome, exposure to cold, night workers, fright, anasarca.

*Pallor > anaemia is common in hypopituitarism and chronic renal failure (CRF).

Q. How will you tackle a case of anaemia?

- Important *history* from the patient:
  - H/o chronic blood loss (bleeding peptic ulcer, haemorrhoids, menorrhagia), bleeding tendencies.
  - Malabsorption (diarrhoea/steatorrhoea), intake of nutritious foods, worm infestations, exposure to drugs/chemicals/radiation.
  - Anorexia, significant weight loss, bowel habits.
- Common *symptoms/signs* attributable to anaemia:
  - *Symptoms:* Fatigue, weakness, giddiness, fainting, anorexia, weakness, tinnitus, ankle oedema, palpitation, angina pain, breathlessness, insomnia, paraesthesia, intermittent claudication, lack of concentration.
  - *Signs:* Pallor, bipedal oedema, tachycardia and cardiac dilatation.
- Meticulous *clinical examination* with a target to hit the aetiology.
- Corroborated by *investigations:*
  - Peripheral blood film (RBC morphology, reticulocytes), Hb concentration, RBC count.

- Blood indices: MCV, MCH, MCHC.
- Serum values: serum iron, TIBC, serum ferritin.
- Stool examination for occult blood test and detection of hookworm ova.
- Upper GI endoscopy, proctoscopy.
- Radiology: USG abdomen, chest X-ray, X-ray skull (e.g., multiple myeloma), CT scan of chest or abdomen in search of malignancy.
- Bone marrow examination.
- Specific test depending on type of anaemia (e.g., ferrokinetics in iron deficiency anaemia, serum level of vitamin B_{12} and folate in megaloblastic anaemia; special haematological tests like Coombs' test, osmotic fragility, Hb-electrophoresis).

*MCV—Mean corpuscular volume, MCH—Mean corpuscular haemoglobin, MCHC—Mean corpuscular haemoglobin concentration, TIBC—Total iron binding capacity.
**Manifestation of acute blood loss is not anaemia (rather tachycardia and postural hypotension are common) though anaemia develops (as a result of haemodilution) in next 24–36 hours.

Q. Do you know the working classification of anaemia?

Working classification of anaemia goes like this:

- Based on morphology—normocytic, microcytic, macrocytic
- Based on aetiology:
  - Blood loss, which may be acute or chronic
  - Inadequate production of RBC
  - Excessive destruction of RBC.

Q. Do you know causes of microcytic hypochromic and macrocytic anaemia?

- *Microcytic hypochromic anaemia:* Iron deficiency anaemia, thalassaemia, sideroblastic anaemia, anaemia of chronic diseases (e.g., rheumatoid arthritis), sometimes in lead poisoning.
- *Macrocytic anaemia:*
  - *Megaloblastic:* Vitamin B_{12} or folate deficiency.
  - *Normoblastic:* Pregnancy, alcoholism, chronic liver disease, myxoedema, haemolysis or acute blood loss, aplastic anaemia.

*Microcyte: <70 cubic micron, macrocyte: >100 cubic micron, normal RBC (MCV): 87±7 cubic micron; normal lifespan of RBC is 120 days.

Q. Common causes of anaemia in India.

Common causes of anaemia in this part of the world are:

- Nutritional anaemia
- Chronic blood loss (bleeding peptic ulcer/haemorrhoids/fibroid)—commonest cause globally
- Chronic malaria, chronic kala-azar, tuberculosis
- Thalassaemia
- Hookworm infestation
- Tropical sprue.

Q. Causes of iron deficiency anaemia.

Iron deficiency anaemia results from:

- Nutritional deficiency (i.e., dietary iron deficiency)
- Bleeding peptic ulcer/haemorrhoids/menorrhagia
- Gastric erosion (NSAID-induced)
- Hookworm infestation (schistosomiasis too)
- Malabsorption syndrome
- Anaemia of chronic diseases (autoimmune diseases, malignancy)
- Carcinoma of stomach, lung, colon; ulcerative colitis
- Pregnancy, lactation and adolescence.

Q. What are the clinical features of iron deficiency anaemia?

Common clinical features of iron deficiency anaemia are:

1. H/o pica (eating of non-nutrient items like clay, ice, cornstarch)
2. Pallor
3. Glossitis (pale and smooth tongue)
4. Angular stomatitis, cheilosis (Fig. 2.9)
5. Brittle nails/hairs, *koilonychia*
6. Dysphagia (Plummer-Vinson syndrome or Patterson-Kelly syndrome)
7. Mild splenomegaly.

NB: In iron deficiency anaemia: Serum iron as well as ferrtin is reduced, and TIBC (total iron binding capacity) is increased.

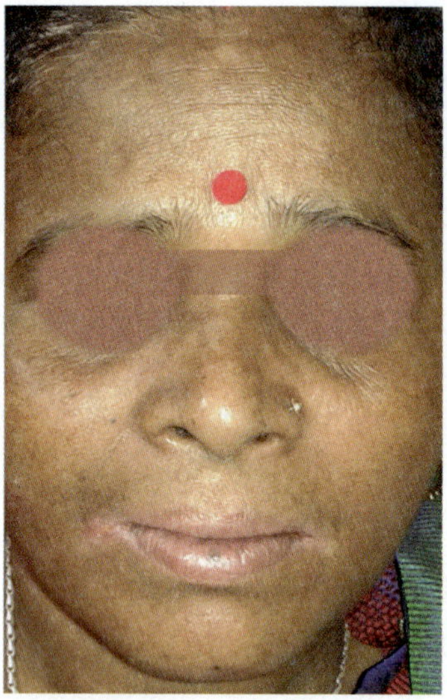

Fig. 2.9: Angular stomatitis and cheilosis from iron deficiency anaemia

Q. What is dimorphic anaemia?

- When microcytes and macrocytes both are circulating in the blood, it is known as dimorphic anaemia. It is due to:
  - Combined iron and vitamin B_{12}/folic acid deficiency
  - Pregnancy
  - Hookworm anaemia with nutritional deficiency.

Q. What is refractory anaemia?

- When anaemia is unresponsive to specific treatment given for optimal period is known as refractory anaemia. The common causes are:
  - Aplastic anaemia
  - Sideroblastic anaemia
  - Myelodysplastic syndrome resulting in refractory anaemia
  - Anaemia due to leukaemia or aleukaemic leukaemia
  - Thalassaemia.

Q. What are the cardiovascular features in severe anaemia?

The features are:

- Tachycardia, capillary pulsation
- Water-hammer pulse
- Cervical venous hum
- Cardiomegaly (cardiac enlargement) and signs of heart failure (later), hyperdynamic apex, haemic murmur over pulmonary area, mitral systolic murmur due to functional mitral regurgitation (MR), rarely mid-diastolic murmur in mitral area secondary to increased blood flow.

NB: Tachycardia and systolic flow murmur are usually evident when Hb <7.5 g/dL.

Q. Why there is anaemia in cirrhosis, malaria, kala-azar and chronic renal failure (CRF)?

- *Cirrhosis of liver:*
  - Haematemesis and/or melaena
  - Anorexia developing into malnutrition
  - Malabsorption
  - Hypersplenism
  - Haemolysis in alcoholic cirrhosis.
- *Malaria:*
  - Haemolysis
  - Impaired erythropoiesis
  - Splenomegaly with hypersplenism
  - Folate deficiency (increased demand).
- *Kala-azar:*
  - Hypoproteinaemia (malnutrition), bleeding, haemodilution
  - Bone marrow depression (due to proliferation of reticulo-endothelial cells)
  - Haemolysis (rare)
  - Hypersplenism.
- *Chronic renal failure (CRF):*
  - Decreased erythropoiesis due to relative deficiency of erythropoietin
  - Anorexia-induced reduced dietary intake
  - Decreased red cell survival
  - Reduced intestinal absorption of iron
  - Diminished erythropoiesis as a result of uraemic toxins
  - Increased blood loss due to abnormal platelet function and increased capillary fragility
  - Vitamin B_{12} and folic acid deficiency.

Q. Enumerate causes of elevated ESR.

- Normal ESR in male is 0–15 mm/hr and in women it is 0–20 mm/hr. ESR is increased in:
  - All acute and chronic infections (particularly tuberculosis)

- Inflammatory disorders e.g., collagen vascular diseases (SLE), rheumatoid arthritis, vasculitis (e.g, temporal arteritis)
- Severe anaemia due to any cause
- Advanced malignancy
- Multiple myeloma
- Pregnancy
- Old age
- Acute rheumatic carditis (i.e., from acute rheumatic fever).

Q. Describe causes of low ESR.

- Low ESR is due to low plasma protein or abnormal red cells making rouleaux formation impossible, and is due to:
  - Polycythemia
  - Congestive cardiac failure (CCF)
  - Sickle cell anaemia
  - Spherocytosis
  - Congenital fibrinogen deficiency

POLYCYTHEMIA

Q. Sites to be examined in polycythemia (ruddy cyanosis).

- It is to be examined *in the same way* as done for detection of anaemia (i.e., *same sites are to be examined).*
- Polycythemia is the increase in red blood cells above normal.
- The patients feature with facial plethora, suffused conjunctiva, increased redness of lower palpebral conjunctiva, cherry-red tongue, red nose and ear lobes, and palmar erythema. The mucous membrane turns dusky-red.

Q. Enumerate common causes of polycythemia.

Common causes of polycythemia are:

- High altitude, severe dehydration
- COPD (commonest case in a tertiary care hospital)
- Cyanotic congenital heart diseases, right-to-left shunt in the heart
- Polycythemia vera
- Abnormal haemoglobin
- Inappropriate erythropoietin secretion by tumours of liver (hepatoma), kidney (hypernephroma) or uterus (fibroid), and pheochromocytoma.

NB: Polycythemia is of two types: Absolute and relative. *Absolute polycythemia* is divided into primary or secondary types. Polycythemia vera is **primary polycythemia** (there is spontaneous proliferation of RBCs in the bone marrow). **Secondary polycythemia** is induced by physiologic changes that increase the body's demand for oxygen, like cyanotic congenital heart diseases, living at high altitudes, lung diseases, or increased levels of erythropoietin production; secondary polycythemia is often associated with cyanosis and clubbing e.g., cyanotic congenital heart diseases. Dehydration is the commonest cause of *relative polycythemia.*

Remember, a polycythmia patient can become cyanosed at normal arterial saturation.

Q. What are the complications of polycythemia?

They are:

- Thrombotic episodes
- Symptoms of hyperviscosity—headache, dizziness blurring of vision
- Peptic ulceration
- Hyperuricemia and gout.

CYANOSIS

Q. Can you define cyanosis?

- It is the bluish discolouration of skin and mucous membrane due to presence of increase amount of reduced haemoglobin (i.e., deoxygenated haemoglobin >5 g/dL), or of haemoglobin derivatives (e.g., sulphaemoglobin and methaemoglobin) in the capillary blood. Cyanosis is a grave sign and warrants immediate intervention.
- Cyanosis is basically of *two types: Central and peripheral.*
- Other less common types of cyanosis are enterogenous, mixed and differential.

Q. Do you know the mechanism, causes and sites to be examined in peripheral cyanosis?

- Mechanism *(stagnant as well as over-utilisation hypoxia)*—Here, *arterial PaO_2 is normal* but there is oxygen unsaturation at venous end of capillary. The mechanisms responsible for *slow speed of circulation* leading to extraction of oxygen from normally saturated arterial blood are:
  - Reduced cardiac output, and
  - Peripheral vasoconstriction.
- *Causes:*
  1. Exposure to cold air or water (possibly most common cause); frost bite
  2. Congestive cardiac failure (CCF)
  3. Peripheral circulatory failure or shock due to any cause
  4. Raynaud's phenomenon (only seen in fingers and toes)
  5. Venous obstruction produces local cyanosis (e.g., superior vena caval syndrome)
  6. Arterial obstruction (e.g., peripheral vascular disease like Buerger's disease) (Fig. 2.10)
  7. Hyperviscosity syndrome (e.g., multiple myeloma, polycythemia)
  8. *Others:* Cryoglobulinaemia, septicaemia, mitral stenosis (i.e., mitral facies, especially lips, cheeks, tip of nose).
- Sites to be examined for peripheral cyanosis (in good natural light):
  - Tip of the nose
  - Ear lobules
  - Outer aspect of lips, chin, cheek

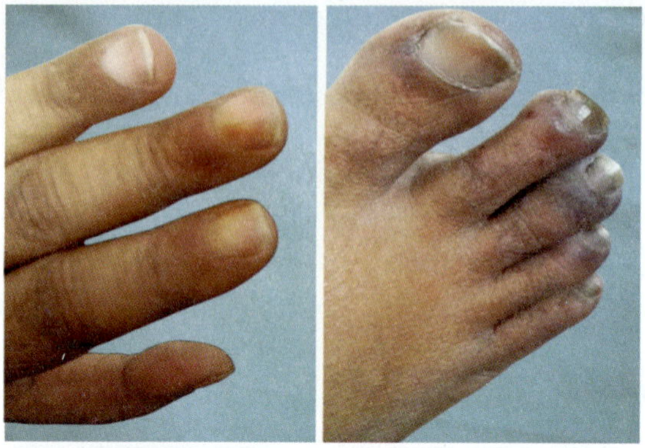

Fig. 2.10: A patient with 'Nicotine stain' in fingers as an imprint of chronic smoking who subsequently developed Buerger's disease (where the blood vessels are blocked leading to gangrene of toes as a result of chronic smoking)

- Tip of fingers and toes
- Nail-bed of fingers and toes
- Palms and soles.

Q. Do you know the mechanism, causes and sites to be looked in central cyanosis?

- Mechanism *(hypoxic hypoxia):* Usually present when the arterial oxygen saturation goes below 85% as a result of marked reduction of oxygen tension in the arterial blood *(i.e., arterial PaO_2 is reduced)*, and is due to:
  - Imperfect oxygenation of blood in lung, or
  - Admixture of venous and arterial blood.
- Causes:
  1. Cyanotic congenital heart disease (e.g., Fallot's tetralogy)
  2. Acute pulmonary oedema (from acute LVF)—most common 'cardiac' cause
  3. COPD, acute severe asthma
  4. Eisenmenger's syndrome (ASD, VSD, PDA with reversal of shunt)
  5. Interstitial lung disease (fibrosing alveolitis)
  6. Tension pneumothorax
  7. Hypoventilatory syndrome: Respiratory muscle paralysis, respiratory centre depression (e.g., opium poisoning)
  8. *Others:* Cor pulmonale, type 2 respiratory failure, high altitude pulmonary oedema, ARDS, lobar pneumonia, acute pulmonary thromboembolism, pulmonary arteriovenous (AV) fistula, acute laryngeal oedema, high altitude (usually at a height of 13000 feet), polycythemia (red cyanosis).

*LVF—Left ventricular failure, ASD—Atrial septal defect, VSD—Ventricular septal defect, PDA—Patent ductus arteriosus, ARDS—Acute respiratory distress syndrome

- Sites to be examined for central cyanosis (in good natural light):
  - Tongue (especially, the margins and the undersurface)
  - Inner aspect of lips
  - Mucous membrane of gum, soft palate and cheeks

- Lower palpebral conjunctiva
- *Plus,* the sites mentioned in peripheral cyanosis (that means, patients with central cyanosis will also be cyanosed peripherally).

Q. What are the differential diagnoses (D/D) of cyanosis?

D/D of cyanosis are:

- Carbon monoxide poisoning—cherry-red flush
- Argyria—slatey-grey hue of silver poisoning
- Osteogenesis imperfecta—only the sclera is blue
- Amiodarone may produce bluish hue in skin due to deposition of blue lipofuscin (ceruloderma).

NB: Argyria and amiodarone-induced blue skin are known as 'pseudocyanosis'. Blue tongue may be seen after consumption of blackberry fruit (Fig. 2.11).

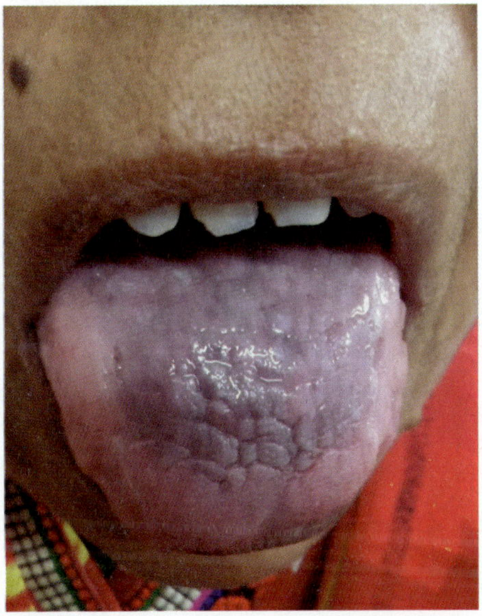

Fig. 2.11: Blue tongue and teeth after taking blackberry fruit (pseudocyanosis)

Q. Do you know any other sites to be seen for central cyanosis?

Nasal mucous membrane, rectal mucous membrane and retina turn blue in a case of central cyanosis though these sites are not routinely looked for.

Q. What are enterogenous, mixed and differential cyanosis?

- ***Enterogenous cyanosis:*** Cyanosis produced due to excessive sulphaemoglobin (>0.5 g/dL) and methaemoglobin (> 1.5 g/dL) in blood is enterogenous cyanosis. It is often considered a variety of central cyanosis. Diagnosis is confirmed by spectroscopic examination of blood. The causes responsible are:
  - Hereditary haemoglobin M disease
  - *Drugs:* Nitrates and nitrites (sodium nitroprusside), dapsone, sulphonamides

- Poisoning by aniline dyes, often added in sweets
- Carboxyhaemoglobinaemia (a cherry-red flush in smokers, and not true cyanosis).

❍ ***Mixed cyanosis*** (i.e., central plus peripheral cyanosis):
- CCF due to left-sided heart failure
- AMI (cardiogenic shock producing *peripheral cyanosis*) with acute LVF (gives rise to *central cyanosis*)
- Rarely, in polycythemia.

❍ ***Differential cyanosis***
- *Hands red (i.e., less blue) and feet blue:* Seen in PDA with reversal of shunt due to pulmonary hypertension
- *Hands blue and feet red (i.e., less blue):* Seen in transposition of great vessels with PDA.

Q. How will you differentiate central from peripheral cyanosis?

Features	*Central cyanosis*	*Peripheral cyanosis*
• Mechanism	Diminish arterial O_2 saturation	Diminished flow of blood in the local part
• Distribution	As described; Warm mucous membrane with blue tongue. Both peripheral and central part	Extremities involved; tongue unaffected. Only peripheral part
• Handshake (i.e., extremities)	Warm	Cold
• Hand rubbing	No alteration	Reduces/abolishes cyanosis
• Clubbing and polycythemia	Usually associated	Not associated
• Exercise	Worsen cyanosis	No change
• O_2 therapy for 10 minutes	May improve	No response
• Dyspnoea	Often breathless	No respiratory distress
• Arterial O_2 saturation	<85%	Normal arterial saturation

Q. How to differentiate cardiac cause of cyanosis from respiratory cyanosis?

Features	*Cardiac cyanosis (e.g., LVF)*	*Respiratory cyanosis (e.g., type 2 respiratory failure)*
• Periphery	Cold peripheries due to vasoconstriction	Warm peripheries due to CO_2-induced vasodilatation
• Pulse	Low volume	Bounding (high volume)
• O_2 therapy	Minimal response	Good response
• Auscultation	Mainly crackles	Mainly wheezes

Q. What is the relationship of cyanosis with hypoxia?

Variations in hypoxia and cyanosis	*Pathological conditions*
• Cyanosis with hypoxaemia	If reduced Hb is >5 g/dL
• Hypoxaemia without cyanosis	Severe anaemia (Hb <5 g/dL) masks cyanosis, and that is why a severely anaemic patient is not cyanosed
• Cyanosis without hypoxaemia	Polycythemia vera (red cyanosis)

JAUNDICE

Q. Can you define jaundice?

It is the yellowish discolouration of skin and mucous membrane due to excess bilirubin >3 mg/dL present in the blood. *Jaundice is clinically classified as mild, moderate and severe types.*

Q. What is icterus?

It is synonymous with jaundice.

Q. What are the sites to be looked for jaundice?

- Sites to be examined (in bright natural daylight):
  - Upper bulbar conjunctiva—retract the upper eyelids upwards and ask the patient to look downwards (both eyes at a time) (Fig. 2.12)
  - Undersurface of tongue
  - Palate (especially, the soft palate)
  - Palms and soles
  - General skin surface.

NB: Earliest jaundice is seen in undersurface of tongue (highly vascular area).

> * In the daytime, *take the patient in front of an open window*. Jaundice should always be examined in broad daylight; mild jaundice may be missed easily, if examined at night. Remember that in artificial light mild jaundice may be missed or severely anaemic patient may mimic jaundice (keep it in mind while examining jaundice at night). *Never put a lighted torch in the oral cavity to diagnose anaemia, cyanosis or jaundice.*
>
> **'Artificial eye' remains white in the presence of jaundice (Fig. 2.13).

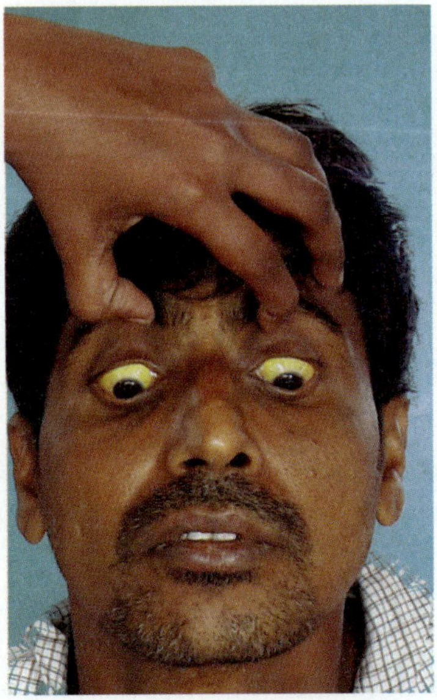

Fig. 2.12: Clinical examination of jaundice (upper bulbar conjunctiva)

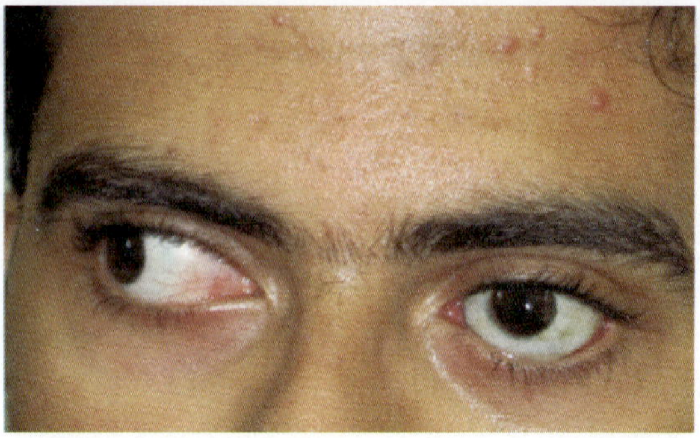

Fig. 2.13: Artificial eye in a normal healthy person: The left eye is artificial which is lustreless with no ocular movement and absent light reflex

Q. What is latent jaundice and its common causes?

- Normal serum bilirubin level is 0.3–1.0 mg/dL (conjugated: 0.1–0.3 mg/dL, and unconjugated fraction: 0.2–0.7 mg/dL). Clinical jaundice (i.e., scleral icterus) is seen when serum bilirubin crosses 3 mg/dL. So, latent jaundice (clinically non-evident subclinical jaundice) is found when serum bilirubin is in between 1 and 3 mg/dL.
- Causes—CCF, mitral stenosis (i.e., passive venous congestion in liver), AMI, pernicious anaemia, pulmonary thromboembolism and acute pancreatitis may present with latent jaundice, which is only detected by serum analysis.

Q. Why upper bulbar conjunctiva is chosen to see jaundice?

Jaundice is conventionally seen in upper bulbar conjunctiva due to following facts (Fig. 2.14):

- Bilirubin has strong affinity for elastic tissue and sclera contains a lot of it.
- Sclera has a white background, which helps to detect jaundice.

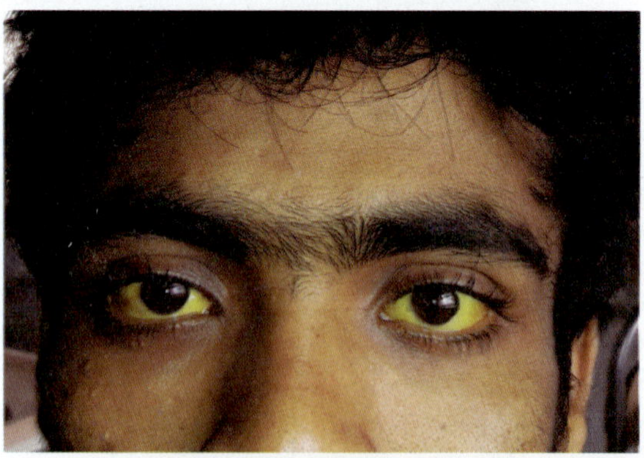

Fig. 2.14: Jaundice is unequivocally displayed in bulbar conjunctiva

Q. What are the differential diagnoses (D/D) of jaundice?

D/D of jaundice are:

- Carotenaemia (carotenoderma): Skin (palms, soles, nasolabial folds) is orange-yellow in colour but sclera and mucous membrane are unaffected. It is commonly seen in myxoedema, diabetes, anorexia nervosa, castrated male, and persons taking large quantities of carrots, papaya, mango, peaches, squash and oranges; they have increase amount of carotene in their blood.

- Quinacrine and mepacrine toxicity (previously used in malaria): Skin, urine, eyes (only the portion exposed to light) are yellow.
- Muddy sclera: Exposed region of sclera looks yellow, non-pathological.
- Diffuse xanthomatosis: Skin may look yellowish-orange.
- Old subarachnoid haemorrhage: Conjunctiva looks yellowish.

Q. How to classify jaundice?

- *Clinical classification:*
  - Mild (<6 mg/dL)
  - Moderate (6–15 mg/dL)
  - Severe (>15 mg/dL).
- *Aetiological or pathological classification:*
  - Haemolytic
  - Hepatocellular
  - Obstructive
    - Intrahepatic (medical)
    - Extrahepatic (surgical).
- *Older classification:*
  - Pre-hepatic (haemolytic or congenital hyperbilirubinaemia)
  - Hepatic (hepatocellular)
  - Post-hepatic (obstructive).
- *Classified on chemical nature of bilirubin:*
  - Conjugated hyperbilirubinaemia
  - Unconjugated hyperbilirubinaemia.

Q. Enumerate the characteristics of haemolytic jaundice.

Haemolytic jaundice is characterised by:

- Freshly voided *urine* is of normal colour *(i.e., acholuric urine)* → kept for sometime in open air → turns dark-yellow due to oxidation of excess urobilinogen to urobilin.
- High-coloured *stool* (excess stercobilinogen is converted to stercobilin).
- *Mild jaundice* (serum bilirubin is usually <6 mg/dL) with lemon-yellow tinge of bulbar conjunctiva; there is predominant unconjugated bilirubin.
- Anaemia (mild, moderate or severe, according to severity of haemolysis).
- Splenomegaly (spleen is regarded as slaughterhouse of RBC in haemolysis).
- Typical facies due to excessive marrow expansion may be there (e.g., chipmunk facies in thalassaemia).
- Reticulocytosis in peripheral blood film examination.
- Chronic cases—leg ulcers and gallstones.

Q. What are the clinical features of obstructive jaundice?

Features of obstructive jaundice are:

- Deep yellow or mustard oil-coloured *urine* due to presence of conjugated bilirubin (in liver, bilirubin is conjugated by enzyme glucuronyl transferase).
- *Stool* is pale or clay coloured (china-clay) due to absence of bile pigment in stool. There is presence of *steatorrhoea* (soft, pale, frothy, bulky, offensive and oily stool which is difficult to flush from the toilet pan but once cleaned, it floats on the water of the pan).
- Usually *deep jaundice* and bulbar conjunctiva looks greenish-yellow due to oxidation of bilirubin to biliverdin (green). Serum bilirubin is predominantly of conjugated variety.
- Severe itching or pruritus with scratch marks in skin and shiny nails. It is due to irritation of free nerve endings by bile salts (sodium taurocholate and sodium glycocholate), or upregulation of opioid receptors and increase level of endogenous opioids (recent view).
- Sinus bradycardia due to inhibition of SA node by bile salts.
- Gall bladder may be palpable; if so, it indicates the site of obstruction in the bile duct and is usually due to carcinoma of the head of pancreas (not due to impacted stone in bile duct resulting from cholecystitis with choledocholithiasis as in that situation, gall bladder will be shrunken and not palpable)—according to *Courvoisier's law.*
- Xanthelasma around the eyes, and xanthoma in the knees or buttocks develop as a result of hypercholesterolaemia due to prolonged cholestasis.
- *Late features*—Weight loss, bleeding tendency with petechiae/purpura/ecchymosis (vitamin K deficiency), night blindness (vitamin A deficiency), osteomalacia/bone pain/fracture of bone (vitamin D deficiency or hepatic osteodystrophy), and muscle cramps (vitamin E deficiency). Remember, lack of bile salts prevent absorption of fat-soluble vitamins like A, D, E and K.
- H/o intermittent fever with chill and rigor, and recurrent abdominal pain with fluctuating jaundice may be present due to acute cholangitis (Charcot's biliary triad). There may be hepatosplenomegaly. Chledocholithiasis may give rise to pain abdomen.

Q. Describe the characteristics of hepatocellular jaundice.

Characteristics of hepatocellular jaundice are:

- *Urine* is yellow in colour.
- *Stool* is high coloured and becomes pale in intrahepatic cholestasis.
- Degree of *jaundice* depends on amount of hepatic injury, and there is orange-yellow tinge of bulbar conjunctiva; both the fractions are elevated but there is predominat conjugated hyperbilirubinaemia.
- Anorexia, nausea, vomiting and fever may be present at the onset (ref: acute viral hepatitis).
- Tender hepatomegaly.
- Variable pruritus.
- Bleeding manifestations due to hepatocellular failure.

Q. Can you do a summary of different types of jaundice?

The summary goes like this:

- *Haemolytic jaundice:* Unconjugated hyperbilirubinaemia, jaundice *plus* anaemia, splenomegaly, and reticulocytosis; increased urobilinogen in urine.
- *Obstructive jaundice:* Conjugated hyperbilirubinaemia, raised alkaline phosphatise, pale stool and pruritus.
- *Hepatocellular jaundice:* Both types of bilirubin are elevated but more so in conjugated variety, tender hepatomegaly with raised transaminases i.e., SGPT and SGOT are elevated (SGPT: Serum glutamic pyruvic transaminase, SGPT: Serum glutamic oxaloacetic transaminase).

*SGPT is nowadays known as ALT (alanine aminotransferase), and SGOT as AST (aspartate aminotransferase).

Q. What are the different causes of jaundice?

Different causes of jaundice are:

- *Pre-hepatic (haemolytic jaundice):* Thalassaemia, falciparum malaria, Viperidae snakebite, Rh-incompatibility, G6PD deficiency (primaquine or sulphonamide-induced), mismatched blood transfusion, sickle cell anaemia.
- *Hepatic (hepatocellular jaundice)*
  - Hepatitis (necro-inflammation of hepatic parenchyma): Viral, autoimmune, alcoholic, drugs (e.g., rifampicin), infections, toxins (e.g., $CuSO_4$ poisoning).
  - Cirrhosis of liver.
  - Right-sided heart failure.
- *Obstructive jaundice:*
  - *Intrahepatic (medical):* Cholestatic viral hepatitis, chronic active hepatitis, primary biliary cirrhosis, alcohol, drugs (e.g., chlorpromazine), sepsis, secondary carcinoma of liver, NASH (non-alcoholic steatohepatitis), lymphoma, sarcoidosis, Dubin-Johnson syndrome.
  - *Extrahepatic (surgical):* Gallstones impacted in bile duct, stricture of bile duct, carcinoma of the head of pancreas, cholangiocarcinoma, sclerosing cholangitis, *Ascaris lumbricoides* infestation in bile duct.

Q. Mention two diseases affecting liver where jaundice is not present.

Jaundice is rarely seen in primary carcinoma of liver (hepatoma) and amoebic liver abscess.

Q. Enumerate causes of predominant unconjugated hyperbilirubinaemia.

Unconjugated hyperbilirubinaemia is commonly seen in:

- Haemolysis
- Ineffective erythropoiesis
- Gilbert's syndrome
- Neonatal jaundice
- Prolonged fasting
- Sepsis.

Q. Causes of fluctuating jaundice.

Fluctuating jaundice is due to:

- Stone impacted in bile duct
- Periampullary carcinoma
- Gilbert's syndrome
- Haemolytic anaemias
- Recurrent pancreatitis.

Q. What do you know about painful versus painless jaundice?

Jaundice may be associated with pain in the abdomen. The different causes are:

- *Painful jaundice:* Viral hepatitis, alcoholic hepatitis, biliary colic, Budd-Chiari syndrome, choledocholithiasis, metastasis in liver, acute pancreatitis.
- *Painless jaundice:* Haemolytic jaundice, cirrhosis, cholangiocarcinoma, carcinoma of the head of pancreas.

Q. Do you know these facts mentioned below?

The basic facts in jaundice are:

- In health, normal colour of urine is given by urochrome and uroerythrin. Bilirubin is absent in urine in health.
- Causes of haemolytic anaemia and haemolytic jaundice are exactly similar.
- Features of *chronic cholestasis* are pruritus, xanthoma, bruising and bone pain, and that of *chronic haemolysis* are anaemia, jaundice and splenomegaly.
- 'Prolonged jaundice' is persistence of jaundice approximately for >6 months.

Q. Describe Murphy's sign and Courvoisier's law.

The signs are described below:

- *Murphy's sign:* There is a catch in breath at the height of inspiration with tenderness and a mass felt there, if right hypochondrium is palpated in a patient suffering from acute cholecystitis. This sign is absent in chronic cholecystitis.
- *Courvoisier's law:* The law says that in a patient of obstructive jaundice, a palpable, smooth and non-tender gall bladder is unlikely to be caused by chronic cholecystitis with choledocholithiasis, and rather it is due to neoplastic obstruction of common bile duct (e.g., carcinoma of the head of pancreas). In chronic cholecystitis, gall bladder is small and contracted.

CLUBBING

Q. Can you define clubbing?

It is the bulbous enlargement of distal portion of fingers and toes, with an increased curvature of antero-posterior as well as transverse diameter of nails due to subungual connective tissue proliferation.

Q. What is Lovibond's angle?

It is:

- Synonymous with *onychodermal angle* (also known as Lovibond's angle), which is around 160°. It is the angle between nail and nail-bed, and is clinically judged by the angle formed between nail and adjacent skin-fold.
- Other names of clubbing are Lovibond's sign and Hippocratic fingers.

Q. How will you examine for clubbing of fingers?

The different steps of examination of clubbing are:

- *First step:* Bring the patient's fingers at your eye level and look tangentially for the onychodermal angle (Fig. 2.15). In clubbing, the angle flattens out and becomes 180° or more.
- *Second step:* Now test for 'fluctuation', which is due to softening at nail-bed. Support patient's pulp of right middle finger on both of your thumbs, and now feel for fluctuation at patient's nail base with both of your index fingers. Remember, there is some amount of fluctuation present in normal fingers (a very subjective sign), and when clubbing is present the nail base may feel spongy.

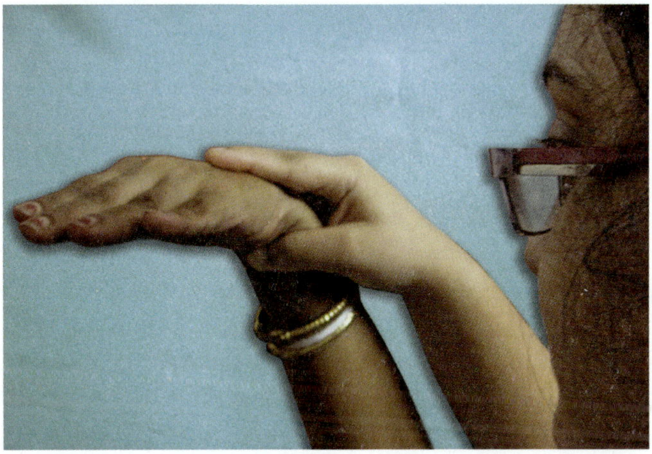

Fig. 2.15: Examining the onychodermal angle tangentially for demonstration of clubbing

Q. Do you know the grades of clubbing?

The different grades of clubbing are:

- *Grade I (1° clubbing):* Increased fluctuation at nail-bed with loss of onychodermal angle.
- *Grade II (2° clubbing):* Grade I *plus* increase in antero-posterior and transverse diameter of nails as well as nails become smooth and glossy with loss of longitudinal ridges.
- *Grade III (3° clubbing):* Grade II *plus* increase in pulp tissue, which gives rise to drumstick (Fig. 2.16) or parrot-beak appearance (Fig. 2.17).
- *Grade IV (4° clubbing):* Grade III *plus* wrist and ankle swelling due to hypertrophic osteoarthropathy (HOA).

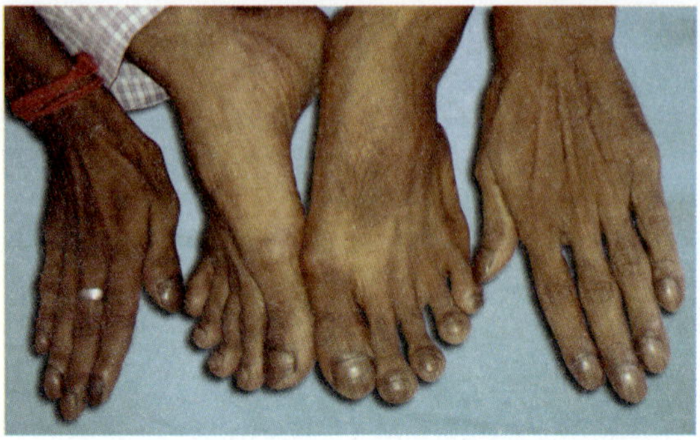

Fig. 2.16: Clubbing (drumstick type) and cyanosis of fingers and toes in cyanotic congenital heart disease

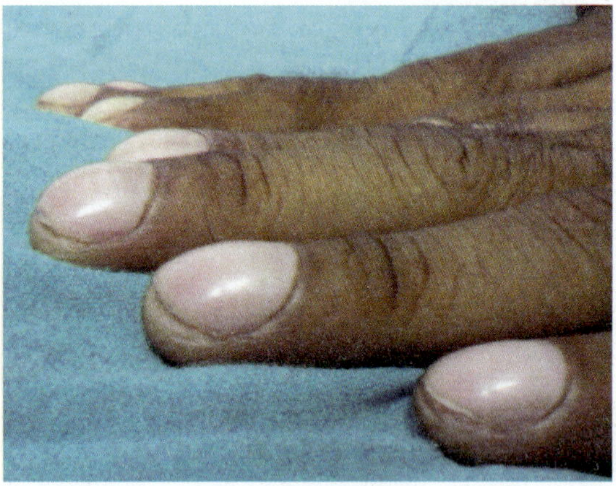

Fig. 2.17: Clubbing (parrot-beak type) in bronchogenic carcinoma

Q. What are the possible mechanisms for development of clubbing?

Clubbing develops due to proliferation of subungual connective tissue, interstitial oedema, and dilatation of arterioles and capillaries at the nail-bed. The different hypothesis are:

- *Anoxic:* It is the most important theory. There is increase in capillary permeability which leads to interstitial oedema (e.g., Fallot's tetralogy). Moreover, arterial hypoxia increases hypervascularity and opens up the anastomotic channels in the nail-bed, which leads to overgrowth of soft tissues.
- *Toxic:* Example is subacute bacterial endocarditis (SBE).
- *Reflex:* Clubbing in bronchogenic carcinoma may improve after vagotomy.
- *Metabolic and humoral (circulating vasodilators):* Example is thyrotoxicosis (thyroid actropachy), acromegaly, etc.
- *Pressure changes:* Between radial and digital arteries.
- Hereditary predisposition.
- *Reduced ferritin:* Ferritin may escape oxidation in lungs which may lead to dilatation of AV anastomosis.

- *Trapping of megakaryocytes and platelet clumps (most recent and accepted view):* Release locally platelet-derived growth factor (PDGF) which increases capillary permeability and tissue proliferation.

Q. Enumerate different causes of clubbing.

Systems involved	*Different diseases*
1. Cardiac	Cyanotic congenital heart disease (e.g., Fallot's tetralogy), subacute bacterial endocarditis (SBE), atrial myxoma, Eisenmenger's syndrome, primary pulmonary hypertension
2. Respiratory	Bronchiectasis, lung abscess, bronchogenic carcinoma, fibrosing alveolitis, empyema thoracis, mesothelioma, pulmonary arteriovenous (AV) fistula, cystic fibrosis, fibrocaseous cavitary tuberculosis (rare)
3. GI tract	Ulcerative colitis, Crohn's disease, malabsorption syndrome, polyposis coli, coeliac disease
4. Hepatobiliary	Biliary cirrhosis, hepato-pulmonary syndrome
5. Genetic	May be familial (autosomal dominant, rare)
6. Normal	Normally seen in some people (idiopathic)

* Commonest cause in young—bronchiectasis, and in elderly—bronchogenic carcinoma.

** COPD per se does not give rise to clubbing but if present, it raises the suspicion of bronchogenic carcinoma or bronchiectasis.

*** Examine both hands and toes in any case of clubbing.

Q. Do you know Schamroth's sign?

Approximate two fingers of two hands, preferably thumbs or ring fingers of both hands, face to face and observe the diamond-shaped area formed between two nails and the proximal nail-folds. In clubbing, this diamond-shaped area is obliterated, and is known as Schamroth's sign or window sign.

Q. Do you know different presentations of clubbing?

Variations in clubbing	*Conditions associated with*
• Different types	*Drumstick* (e.g., Fallot's tetralogy and bronchiectasis), and *parrot-beak* type (bronchogenic carcinoma)
• 'Acute' clubbing	Clubbing develops very rapidly within 10–14 days as in lung abscess and empyema thoracis
• Most 'reliable' sign of clubbing	Loss of onychodermal angle
• First affected finger in clubbing	Usually index finger
• Unilateral clubbing	Presubclavian coarctation of aorta, Pancoast's tumour, cervical rib, prolonged hemiplegia, erythromelalgia, AV (arteriovenous) fistula of brachial vessels, aneurysm of subclavian artery, AV fistula made for haemodialysis
• Unidigital clubbing	Local injury, tophaceous gout, sarcoidosis, hereditary
• Limited to upper extremity	Chronic phlebitis due to chronic IV drug addiction
• Limited to lower extremity	• PDA with reversal of shunt *(differential clubbing)* • Infected abdominal aortic aneurysm
• Painful clubbing	Bronchogenic carcinoma, lung abscess, SBE
• Reversible clubbing	Lung abscess, empyema thoracis

• Pseudoclubbing	Due to subperiosteal bone resorption of terminal phalanges (with preservation of onychodermal angle): Seen in scleroderma, leprosy, acromegaly, hyperparathyroidism, working with vinyl chloride
• Uncommon causes of clubbing	Thyrotoxicosis (i.e., thyroid acropachy), asbestosis, sarcoidosis, portal cirrhosis, occupational (e.g., Jackhammer operators), Whipple's disease

NB: Chronic paronychia may be confused with clubbing.

Q. What is hypertrophic osteoarthropathy (HOA)?

HPO is:

- It is the 'subperiosteal new bone formation' with thickening of periosteum at lower end of radius, ulna, tibia and fibula in a patient of clubbing. The patient complains of (C/o) pain and swelling of wrist (commonest) and ankle, and even elbow and knee may be affected. It is commonly seen in bronchogenic carcinoma and probably due to release of vascular endothelial growth factor (VEGF) in the circulation. Familial HOA is known as pachydermoperiostitis.
- Always look for any swelling and/or tenderness in wrist or ankle of a patient of clubbing, and if present, it is of 4° clubbing.

Q. Do you know the interrelationship between clubbing and cyanosis?

Variations in cyanosis and clubbing	*Conditions associated with*
• Cyanosis with clubbing	Cyanotic congenital heart disease, fibrosing alveolitis, bilateral extensive bronchiectasis, cystic fibrosis, Eisenmenger's syndrome, pulmonary AV fistula
• Cyanosis without clubbing	Peripheral cyanosis and acutely developing central cyanosis
• Clubbing without cyanosis	SBE, ulcerative colitis, lung abscess, bronchogenic carcinoma

KOILONYCHIA

Q. Can you define koilonychia?

- This is the 'spoon-shaped deformity' of nails commonly found in chronic iron deficiency anaemia.
- Toe nails are affected earlier than finger nails.

Q. How to examine for koilonychia?

As in examination for clubbing, bring the patient's fingers at your eye level and look tangentially. See and palpate the nails for flattening or concavity.

Q. What are the causes of koilonychia?

Causes of koilonychias are:

1. Iron deficiency anaemia (long-standing)—commonest
2. Idiopathic or familial
3. Onycholysis due to any cause (e.g., trauma)
4. Overuse of detergent or solvent (e.g., nail polish remover).

Q. Do you know different stages of koilonychia?

Different stages of koilonychias are:

- *First stage:* 'Stage of brittleness' (nails become brittle and rough).
- *Second stage:* 'Stage of flattening' (*platonychia*; nails are thin and flat).
- *Third stage:* 'Stage of spooning' (nails become concave).

SKIN, HAIRS AND NAILS

Q. Enumerate different 'nail changes' in clinical medicine.

Nail abnormalities	*Clinical abnormalities*
• Pitting (thimble) nails	Psoriasis (Fig. 2.18), atopic eczema, alopecia areata, trauma, nail biters (bitten nails are found in persons with anxious personality)
• Red lunula (red-half moon)	Congestive cardiac failure (CCF)
• Yellow nails	In 'yellow nail syndrome': other components of this syndrome are lymphoedema and pleural effusion (Fig. 2.19)
• Blue lunula (azure arcs)	$CuSO_4$ poisoning, Wilson's disease, cyanosis, zidovudine therapy, ochronosis, argyria (silver poisoning)
• Green nail	Pseudomonas infection (severe)
• Black nail	Peutz-Jeghers syndrome, hair dyes, melanoma

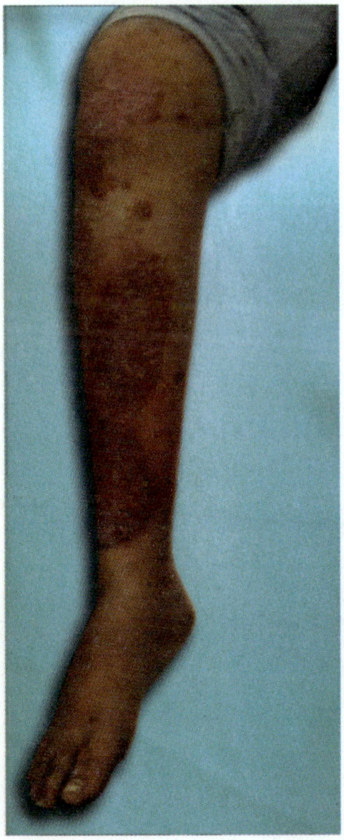

Fig. 2.18: Red, scaly, sharply defined plaques in extensor surfaces of leg and knee in psoriasis

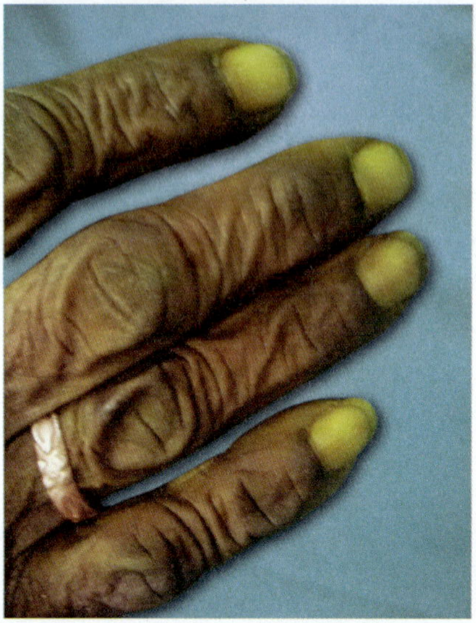

Fig. 2.19: Yellow nails (very rarely seen in a condition called yellow nail syndrome with pleural effusion)

• Shiny nails	Indirect evidence of severe pruritus
• Koilonychia	Concave nails in chronic iron deficiency anaemia
• Leuconychia (white nails; also Terry's nail)	Hypoalbunaemia from cirrhosis, nephrotic syndrome, PEM, severe malnutrition (Fig. 2.20)
• Paronychia (whitlow)	Swollen and inflamed nail-bed are found in working in wet conditions, diabetes, repeated trauma
• Platonychia (flat nails)	Chronic iron deficiency anaemia, hereditary
• Clubbing (convex nail)	Bronchiectasis, bronchogenic carcinoma, SBE

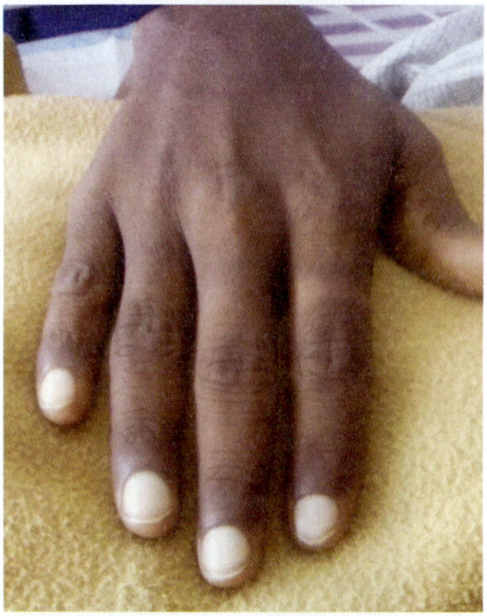

Fig. 2.20: White nails (leuconychia or Terry's nails) in cirrhosis of liver

• Onycholysis	Trauma, psoriasis (Fig. 2.21), candidiasis, ringworm infection, lichen planus, Graves' disease (Plummer's nail), idiopathic
• Beau's line	Transverse ridges develop during recovery from severe systemic illness and malnutrition e.g., typhoid fever, chronic illness (e.g., chronic infection) (Fig. 2.22)

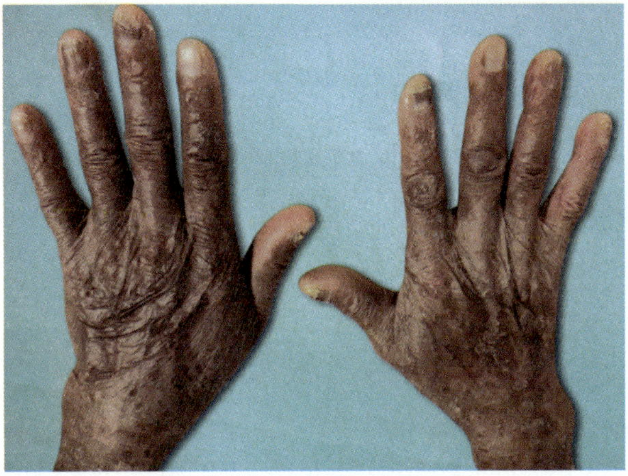

Fig. 2.21: Psoriasis with nail dystrophy (mainly causes onycholysis)

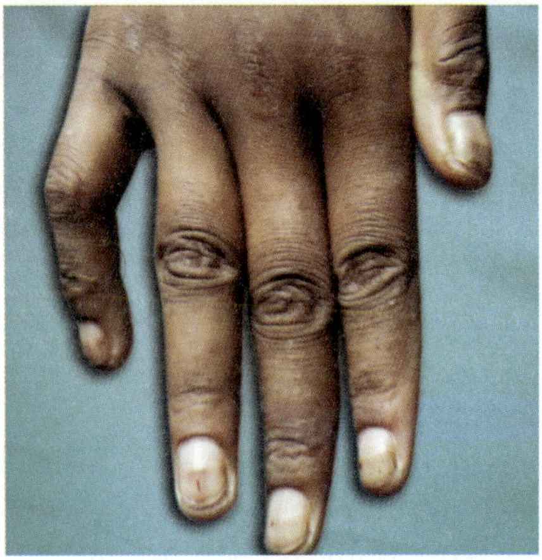

Fig. 2.22: Beau's line—transverse ridges in nails developing during recovery from any febrile illness

• Horder's line (splinter haemorrhage)	Linear longitudinal haemorrhage under the nail is found in trauma, SBE, trichinosis, leukaemia, scurvy, septicaemia, vasculitis
• Mees' line	Transverse white band (1–2 mm wide) above lunula is seen in chronic arsenic poisoning
• Muehrcke's lines	A pair of transverse white lines are seen in hypoalbuminaemia, which disappears on pressure
• Hypertrophy of nails	Chronic fungal infection
• Missing (absent) nail	In nail-patella syndrome (presents as nephrotic syndrome), congonital ectodermal defect
• Onychomycosis	Fungal infection of nails are found in candidiasis and ringworm infection (tinea unguium)—discolouration of nails like white, yellow, brown, black patches or streaks are seen (Fig. 2.23)

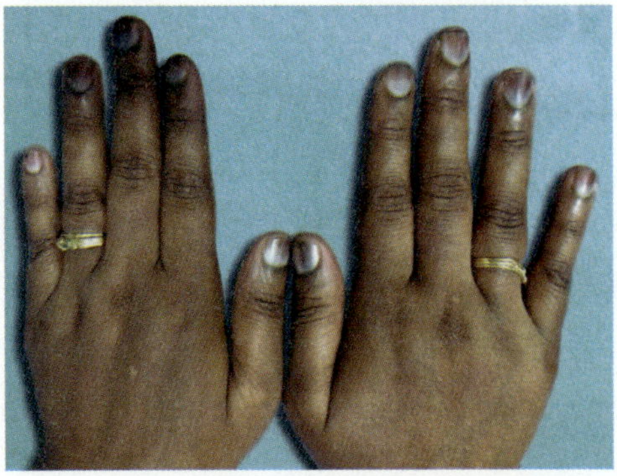

Fig. 2.23: Chromonychia—coloured nail

• Nail-fold thrombi and nail-bed infarct	Vasculitis especially in scleroderma
• Nail-fold telangiectasia	Scleroderma, dermatomyositis, SLE
• Onychorrhexis (brittle nails)	Fungal infection, psoriasis, iron deficiency anaemia
• Wider nail	Acromegaly
• Long narrow nail	Hypopituitarism
• Subungual fibroma (Koenen's)	Tuberous sclerosis (or epiloia)
• Half-and-half nail (Lindsay nail)	Proximal half white, distal half pink with distinct line of separation—seen in chronic renal failure (CRF)
• Plummer's nail	Separation of distal margin of nail from nail-bed in Graves' disease
• Ridges in nails	Transverse: Psoriasis, trauma, eczema, Beau's line Longitudinal: Ageing, trauma, onychomycosis, psoriasis

Q. Do you know the rate of growth of nail?

Regarding the rate of growth of nail:

- Nail grows at a rate of 0.1 mm/day (3 mm/month). Finger nails take 3–6 months to grow out completely, while toe nails may require 12–18 months. So, Beau's line may allow estimation of date of illness of a person.
- Finger nails grow much faster than toe nails. In psoriasis, rapid growth of nail plate occurs.
- Growth of nail is faster in winter than in summer, and in long fingers than in small fingers.

Q. Can you enumerate causes of alopecia?

Different causes of alopecia (loss of hair) are:

- *Adults have two types of hair: Vellus* and *terminal*. Vellus hair is short, soft, fine and usually colourless, while terminal hair is long, coarse, dark sometimes curly; *lanugo hair* is foetal hair. There are three phases in the cycle of hair growth: Anagen (growth), catagen (resting) and telogen (shedding). The rate of hair growth is about 1.25 cm or 0.5 inches/month, or about 15 cm or 6 inches/year. The average daily hair loss from human scalp is 20–100.
- The anagen-catagen-telogen cycle lasts up to 5 years for scalp hair; eyebrow, axillary and pubic hair have a lesser duration cycle than scalp hair. Pubic hair appears two years earlier the appearance of axillary hair and moustache (in boys).
- *Alopecia*: It is the partial or complete loss of hair, especially on the scalp. It is of two types:
  - *Scarring or cicatricial (i.e., permanent loss of hair follicle)*
    - Discoid lupus erythematosus (DLE) (Fig. 2.24), scleroderma, lichen planus, 'pseudopelade', bacterial folliculitis, folliculitis decalvans, sarcoidosis, burn, irradiation.
  - *Non-scarring (temporary loss of hair follicle)*
    - Androgenic alopecia (male-pattern of baldness), alopecia areata (Fig. 2.25), telogen effluvium, postpartum alopecia, SLE, tinea capitis, bullous pemphigoid, diabetes, enteric fever, hypothyroid, HIV infection, anticancer chemotherapy.

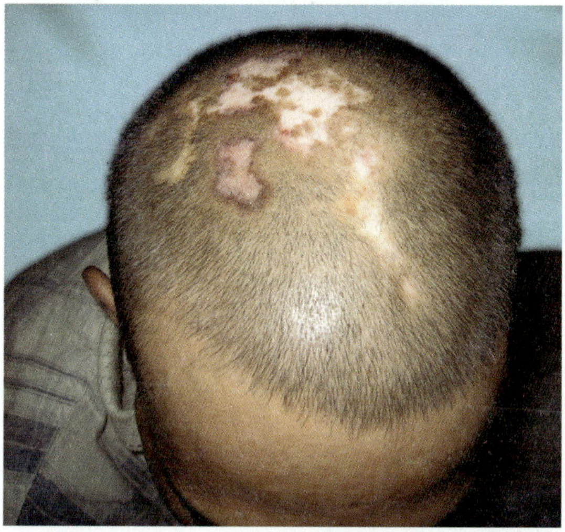

Fig. 2.24: Discoid lupus erythematosus (DLE)—erythematous, scaly plaques with prominent follicular plugging and scarring. There is cicatricial alopecia over the lesions

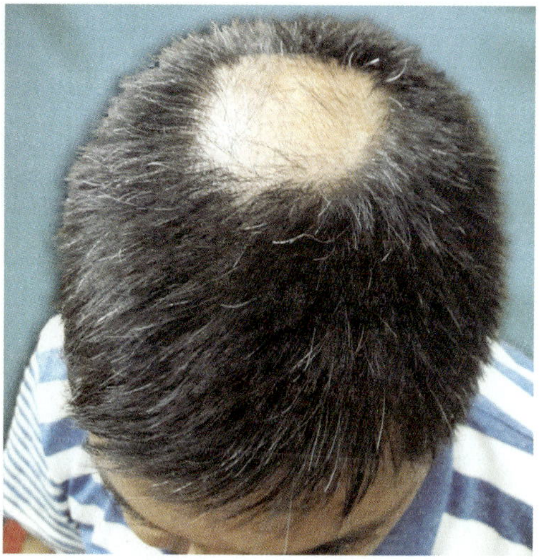

Fig. 2.25: Alopecia areata (localised loss of hairs) in scalp

Q. Do you know madarosis?

It is the loss of hair in lateral one-third of eyebrows, and is commonly due to:

- Leprosy
- Myxoedema (Fig. 2.26)
- Amyloidosis
- Neurodermatitis.

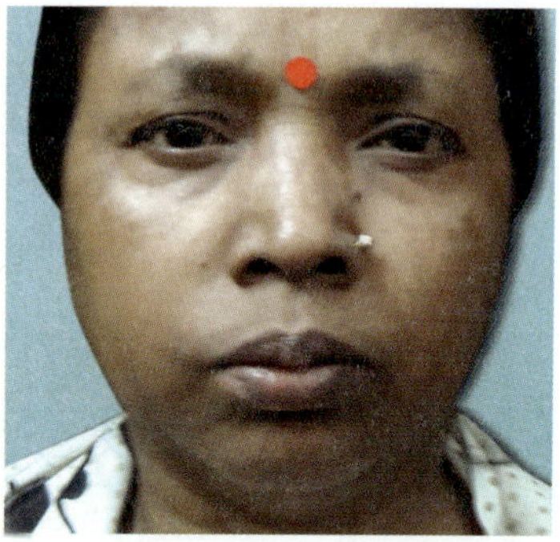

Fig. 2.26: Myxoedema with madarosis i.e., loss of lateral 1/3rd of eyebrows is present bilaterally

Q. What is hirsutism?

It is the growth of terminal hair in women in a pattern characteristic of men. Hirsutism may be present with or without *virilisation;* signs of virilisation are—frontal baldness, acne, seborrhoea, broad shoulders, clitoromegaly, coarse voice, and increased libido (Fig. 2.27). The common causes of hirsutism are:

- Familial
- Idiopathic or simple hirsutism
- Cushing's syndrome
- Polycystic ovarian disease (PCOD)
- Congenital adrenal hyperplasia
- *Drugs:* Minoxidil, diazoxide, phenytoin, androgens, psoralens, corticosteroids
- *Others:* Hyperprolactinaemia, acromegaly, adrenal tumour, virilising ovarian tumour, menopause, obesity.

*Remember, most of the hairy women have no underlying disease.

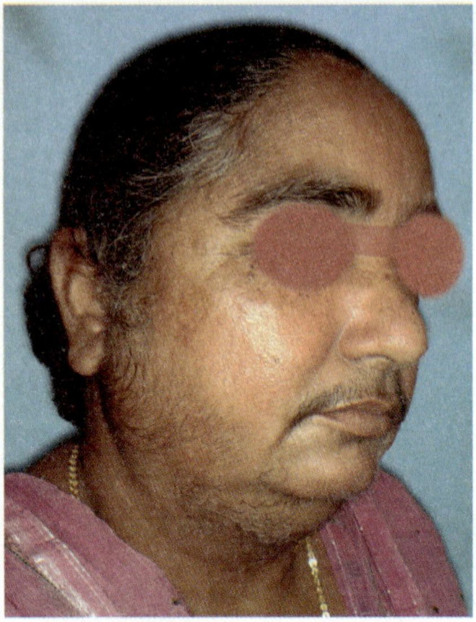

Fig. 2.27: Hirsutism (patient has features of virilisation too)

Q. What is hypertrichosis?

- It is the excessive hair growth in both sexes in a generalised or localised pattern, and is commonly due to malnutrition, hypothyroid, underlying malignancy, Cushing's syndrome, Hurler's syndrome, porphyria cutanea tarda, anorexia nervosa and drugs (mentioned above).
- Hairy ears (hypertrichosis) in a male are Y-linked manifestation.

Q. What are the causes of premature graying of hair?

- Ageing gives rise to natural graying of hairs (canities).
- *Premature graying:* Hereditary, albinism, over vitiligo patches, thyrotoxicosis, pernicious anaemia, diabetes mellitus, Waardenburg syndrome, chloroquine toxicity.

Q. What are the causes of excessive sweating, 'night sweats' and 'cold and clammy' skin in clinical medicine?

Sweat glands are supplied by post-ganglionic sympathetic fibres though they are cholinergic in nature i.e., pilocarpine increases flow of sweat and atropine reduces sweating.

Variations in sweating	*Disease entities*
• Excessive sweating	Familial or idiopathic, pyrexia, anxiety neurosis, AMI, thyrotoxicosis, hypoglycaemia, pheochromocytoma, acromegaly, arecoline sensitivity (present in betel-nut), intense pain, psychoneurosis, obesity, drugs (e.g., insulin, antipyretics, sildenafil)
• Drenching sweat	Hypoglycaemia, AMI, arecoline hypersensitivity
• 'Night sweats' (drenching sweats that require changing of bedclothes)	Tuberculosis, lymphoma, giant cell arteritis, chronic myeloid leukaemia (CML), brucellosis, nocturnal hypoglycaemia, AIDS, menopausal syndrome, amoebic liver abscess, infective endocarditis

• 'Cold and clammy' skin	Sweating associated with cutaneous vasoconstriction (clammy means sticky sweat) is characteristic of shock, AMI, hypoglycaemia, vasovagal attack, alcohol withdrawal, and dumping syndrome

Q. Enumerate causes of hyperpigmentation and hypopigmentation.

Variations in pigmentation	*Conditions associated*
• Hyperpigmentation of skin [i.e., excessive pigmentation of skin]	Familial/racial, sunburn, Addison's disease (Fig. 2.28), haemochromatosis, chronic kala-azar, cirrhosis, uraemia, acanthosis nigricans, pellagra, chloasma/melasma, pregnancy, primary biliary cirrhosis, drugs (clofazimine, psoralens, bleomycin, busulphan), alkaptonuria, paraneoplastic syndrome, scleroderma, melanoma, malnutrition
• Hypopigmentation (hypomelanosis) of skin [i.e., inadequate pigmentation of skin]	Tuberculoid leprosy, vitiligo, albinism, pityriasis alba, pityriasis versicolor (Fig. 2.29), tuberous sclerosis (leafy macules), psoriasis (Fig. 2.30), phenylketonuria, piebaldism (manifested by a forelock of white hair), post-burn, prolonged chloroquine therapy, chemical toxicity, nevus anaemicus

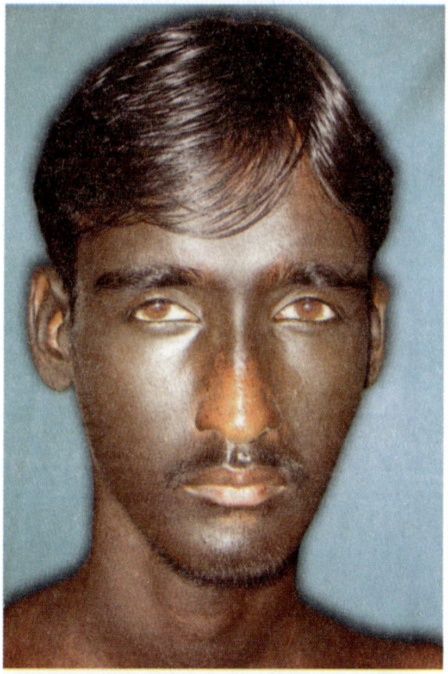

Fig. 2.28: Hyperpigmentation of face in Addison's disease

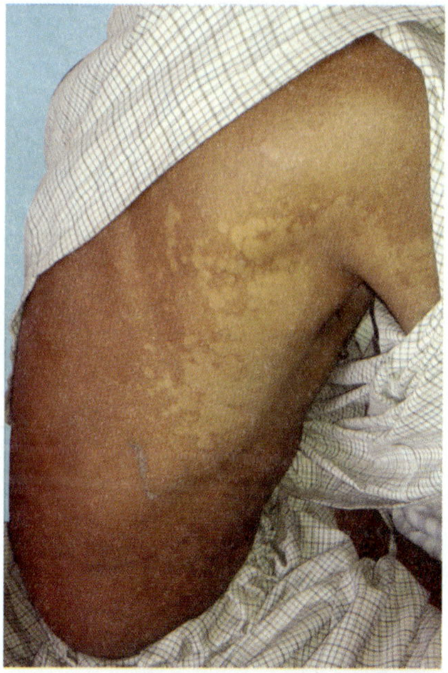

Fig. 2.29: Pityriasis versicolor producing hypopigmentation in a large area

NB: Vitiligo (smooth, white patches on various parts of the body, caused by the loss of the natural pigment) may be idiopathic (Fig. 2.31), or may be present in autoimmune diseases (Fig. 2.32) e.g., Hashimoto's thyroiditis, pernicious anaemia, type 1 diabetes mellitus, Addison's disease or SLE.

Generalised hyperpigmentation occurs in Addison's disease and haemochromatosis; others are *patchy* hyperpigmentation. *Generalised* hypopigmentation is seen in albinism (Fig. 2.33), while others are *patchy* hypopigmentation.

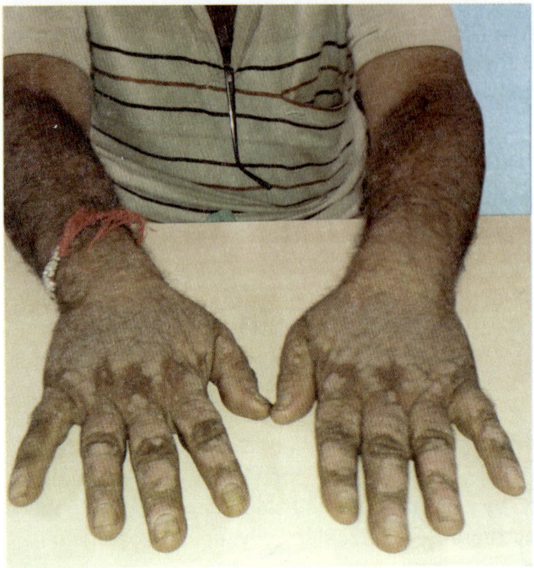

Fig. 2.30: Psoriasis affecting dorsum of hand and fingers mimicking hypopigmentation

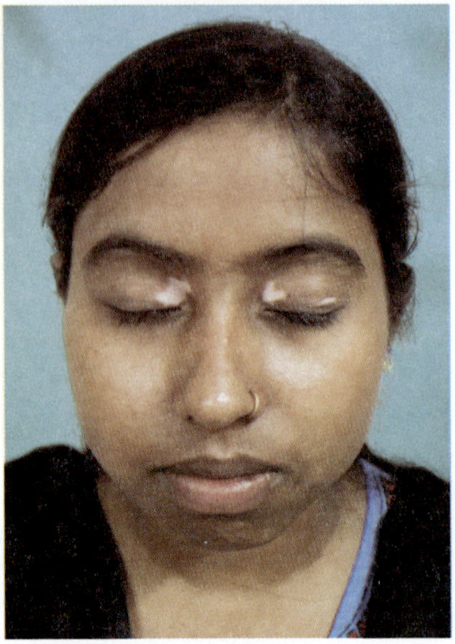

Fig. 2.31: Vitiligo (leucoderma) of upper eyelids

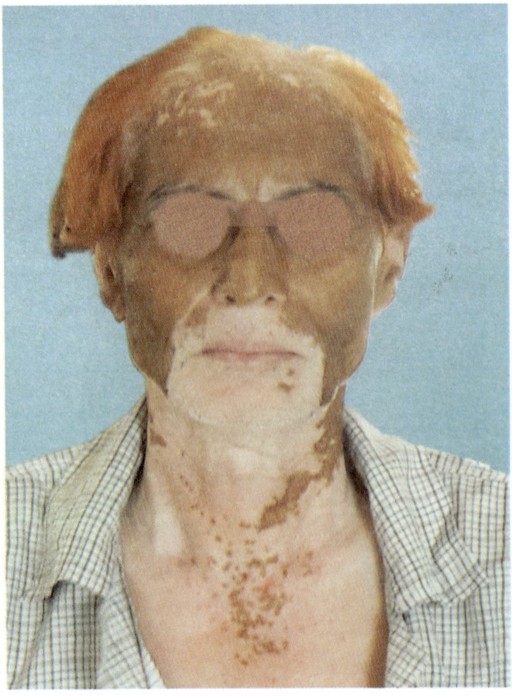

Fig. 2.32: Vitiligo (leucoderma) involving major aspect of body and part of face

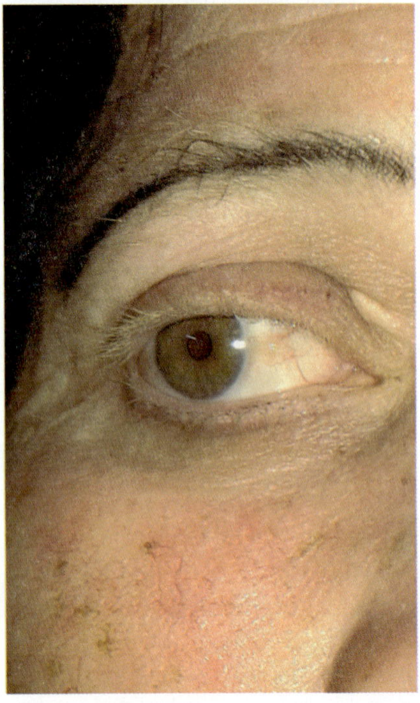

Fig. 2.33: Albinism (congenital disorder with complete or partial absence of pigment in the skin, hair and eyes) with gray iris and white eyelashes

Q. What are the sites examined at the bedside for pigmentation?

Sites to be examined for pigmentation are:
- Face
- Buccal mucosa, lip, gum, palate and tongue
- Palms (especially the creases) and soles
- *General skin surface:* Pressure points (e.g., elbow, knee) and normally pigmented areas (e.g., areola, knuckles, genitals, recent scars).

Q. Can you enumerate causes of pigmentation in oral cavity?

Pigmentation in oral cavity is commonly due to:
- Racial
- Addison's disease
- Peutz-Jeghers syndrome
- Haemochromatosis
- Chloasma
- Malabsorption syndrome
- *Others:* Chronic lead poisoning (Burtonian line), amalgam tattoo, melanotic macule, 'black hairy tongue', busulphan-induced.

*Remember specific sites of pigmentation for a particular disease: Kala-azar—around mouth, temple, forehead; Addison's disease–described in the sites examined at bedside (see before); chloasma/melasma—malar prominence, bridge of the nose, moustache area; haemochromatosis—face, neck, lower forearms, lower legs, genitals; Peutz-Jeghers syndrome–perioral; acanthosis nigricans—sides of neck, axilla, groin (Fig. 2.34).

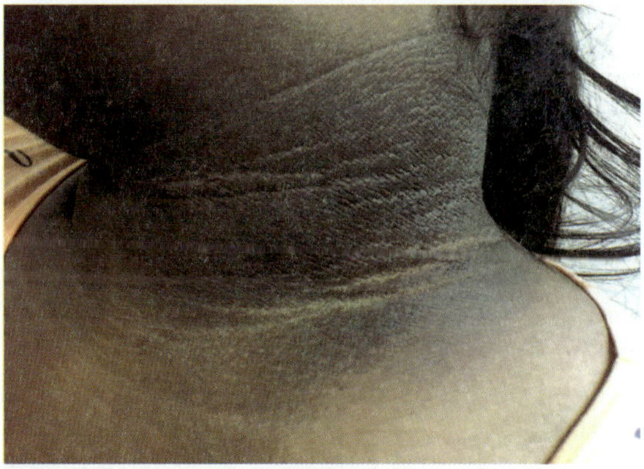

Fig. 2.34: Acanthosis nigricans—dark patches of skin with a thick, velvety texture in an obese diabetic

Q. What are the causes of plethoric face or 'flushed face appearance'?

Facial plethora is seen in:
- Chronic alcoholism
- Cushing's syndrome
- Superior vena caval (SVC) syndrome
- Polycythemia vera
- Carcinoid syndrome

- Myxoedema
- Systemic mastocytosis
- *Others:* Mitral stenosis, thyrotoxicosis, menopause, embarrassment, pyrexia, high altitude, pheochromocytoma, long-term use of corticosteroid (Fig. 2.35), patient on disulfiram (antabuse) therapy taking alcohol, normal variation.

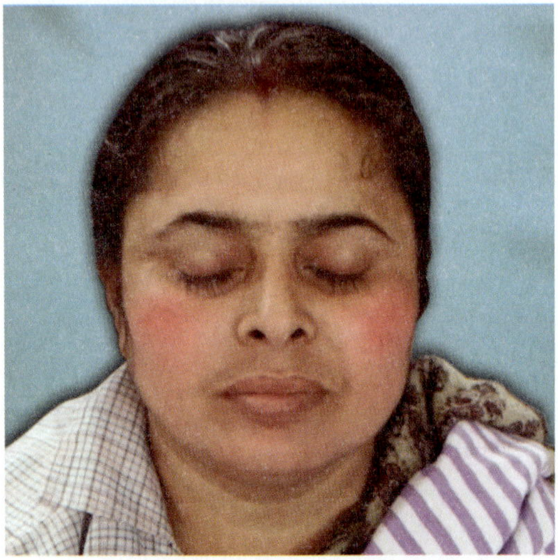

Fig. 2.35: Malar flush due to prolonged use of corticosteroid locally

Q. Colour (pigmentary) changes in skin.

Different colours of skin encountered in clinical medicine are:

- *Yellowish:* Jaundice
- *Bluish:* Cyanosis
- *Pallor:* Anaemia, hypopituitarism
- *Blackish:* Addison's disease
- *Orange-yellowish:* Carotenaemia (e.g., myxoedema).

Q. Few terminology used in dermatology.

These are the language commonly used by the dermatologists. They are:

1. *Macule:* Localised discolouration in skin, which is neither raised nor depressed and of a size of <1 cm; a big macule is known as 'Patch' (>1 cm).
2. *Papule:* Palpable solid elevation of skin (<5 mm); a big papule of >5 mm spread horizontally is called 'Plaque'.
3. *Maculopapular:* Features of both macule and papule.
4. *Vesicle:* Small (<5 mm), clear fluid-containing elevated lesion in skin, whereas 'bulla' is large vesicle (>5 mm); 'pustules' are vesicles filled with pus. 'Nodules' are solid elevation in skin of >5 mm in diameter.
5. *Scale:* Excess of loose, desquamated epithelium (stratum corneum).
6. *Crust:* Dried-up exudates, which may be yellow (serous crust), or red (haemorrhagic crust).

7. *Erosion:* Loss of epidermis without associated loss of dermis.
8. *Excoriation:* Loss of skin substance by 'scratching'.
9. *Sclerosis:* Induration of skin.
10. *Lichenification:* Distinctive thickening of epidermis with exaggerated skin-fold markings, caused by rubbing.
11. *Erythema:* Superficial reddening of the skin, usually in patches.
12. *Ulcer:* Loss of epidermis, dermis, and even the subcutaneous tissue.
13. *Urticaria (hives):* Intensely pruritic, raised *wheals*, with or without oedema of the deeper cutis.
14. *Scar:* Areas of fibrous tissue which replace normal skin after injury.
15. *Morbilliform:* Generalised, small erythematous macules and/or papules that look like skin lesions of measles.
16. *Telangiectasia:* Cluster of dilated superficial blood vessels seen on skin surface.

Q. Common causes of vesicles/bullae in skin.

1. Varicella infection i.e., chickenpox (vesicles) (Fig. 2.36).
2. Pemphigus vulgaris (Figs 2.37 and 2.38).
3. Bullous pemphigoid.
4. Stevens-Johnson syndrome.
5. Toxic epidermal necrolysis (Fig. 2.39).
6. Bullous impetigo.
7. Herpes zoster infection (Figs 2.40 and 2.41).

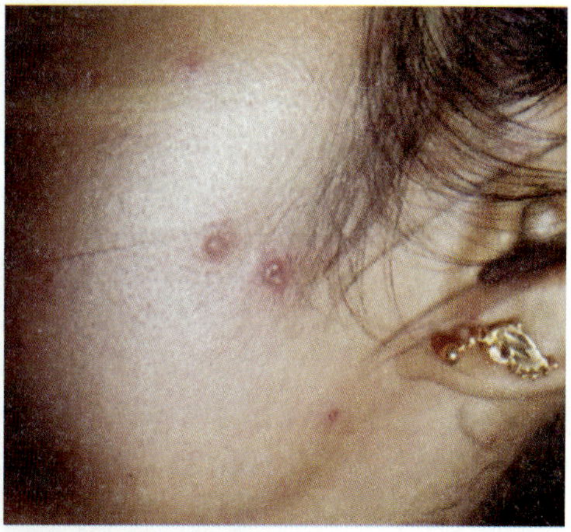

Fig. 2.36: Vesicles of chickenpox over the face

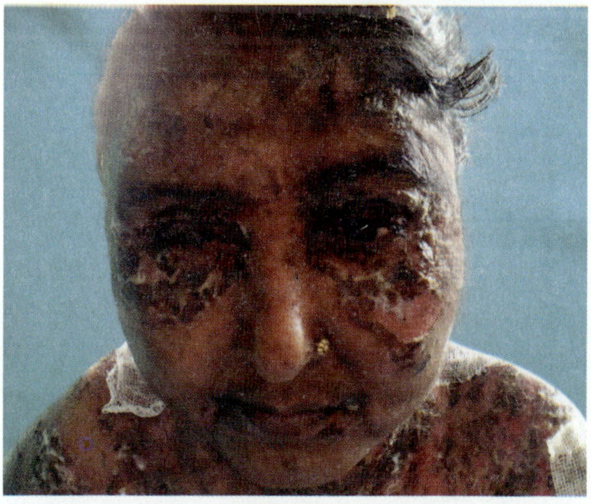

Fig. 2.37: Pemphigus vulgaris—bulla (i.e., the blisters) are ruptured with denudation of skin of face and upper chest

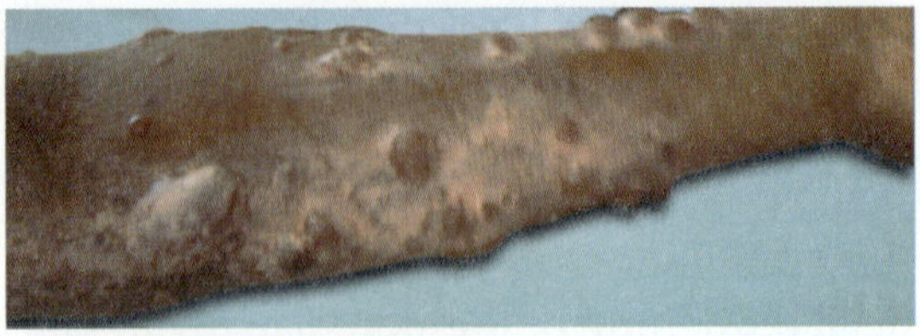

Fig. 2.38: Pemphigus vulgaris with multiple bullae in upper limb (painted with lotio calamine)

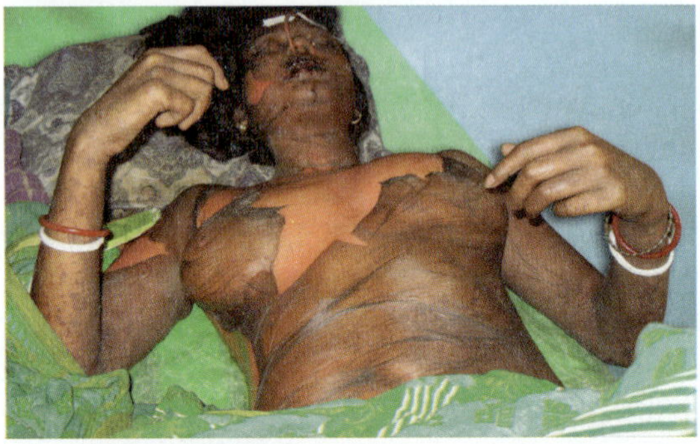

Fig. 2.39: Toxic epidermal necrolysis (TEN)—a potentially life-threatening dermatological condition with skin peeling (more dangerous than Stevens-Johnson syndrome), commonly drug-induced

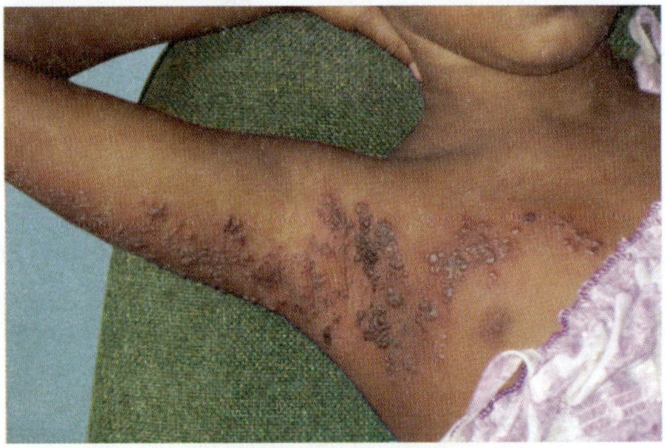

Fig. 2.40: Multiple vesicles are seen in herpes zoster infection (shingles) due to reactivation of latent varicella zoster virus (chickenpox)

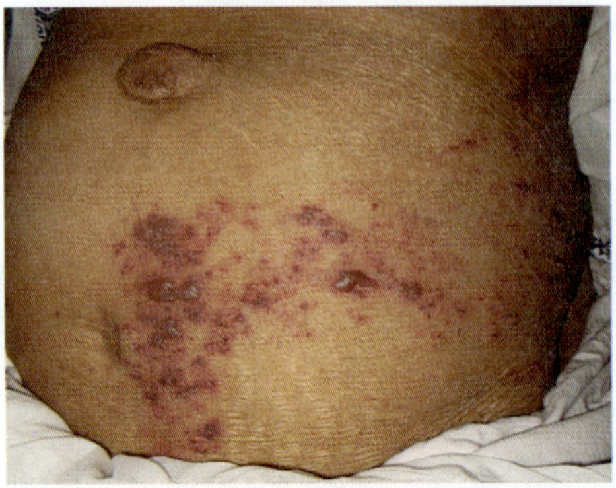

Fig. 2.41: Herpes zoster infection (shingles) with multiple vesicles affecting abdominal dermatomes

Q. Skin (the mirror of systemic diseases) in different disorders.

A. *Skin manifestations in internal malignancy:*

- Acanthosis nigricans (adenocarcinoma of stomach)
- Dermatomyositis (malignancy of ovary, lung, breast, and GI tract)
- Clubbing with HOA (bronchogenic carcinoma leading to pachydermoperiostitis)
- Pruritus, generalised (lymphomas, leukaemias, polycythemia vera)
- Migratory thrombophlebitis (carcinoma of the pancreas): Trousseau's sign
- Ichthyosis (lymphomas)
- Erythema multiforme or exfoliative dermatitis (lymphomas) (Fig. 2.42)
- Hypertrichosis lanuginosa (adenocarcinoma of GI tract)
- Pellagra-like skin lesions (carcinoid syndrome)
- Palmoplantar keratoderma (Tylosis—in oesophageal carcinoma)
- Blistering disorders (paraneoplastic bullous pemphigoid)
- Pyoderma gangrenosum (leukaemias, multiple myeloma)
- *Others:* Malignant infiltration of skin by nodules, ulcers; functional disturbance manifested by pigmentation, purpura, etc.

B. *Systemic diseases manifested by generalised pruritus:*

- Obstructive jaundice (i.e., cholestasis)
- Chronic renal failure (uraemia)
- Diabetes mellitus
- Polycythemia vera (especially, after a hot bath)
- Lymphomas (Hodgkin's disease), leukaemias, multiple myeloma
- Systemic mastocytosis

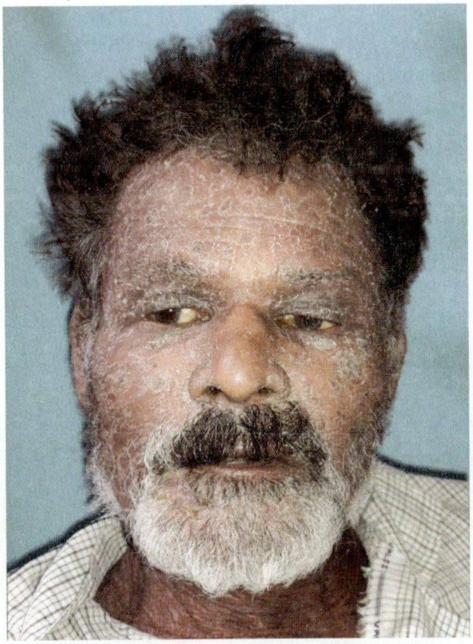

Fig. 2.42: Erythroderma or exfoliative dermatitis from lymphoma

- Carcinoid syndrome
- *Others:* Pregnancy (last trimester), psychological, thyrotoxicosis, old age, drug reactions.

C. *Dermatological manifestations in cardiovascular system (CVS):*
- Osler's node, splinter haemorrhage, Janeway's spot, pallor, clubbing, petechiae/ purpura, nail-fold thrombi: Seen in infective endocarditis
- Erythema marginatum, subcutaneous nodules, erythema nodosum: Seen in acute rheumatic fever.

NB: Xanthelasma (often associated with hypercholesterolaemia) is a clinical window for coronary heart disease (Fig. 2.43).

D. *Dermatological manifestations in neurological disorders:*
- Features of different congenital neuro-cutaneous syndromes like café-au-lait spots, neurofibroma (Fig. 2.44), axillary freckles are found in von Recklinghausen's disease; capillary haemangioma in face is seen in Sturge-Weber syndrome; adenoma sebaceum and shagreen patches are seen in tuberous sclerosis.
- Seborrhoea (facial) in post-encephalitic parkinsonism
- Hypopigmented macules, patches, plaques, or nodules are seen in leprosy, which may give rise to peripheral neuropathy
- Telangiectasia is common in ataxia-telangiectasia and hereditary haemorrhagic telangiectasis (Rendu-Weber-Osler disease).

E. *Dermatological manifestations in pulmonary disorders:*
- Warm and moist hand: Type II respiratory failure
- Erythema nodosum: Tuberculosis, sarcoidosis
- Clubbing and nicotine stain in fingers: Bronchogenic carcinoma
- Flushing of face with facial oedema: SVC syndrome
- Cold abscess with sinuses (e.g., in axilla): Tuberculous lymphadenitis.

F. *Dermatological manifestations in GI tract disorders:*
- Palmar erythema, spider naevi, muddy skin with diffuse pigmentation, petechiae/ purpura/ecchymosis: Cirrhosis of liver
- Tylosis (hyperkeratosis of palms and soles): Carcinoma of the oesophagus
- Migratory thrombophlebitis: Carcinoma of the pancreas
- Pyoderma gangrenosum: Ulcerative colitis

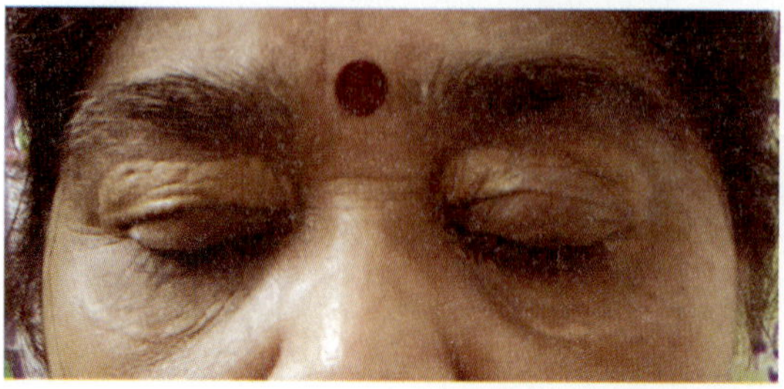

Fig. 2.43: Xanthelasma encircling the eyeball where the patient has hypercholesterolaemia, H/o IHD and hypothyroidism

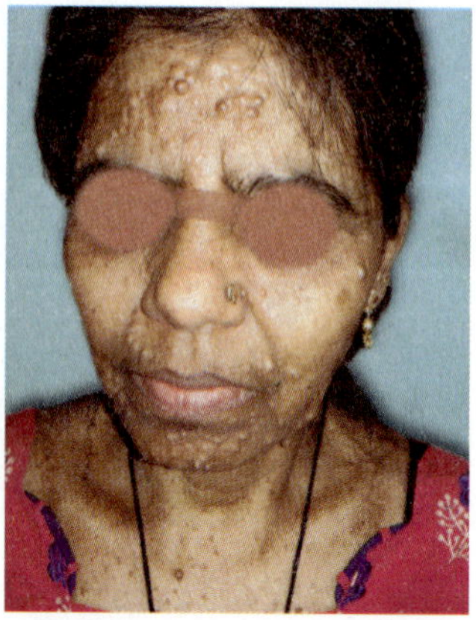

Fig. 2.44: Multiple neurofibroma

- Cullen's sign (bluish discolouration around umbilicus) and Grey Turner's sign (bluish-red discolouration of abdominal skin in flanks): Haemoperitoneum from any cause (e.g., acute pancreatitis)
- Telangiectasia: Hereditary haemorrhagic telangiectasis (Rendu-Weber-Osler disease) may be a cause of haematemesis
- Perioral pigmentation: Peutz-Jeghers syndrome (having polyps in intestine, which may lead to haematochezia).

G. *Dermatological manifestations in haematological diseases:*

- Petechiae, purpura, ecchymosis (even painful): Leukaemias, coagulation disorders (Fig. 2.45)
- Urticaria: Polycythemia vera.

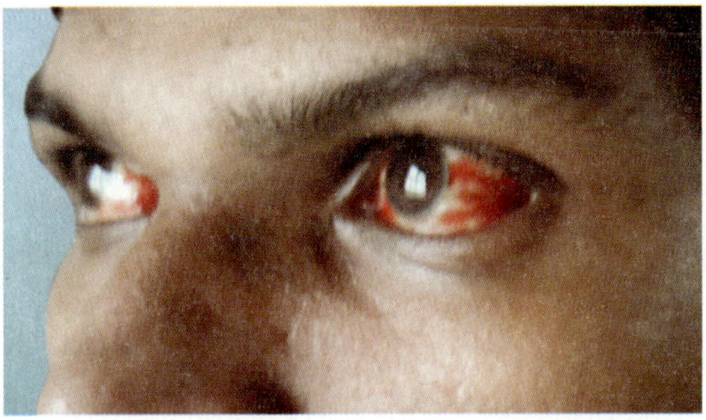

Fig. 2.45: Subconjunctival haemorrhage due to coagulation disorders

H. *Dermatological manifestations in rheumatic disorders:*

- Features of vasculitis:
  - Large arteries: Digital gangrene
  - Small arteries: Palpable purpura, morbilliform eruptions, urticaria
  - Arterioles and very small arteries: Digital infarction, digital ulceration, nail-fold thrombi, pulp atrophy, splinter haemorrhage, Raynaud's phenomenon.
- Butterfly rash in face, panniculitis, periungual erythema, telangiectasia, features of vasculitis: SLE
- Tight skin, salt-pepper appearance (Fig. 2.46), pulp atrophy (Fig. 2.47), dilated nail-fold capillary loops, digital ulcer, calcinosis cutis: Scleroderma (i.e., progressive systemic sclerosis or PSS)
- Livedo reticularis: Anticardiolipin antibody syndrome
- Heliotrope rash in face (Fig. 2.48), Gottron's papule over knuckles: Dermatomyositis
- Loose and lax skin: Ehlers-Danlos syndrome (Fig. 2.49)

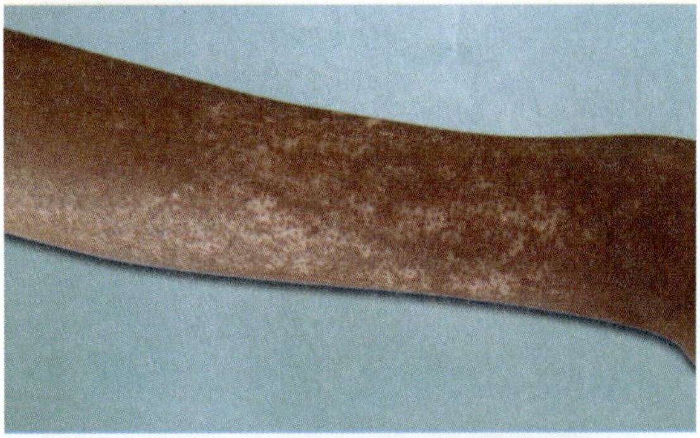

Fig. 2.46: Pigmented (pepper) and depigmented (salt) skin in forearm of a patient suffering from scleroderma giving the salt-pepper appearance

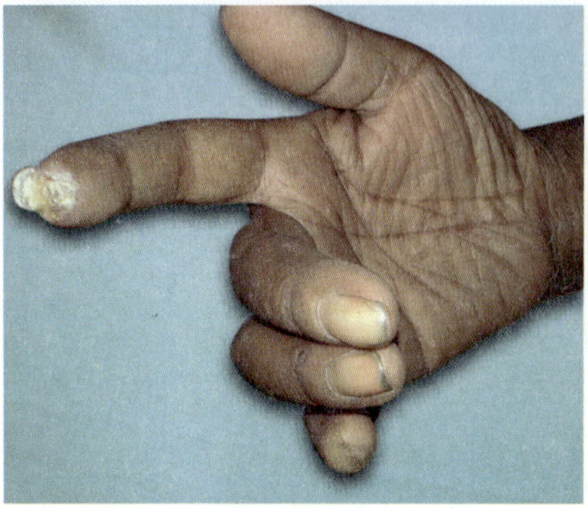

Fig. 2.47: Excoriation of skin in tip of right index finger with pulp atrophy—feature of vasculitis

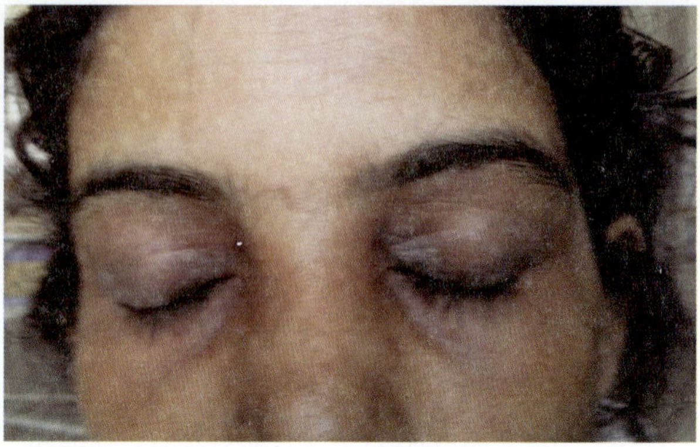

Fig. 2.48: The 'heliotrope rash'—lilac or purple-coloured rash around the eyes with oedema of eyelids seen in dermatomyositis

- Pyoderma gangrenosum: Rheumatoid arthritis
- Tophi deposited in skin: Gout (Fig. 2.50)
- Keratoderma blennorrhagica, circinate balanitis: Reactive arthritis.

Q. What are the different sexually transmitted infections?

Sexually transmitted infections (STIs) are also known as sexually transmitted diseases (STDs) and venereal diseases (VDs). These infections are commonly spread by sex, especially by vaginal intercourse, anal sex or oral sex. Safer sex (e.g., use of condom) and having a smaller number of sexual partners decrease the risk of STDs. The different STDs are:

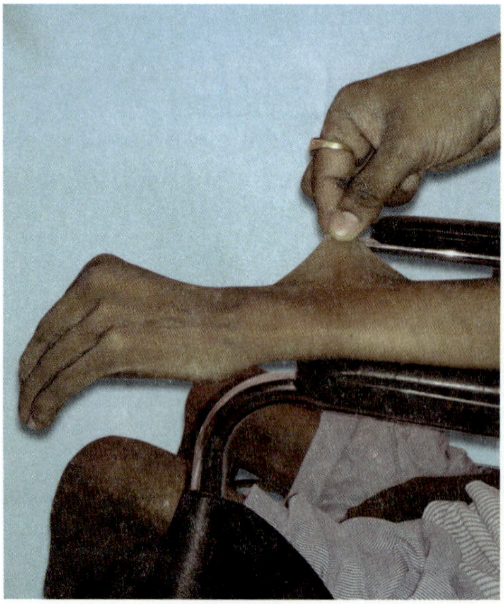

Fig. 2.49: Stretchy skin is noted in Ehlers-Danlos syndrome; other components are loose-jointedness and abnormal scar formation

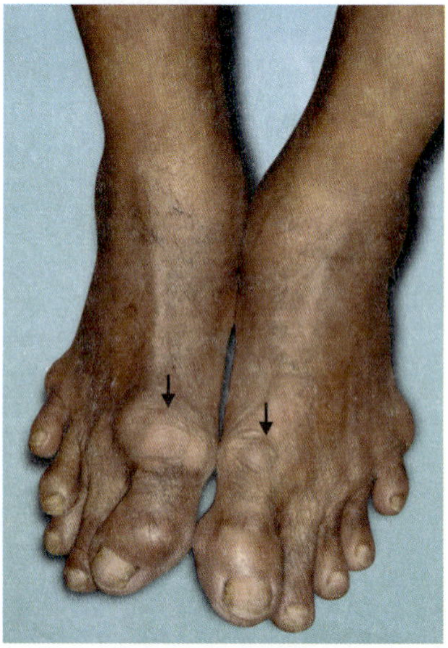

Fig. 2.50: Gouty tophi over both 1st metatarsophalangeal joints

Bacterial

- Chancroid (*Haemophilus ducreyi*)
- Gonorrhoea (*Neisseria gonorrhoeae*)
- Syphilis (*Treponema pallidum*)
- Chlamydia (*Chlamydia trachomatis*)
- Granuloma inguinale (*Klebsiella granulomatis*).

Viral

- Viral hepatitis (hepatitis B virus and rarely hepatitis C virus)
- HIV (human immunodeficiency virus)
- Herpes simplex (herpes simplex virus 1 and 2; produces genital herpes)
- HPV (human papillomavirus)—responsible for cervical carcinoma and genital warts
- Molluscum contagiosum virus.

Fungal

- Candidiasis (yeast infection).

Parasites

- "pubic lice" (Pthirus pubis)
- Scabies (*Sarcoptes scabiei*).

Protozoal

- Trichomoniasis (*Trichomonas vaginalis*).

FACIES

Q. What is facies?

Facies is the 'expression in the face' of the patient, which may sometimes indicate aetiological diagnosis of a disease. The 'facial expression/appearance' may be anxious, sad, calm, flushes, pyrexial, toxic, dehydrated, or may show some features specific for a disease (e.g., parkinsonism, myxoedema). Reading of face in clinical medicine is very important as face is regarded as 'mirror of the mind'.

Q. Can you describe some common disease-specific facies?

The disease-specific diagnostic facies are:

- *Cushing's syndrome:* The face looks bloated and rounded, like the full moon, and is known as 'Moon face'. The face is dusky and plethoric, and may have hirsutism and acne.
- *Acromegaly:* Enlarged face with prognathism (prominent lower jaw), wide-spaced teeth, frontal bossing, prominent supraorbital ridges, large nose and ears, thick lips, bushy eyebrows with hyperhidrosis, and macroglossia; deep and husky voice.
- *Thyrotoxicosis:* Staring and anxious look, exophthalmos with lid retraction, sclera visible around cornea, moist facial skin with malar flush.
- *Myxoedema:* Dull, expressionless, puffy face (periorbital puffiness with baggy lower eyelids), and dry, rough skin with madarosis; facial pallor (may have malar flush), thick lips with macroglossia; hoarseness of voice with bradylalia (Fig. 2.26).

- *Cretinism:* Dull, expressionless, idiotic face with depressed bridge of the nose along with big nostrils; large head with hypertelorism; thick lips with large, fissured protruded tongue (Fig. 2.51).

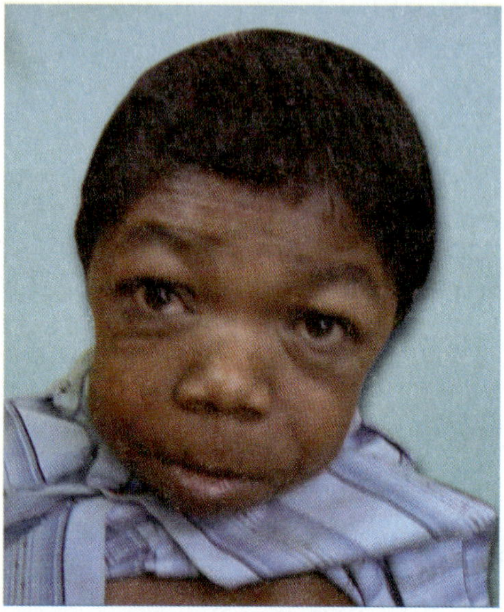

Fig. 2.51: Cretinism with a gruesome facies; depressed bridge of the nose with broad and flat nose are evident

- *Hepatic facies:* Shrunken eyes with hollowed temporal fossa, pinched-up nose, malar prominence (prominent zygoma), parched lips, sallow and dry face with muddy complexion (blending of pallor, jaundice and melanosis), icteric tinge of conjunctiva (i.e., jaundice); bilateral parotid swelling, especially in alcoholics (Fig. 2.52). It is characteristically seen in chronic liver disease (e.g., cirrhosis of liver).
- *Leonine facies:* Deep lines in forehead, depressed bridge of the nose, broad nose with nasal collapse (i.e., saddle nose), thick eyebrows with madarosis, thick skin of face/forehead/infiltrated ear lobes, may have perforation of nasal septum. This is found in lepromatous leprosy (Fig. 2.53).

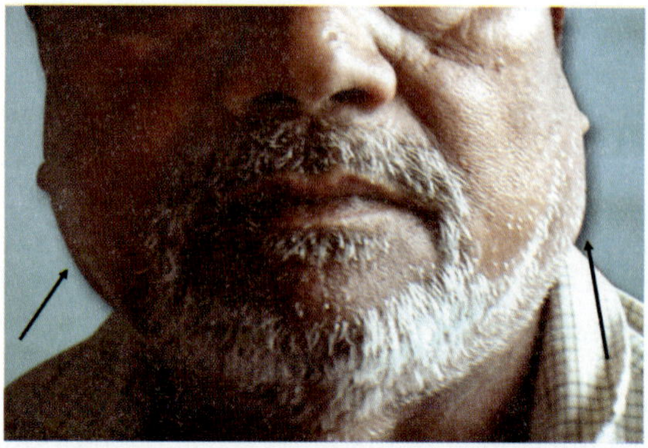

Fig. 2.52: Bilateral parotid swelling in a case of alcoholic cirrhosis

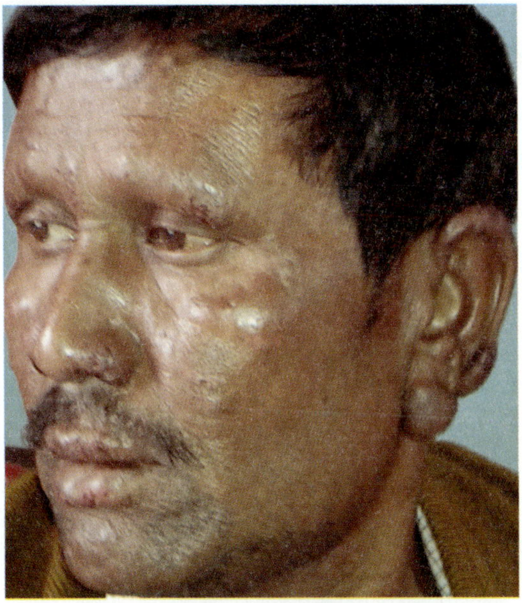

Fig. 2.53: Leonine face (i.e., lion-like face) with infiltrated thick skin of face and ear lobes in leprosy

- *Dehydration (facies Hippocraticus):* Shrunken eyes with hollowed temporal fossa, face is drawn, pinched-up nose, parched lips, tongue is dry and coated, soft eyeballs, and skin is dry and wrinkled (Fig. 2.54).
- *Thalassaemia (mongoloid):* Frontal bossing, depressed bridge of the nose, hypertelorism (widely set eyes due to hyperplasia of lesser wing of sphenoid) with apparent mongoloid slant of eyes, malar prominence, dental malocclusion with prominent upper incisors, and varying degree of jaundice and pallor. This type of face is often called 'chipmunk facies'.

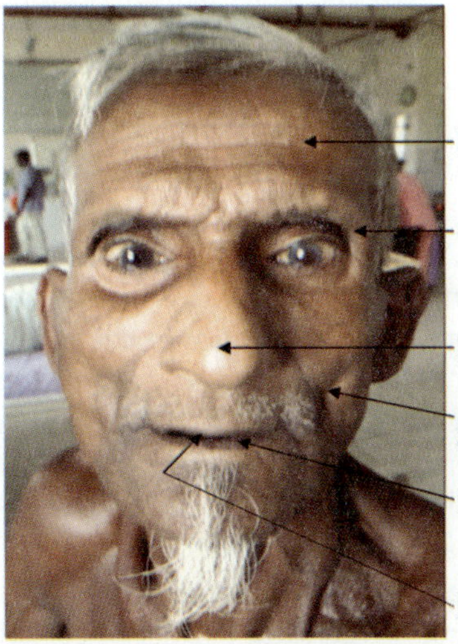

Fig. 2.54: A face of dehydration (facies Hippocraticus)

- *Down's syndrome (mongolism):* Small, round and flat face, brachycephaly, upwards-slanting eyes (oblique orbital fissure) with epicanthic folds, small nose with depressed bridge of the nose, small and low set ears, hypertelorism, high arched palate, open mouth with protruded and furrowed tongue, and an idiotic look (Fig. 2.55).

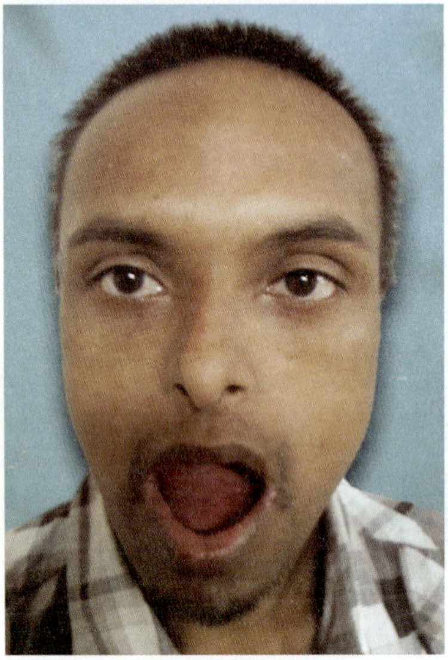

Fig. 2.55: Down's syndrome (mongolism) with an idiotic look; the patient is having a large tongue with angular stomatitis

- *Parkinsonism:* Expressionless, mask-like facies; infrequent blinking with a staring look (reptilian stare); monotonous speech with bradylalia and hypophonia.
- *Nephritic facies:* Pale and puffy face with pronounced periorbital oedema, and narrow palpebral fissure are seen in acute glomerulonephritis. In *nephrotic syndrome*, moon facies is more prominent, especially the periorbital oedema in comparison to nephritic facies.
- *Systemic lupus erythematosus (SLE):* Classical photosensitive 'butterfly' rash over malar areas and bridge of the nose, sparing the nasolabial folds; patchy alopecia with 'lupus hairs' (short and broken hairs) seen above the forehead; painless palatal ulcer (Fig. 2.56).
- *Scleroderma:* Mask-like facies with absence of wrinkling of skin in face and forehead, and pinched-up nose; small mouth (microstomia) with radial furrows around the lips on closing (tobacco-pouch appearance); skin over the face seems taut and shiny with telangiectasia/pigmentation/depigmentation over the face. Typical facies of scleroderma is known as 'mauskopf' (mouse head) appearance (Fig. 2.57).
- *Myotonia:* Frontal baldness, bilateral ptosis (monk-face appearance) with long facial structure ('hatchet face' due to atrophy of temporalis, and 'swan-neck' due to atrophy of sternomastoid muscles); cataract and mental retardation may be noted.
- *Myasthenic face:* Bilateral partial ptosis with wrinkling of forehead; when asked to smile or laugh, there is a 'transverse smile' due to lack of elevation of corners of the mouth as a result of facial muscular weakness, known as 'myasthenic snarl' (Fig. 2.58).

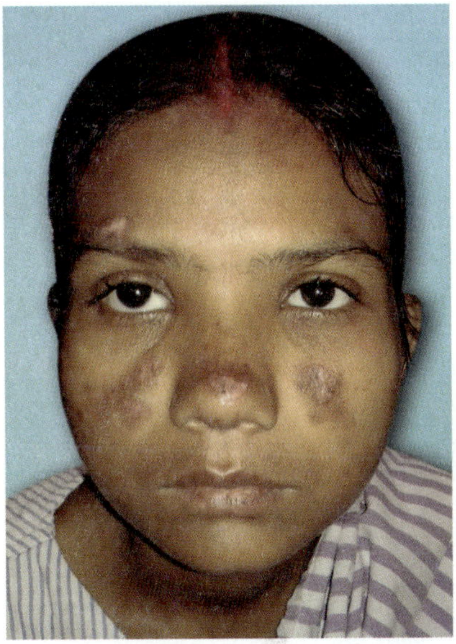

Fig. 2.56: Butterfly rash over face in SLE

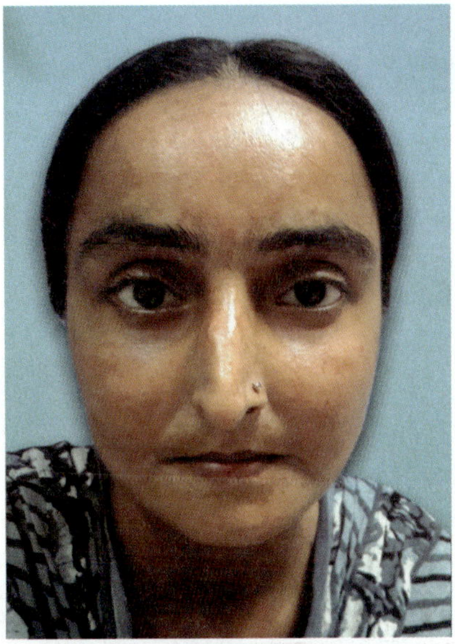

Fig. 2.57: Facies in scleroderma—masked facies, absence of normal wrinkling of skin with taut and shiny skin over face, microstomia and pinched-up nose are evident

- *Bell's palsy:* Facial asymmetry, and asymmetry of blinking and eye closure; wide palpebral fissure and epiphora (on affected side); lack of spontaneous movements of face on affected side, and deviation of angle of the mouth to healthy side when asked to show the upper teeth; Bell's phenomenon is present i.e., eyeball rolls upwards and inwards during attempted forced eye closure on the affected side (Fig. 2.59).

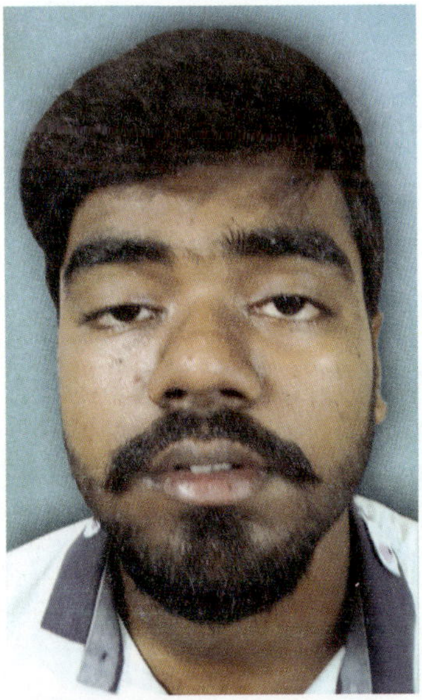

Fig. 2.58: Bilateral partial ptosis from myasthenia gravis

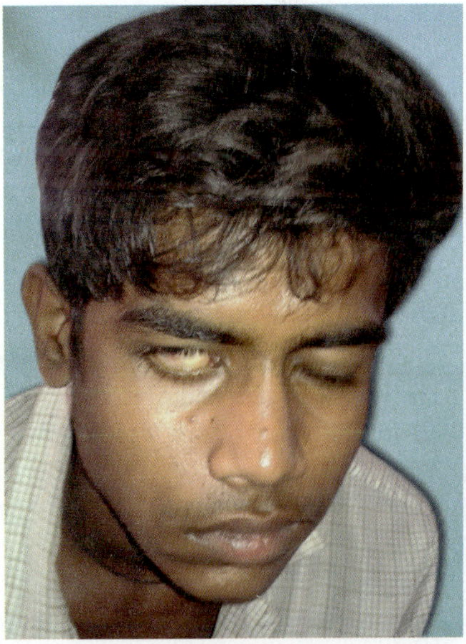

Fig. 2.59: Right-sided Bell's palsy with Bell's phenomenon

- *Polycythemia:* See the section on 'Anaemia'.
- *Mitral facies:* It is the pinkish purple patches on cheeks (especially appreciated in fair-skinned persons, and rare in Indians); low cardiac output in MS produces cyanosis in lips, tip of nose and cheeks, while 'malar flush' is seen due to vasodilatation in malar area.
- *Facies in tetanus:* With 'risus sardonicus' (grimace mimicking 'smile of satan') due to sustained contraction of facial muscles, and blepharospasm; there may be lock jaw (trismus) (Fig. 2.60).

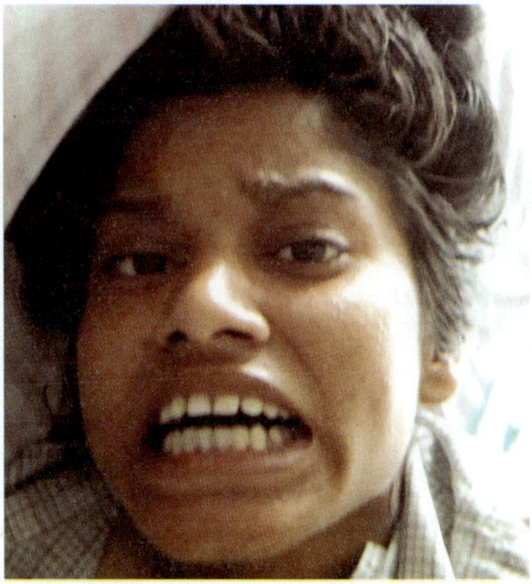

Fig. 2.60: 'Lock jaw' in tetanus with smile of satan (risus sardonicus)

- *Masked facies:* 'Poverty of expression of face' is seen in parkinsonism, scleroderma, bilateral upper motor neuron (UMN) facial nerve palsy, myxoedema, depression, dementia, myasthenia gravis and pseudobulbar palsy. Masked facies is characterised by:
  - Infrequent blinking with staring look
  - Loss of facial expression, and face looks blank and apathetic
  - Widened palpebral fissure.
- *Moon face (i.e., swollen and puffy face):* Face looks bloated and rounded, like the full moon. It is commonly found in Cushing's syndrome, nephrotic syndrome, acute glomerulonephritis, prolonged corticosteroid therapy, myxoedema, SVC syndrome (i.e., obstruction of SVC due to compression by superior mediastinal tumours) (Fig. 2.61), advanced CCF, alcoholism and angioneurotic oedema of face.
- *Hurler syndrome (gargoylism or mucopolysaccharidosis):* Coarse face with low nasal bridge, hypertrichosis, macroglossia, mental retardation and corneal clouding; as a whole, a gruesome and unpleasant face.
- *Tabetic facies (very rare nowadays):* Bilateral partial ptosis with compensatory wrinkling of forehead and elevated eyebrows; associated with Argyll Robertson pupil.

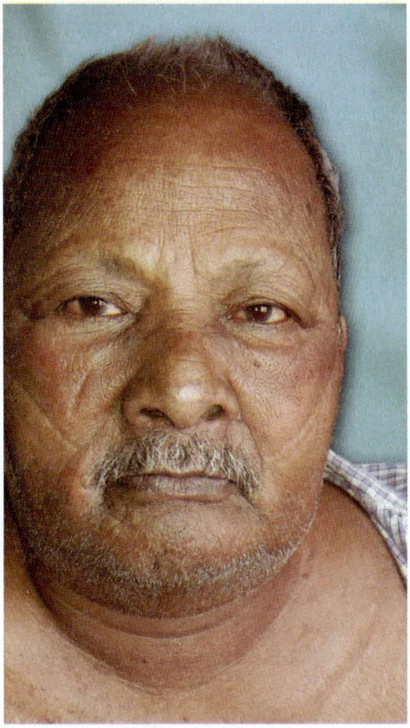

Fig. 2.61: Moon face (round and bloated) in superior mediastinal syndrome; neck and upper chest are full, while facial oedema is easily appreciated by impressions developing by pressure of bed sheet, etc. while lying

- *Facies of COPD (chronic obstructive pulmonary diseases):* Central cyanosis, nasal flare (alae nasi moving outward in inspiration) with 'purse-lip' respiration (inhaling through nose and mouth, and exhaling slowly through pursed lips to overcome shortness of breath).
- *'Bags under the eyes' or baggy lower eyelids:* May not have any clinical value but often seen in chronic alcoholism, myxoedema, insomnia and old age (Fig. 2.62).

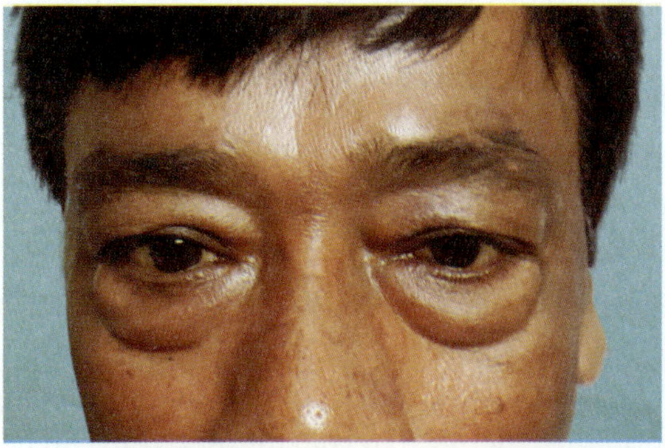

Fig. 2.62: Baggy lower eyelids, which is not of much clinical importance

NB: A student/doctor becomes familiar to a particular facies, if he/she is patient-bound, gives the daily clinical round, and spends some time at the bedside; otherwise, it is very difficult to memorise the facial features.

- If after careful observation of face, no diagnosis is reached, always try to look for the following:
  - Pseudoptosis or partial ptosis
  - Mild exophthalmos
  - Malar flush
  - Masked facies
  - Tongue (e.g., cyanosis, severe anaemia, macroglossia)
  - Small goitre (though not a structure within face), and
  - Ask to show the upper teeth (to note facial palsy).

NECK VESSELS

Q. In the heading of 'neck vessels', what are the structures to be examined?

- Jugular veins (internal jugular veins mainly though external jugular veins are gaining importance too)—*study of neck veins are more important* than that of carotid artery in clinical medicine, and
- Common carotid artery and its branches.

Applied anatomy

Jugular veins: There are two sets of jugular veins i.e., external (runs superficial to sternomastoid muscle) and internal (lies deep into neck, inside the 'carotid sheath'), which ultimately drains into superior vena cava.

Carotid arteries: The right common carotid artery originates from brachiocephalic trunk, and the left from aortic arch, which supply the head and neck with oxygenated blood. The common carotid arteries on both sides are divided into internal and external carotid arteries at the upper border of thyroid cartilage, around the level of C_4 vertebra. The common carotid artery is contained within 'carotid sheath' in neck; 'carotid sheath' contains common carotid as well as internal carotid artery, internal jugular vein and vagus nerve. Within the 'carotid sheath', the carotid artery lies medial to internal jugular vein, and vagus nerve occupies the position in between the two vessels posteriorly. External carotid artery has 8 branches in neck of which superior thyroid artery (sometimes, ascending pharyngeal artery) is the first and superficial temporal artery is the last branch in neck; internal carotid artery has no branch in neck.

In clinical medicine, internal jugular vein gained immense importance as it reflects the right atrial pressure as well as central venous pressure (CVP) because of its direct continuity with the right atrium, and thus it is the task of every clinician to study neck veins at the bedside in each and every patient.

Q. Which vein is important in clinical medicine: Internal or external jugular vein?

It is the *internal jugular vein which is most important* because of its direct continuity with the right atrium but as it is deeply situated, it is difficult to visualise or interpret. In a desperate situation, non-obstructive external jugular vein can be assessed keeping the facts in mind that external jugular vein is:

- A superficial vein, which is prone to kinking, may have valves, and may pierce fascia
- May engorge if the patient wears tight collar (of shirt)
- Does not directly drain into SVC and thus, not a direct reflector of CVP.

Q. Position of the patient before studying neck veins.

A. Facts observed in health when a person remains in:

a. Lying down position—neck veins are visible at neck
b. Sitting position—neck venous column remains invisible
c. At 45° semi-reclined position—upper level of neck venous column is just visible (or invisible) at the root of the neck above the clavicle.

B. Thus, to examine the neck veins, the patient should be reclining supine at 45° (i.e., angle formed by trunk and the level of the bed at waist should be 45°). Neck muscles should be relaxed by applying a 'back-rest' or properly adjusted pillows; patient's head and neck resting on clinician's left forearm does not relax the neck muscles properly, which is a pre-requisite for neck vein examination. Standing on the right side of the patient, one should observe in between two heads of sternomastoid muscle (it is better to observe right-sided neck vein as left-sided innominate vein may be compressed by aortic knob) (Figs 2.63 and 2.64). One may identify the neck vein by these *two methods*:

- Application of abdominal pressure increases venous column in neck (i.e., by hepato-jugular reflux), and
- Venous pulsation over neck can be abolished by application of gentle digital pressure over clavicle.

If at 45° position in bed, neck venous column are visible far above the clavicle, it is said that jugular venous pressure (JVP) is raised. That means, *neck veins are always examined in 45° to standardise reading.*

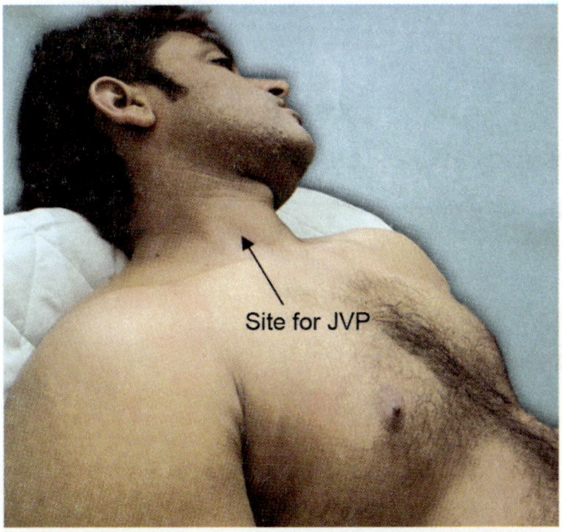

Fig. 2.63: Jugular venous pulse (JVP) examination—right-sided JVP is preferred to the left side

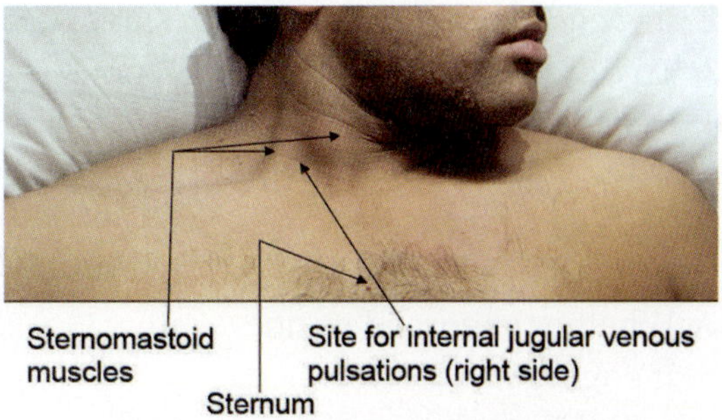

Fig. 2.64: Site for jugular venous pulse (JVP) examination in between two heads of sternomastoid muscle in 45° semi-reclined position

C. If the neck veins are fully engorged in sitting position, do not examine the patient in 45° position (i.e., in that situation, measure JVP in sitting position); similarly, the patient is examined in lying down position when JVP is very low.

Q. How to differentiate arterial and venous pulsations at bedside?

Many a time, the clinician is confused but the following points differentiate arterial from venous pulsations at the bedside.

Venous pulsation (i.e., internal jugular vein)	*Arterial pulsation (i.e., carotid artery)*
1. Wavy; rapid inward movement	1. Jerky; rapid outward movement
2. Better seen than felt	2. Better felt than seen
3. Prominent on expiration	3. No change observed
4. Prominent on lying down	4. No change observed
5. Prominent on application of pressure over abdomen (hepato-jugular reflux)	5. No change observed
6. Has a definite upper level seen at neck	6. No such level seen at neck
7. Two positive waves seen (c-wave is rarely seen)	7. One positive wave seen (i.e., in sinus rhythm)
8. Can be abolished by gentle digital pressure applied above clavicle	8. Arterial pulsation is not affected

Q. What is hepato-jugular reflux?

When pressure is applied over any part of the abdomen by right hand (abdomino-jugular reflux), especially over the right hypochondrium (hepato-jugular reflux), for at least 10 seconds, there is 'transient' rise in JVP as an extra amount of blood from abdomen is added to right side of the heart due to compression of hepatic venous reservoir; the patient should recline in bed at 45°.

A positive hepato-jugular reflux is defined by a 'sustained' rise of >3 cm in JVP for at least 15 seconds after release of the pressure. Its importance (i.e., *positive reflux*) lies in the facts like:

1. Congestive cardiac failure [CCF (overt)].
2. Impending or incipient (early stage) congestive cardiac failure
3. To differentiate arterial from venous pulsations
4. In patients with SVC syndrome (SVC obstruction) or Budd-Chiari syndrome (hepatic vein obstruction), the hepato-jugular reflux is absent or *negative*.

Q. What to be seen in neck veins when examined at bedside?

A. Whether engorged or not
B. If engorged, look for:
   a. Pressure
   b. Pulsations (i.e., waveforms)
   c. Hepato-jugular reflux.

Q. Can you enumerate the diseases with increased and decreased JVP?

Increased JVP		*Decreased JVP*
Engorged and pulsatile 1. CCF (commonest) 2. Chronic constrictive pericarditis, cardiac tamponade, restrictive cardiomyopathy 3. Tricuspid incompetence 4. After massive IV fluid infusion (iatrogenic) or blood transfusion, pregnancy, acute glomerulonephritis 5. Complete heart block 6. Pulmonary thromboembolism (PTE), chronic cor pulmonale	*Engorged and non-pulsatile* 1. Superior mediastinal syndrome (SVC syndrome*) 2. Chronic constrictive pericarditis (rare) 3. After Valsalva manoeuvre ***SVC syndrome:** Obstruction of SVC by superior mediastinal tumours (e.g., carcinoma of bronchus or lymphoma) producing breathlessness, oedema of face and chest, engorged veins over chest, and engorged and non-pulsatile neck veins (Fig. 2.65)	1. Dehydration 2. After massive haemorrhage, or diuretic therapy 3. Hypovolaemic shock

NB: Signs of **'shock'** are: Cold and clammy extremities, tachycardia with thready pulse, tachypnoea with urine output <30 ml/hour, hypotension with systolic BP <90 mm of Hg.

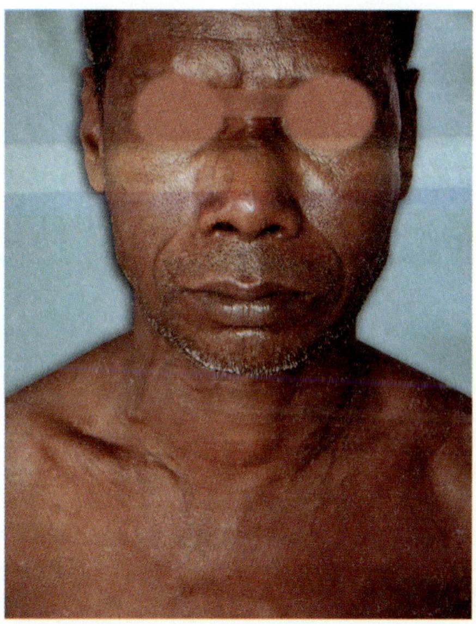

Fig. 2.65: Superior mediastinal syndrome—visible veins over chest (with a blood flow from above downwards) and engorged external jugular vein are seen; it seems that the patient is holding breath at end of inspiration

Q. What is normal JVP?

It is known that regardless of body position (whether lying, supine or reclined), the centre of right atrium lies 5 cm below the sternal angle (the so called 'reference point'). At 45°, the vertical distance from the top of the oscillating venous column and the sternal angle is the JVP, and is normally 3–4 cm (measured at bedside by two scales or postcards). So, normal venous pressure, right atrial pressure, JVP or CVP is, 3 cm + 5 cm = 8 cm of blood or water.

Q. What is Kussmaul's sign?

In health, JVP rises on expiration and falls on inspiration. In conditions like constrictive pericarditis, severe right-sided heart failure, right ventricular infarction and cardiac tamponade (less common), there is paradoxical rise in JVP in inspiration due to non-accommodation of increased venous return to the right heart, which is known as Kussmaul's sign (or, venous pulsus paradoxus).

Q. Different waves in neck venous pulsation and their associations.

There are three positive and two negative waves (descents or troughs) seen in neck veins. *Sequence of events* is like this: *a*-wave (first positive wave) → *c*-wave (second positive wave) → *x*-wave (first negative wave) → *v*-wave (third positive wave) → *y*-wave (second negative wave) (Fig. 2.66).

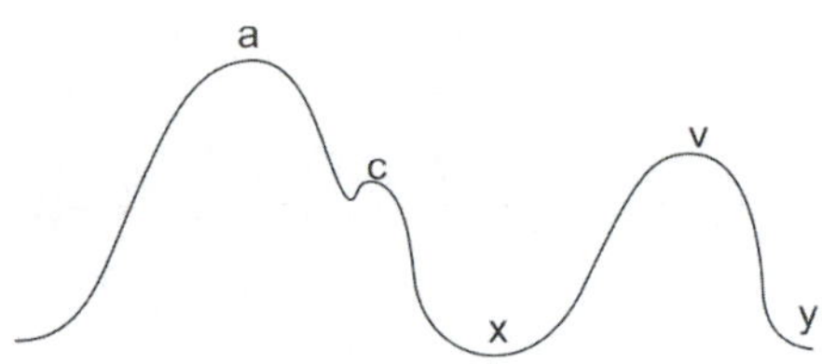

Fig. 2.66: Normal jugular venous waves

Remember, *a*-wave coincides with S_1, *v*-wave with S_2. In health, *a*-wave is larger than *v*-wave, and *x*-descent is more pronounced than *y*-descent.

Waves	*Mechanism*	*Pathology*
1. *a*-wave	Right atrial contraction (most prominent wave in JVP)	1. *a-wave:* • *Absent:* Atrial fibrillation • *Giant a-wave:* Tricuspid stenosis, pulmonary stenosis, pulmonary hypertension • Cannon wave (huge pathological *a*-wave): Complete heart block, junctional rhythm
2. *c*-wave	Closure and bulging of tricuspid valve/carotid impact (small and rarely appreciated)	2. *c-wave:* Of least clinical importance
3. *x*-descent	Atrial relaxation with downward descent of tricuspid valve	3. *Prominent x-descent:* Cardiac tamponade
4. *v*-wave	Passive right atrial filling against closed tricuspid valve during ventricular systole	4. *Large v-wave ('systolic wave' or 'cv'-wave):* Tricuspid incompetence, right ventricular failure
5. *y*-descent	Right ventricular filling with atrial emptying with opening of tricuspid valve	5. *Sharp y-descent:* Constrictive pericarditis

NB: Cannon wave develops when the right atrium contracts against a closed tricuspid valve.

Q. Can you describe the neck venous study in CCF?

The neck veins are engorged and pulsatile. The JVP is raised, the different waves are seen in the neck, and the hepato-jugular reflux is present.

LYMPH NODES

Q. How the lymph nodes are palpated?

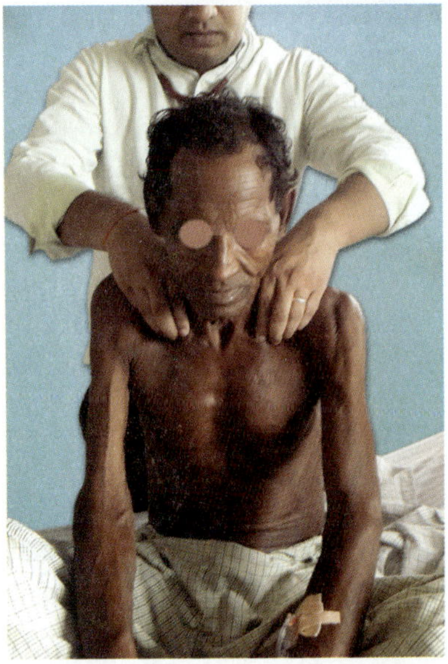

Fig. 2.67: Method of examination of supraclavicular glands (including Virchow's gland and scalene nodes) from behind

Lymph nodes are soft, small and round structures, which are linked to each other by lymphatic channels, and are located throughout the body. There are approximately 400–450 lymph nodes present in normal adults. Lymph nodes are palpated symmetrically *on both the sides* from above downwards. Remember, in health the lymph nodes are not palpable unless enlarged (inguinal nodes are sometime palpable). Muscles and arteries in neck and groin may mislead a clinician.

- *Cervical lymph nodes (neck): Cervical nodes are always palpated from behind* in a sitting or standing patient with neck flexed forward; if one side of neck is palpated, neck should be flexed to that side (Fig. 2.67). Cervical nodes are divided into:
  a. *Upper circular group is palpated from front to back as follows:*
     - Submental (below the chin)
     - Submandibular (below the mandible)
     - Tonsillar (at the angle of mandible)
     - Preauricular (in front of ear)
     - Postauricular (behind the ear over mastoid process)
     - Occipital (below the occiput).
  b. *Lower horizontal or supraclavicular group (palpated from back):* Arbitrarily divided into medial, intermediate and lateral group. Virchow's (medial group of left-sided supraclavicular nodes which lie in between two heads of *left* sternomastoid muscle) and scalene nodes (present above and behind the head of clavicles, deep to sternomastoid in relation to scalenus anterior muscle on *both* sides of neck) need special attention.
  c. *The vertical chain in the middle of neck (palpated from back):* The region is divided by ipsilateral sternomastoid muscle into glands in the (i) anterior triangle, and (ii) posterior triangle.
- *Axillary lymph nodes:* Examination is done in a sitting patient with full relaxation of axillary muscles. There are 5 groups of lymph nodes and all groups are palpated from front except the subscapular group, which is palpated from behind. Patient's hand on the side of examination should be fully relaxed for a proper palpation. There are:
  - Central group
  - Apical group
  - Pectoral (anterior) group
  - Brachial (lateral) group
  - Subscapular (posterior) group.

- *Epitrochlear lymph nodes:* The glands are palpated in the antero-medial region of lower arm (i.e., in between the groove of biceps and brachialis muscles).
- *Mediastinal lymph nodes:* These group of lymph nodes cannot be palpated, rather they are detected by percussion over the sternum. Signs of mediastinal widening by percussion or looking for pressure effects on surrounding structures (like puffy face and engorged veins over chest) give an idea of enlargement of mediastinal group of lymph nodes. Paratracheal, subcarinal, tracheobronchial and hilar lymph nodes constitute mediastinal group.
- *Abdominal lymph nodes:* These groups (pre- and para-aortic, celiac, retroperitoneal and mesenteric group) present as 'lump/mass abdomen', if enlarged; they then feel nodular discrete or matted mass in abdomen.
- *Inguinal lymph nodes:* Horizontal chain lies below and parallel to the inguinal ligament, while vertical chain lies along saphenous vein. The patient is examined in supine position after extending the thighs. This group is commonly enlarged in bare-footed persons.
- *Popliteal lymph nodes:* The glands are palpated in a supine patient with partially flexed knee joint when fingers of both hands of examiner are curled into the popliteal fossa to palpate the glands.

Q. How to palpate scalene node and Virchow's node?

- *Scalene node*
  - Stand behind the sitting patient. Ask him/her to shrug the shoulder, and dip down your palpating index finger behind the head of the clavicle through the clavicular origin of sternomastoid, pressing gently downwards with flexing the patient's neck to that side. These nodes lie anterior to scalenus anterior and deep to sternomastoid muscle. Scalene nodes are enlarged and palpable in bronchogenic carcinoma.
- *Virchow's node (sentinel node)*
  - Stand behind the sitting patient, and make the two heads of left sternomastoid prominent (put your right hand over the right face of the patient and ask him/her to turn the face to right against resistance offered by your hand). Now palpate the gap in between two heads of left sternomastoid by your left index finger. Virchow's node receives lymphatics from:
    - Upper limb (left)
    - Breast (left)
    - Lung (left)
    - Stomach (Troisier's sign)
    - Testes.

NB: Virchow's nodes are enlarged in relation to malignancy of lung, stomach, breast and genitals.

Q. How to describe a lymph node enlargement?

The enlarged lymph node should be described in the following ways:

1. Site (anatomical region)—situation and extent
2. Size

3. Number
4. Margin—discrete or matted
5. Tenderness
6. *Consistency:*
   - Soft (inflammation, cold abscess)
   - Rubbery and elastic (lymphoma)
   - Firm and shotty (syphilis)
   - Rock-hard (malignancy)
7. Surface
8. Mobility—fixity to surrounding structures (e.g., muscles, vessels, viscus) i.e., fixed or mobile
9. Skin changes over the node (sinus, peau d'orange, or signs of inflammation)
10. Rise of local temperature (i.e., indicating inflammation)
11. Lymphangitis: Red, linear, tender lymph vessels radiating proximally, or not
12. Draining area (e.g., in inguinal adenopathy, examine the sole of foot).

Q. When the enlarged nodes are of pathological in nature?

- Lymph nodes are said to be significant in nature (though always needs clinical correlation), when:
  - >1 cm in diameter
  - Firm in consistency
  - Matted (nodes are adherent)
  - Tender on palpation.
- However, in this setting, the clinical context is to be considered as a whole.
- Inguinal nodes ≥2 cm size may be considered significant, and even lower size (≤1 cm) of epitrochlear lymphadenopathy may be considered pathological.
- Hard and fixed nodes are commonly 'malignant' in nature.

Q. Some hard facts about lymph node enlargement one should know.

1. Small, soft, discrete, non-tender nodes are usually 'benign' in nature, whereas hard, fixed, non-tender (sometimes tender) nodes, which are fixed to deeper tissues are 'malignant' in nature.
2. Red flag signs for underlying malignancy include a node >2 cm which is progressively enlarging, associated with weight loss >10%, age >40 years, and especially involving supraclavicular nodes; associated constitutional symptoms like pyrexia, night sweats and weight loss make the clinician more suspicious.
3. 'Tender lymph nodes' are usually infectious or inflammatory in nature.

Q. What is generalised lymphadenopathy?

The definitions of different terminology related to lymhadenopathy are:

- Lymphadenopathy is the inflammatory or non-inflammatory enlargement of lymph nodes.
- 'Localised' (regional) lymphadenopathy is limited to one area (i.e., single anatomical area of lymph node involvement).

- *Generalised lymphadenopathy* is the involvement of 3 or more non-contiguous lymph node areas, and the common causes in clinical practice are:
  - Tuberculosis (disseminated or miliary)
  - Lymphoma [Hodgkin's disease (HD) or non-Hodgkin's lymphoma (NHL)]
  - Leukaemias [acute lymphoblastic (ALL) and chronic lymphocytic leukaemia (CLL)]
  - Secondary metastases to lymph nodes
  - Collagen vascular diseases e.g., SLE
  - HIV and other viral infections [e.g., cytomegalovirus (CMV)]
  - Infectious mononucleosis
  - Chronic lymphadenitis
  - Sarcoidosis
  - *Others:* Filariasis, secondary syphilis, toxoplasmosis, blast crisis of chronic myeloid leukaemia (CML), brucellosis, amyloidosis, drug-induced (phenytoin, hydralazine, cyclosporine A, carbamazepine).

Q. Do you know the causes of region-wise lymphadenopathy?

Regions involved	*Clinical conditions*
• Cervical (Fig. 2.68)	Infection/malignancy/ulcer in oral cavity, scalp infection, infection in ear/eye/nose, and throat for nasopharyngeal carcinoma; tuberculosis, lymphoma, ALL and CLL, metastases from chest/breast/stomach/head and neck, sarcoidosis, infectious mononucleosis, CMV, HIV infection
• Auricular	• *Preauricular:* Conjunctivitis, rodent ulcer (Fig. 2.69), rubella, herpes zoster ophthalmicus • *Postauricular:* Leprosy, sarcoidosis, rubella, otitis media, head/neck malignancy

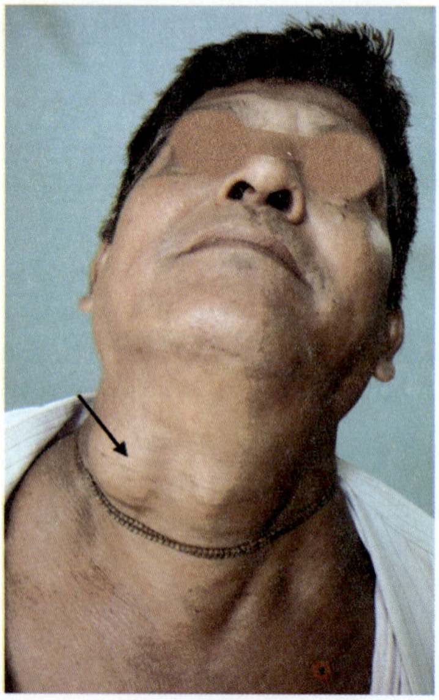

Fig. 2.68: Lymph node swelling in right side of neck

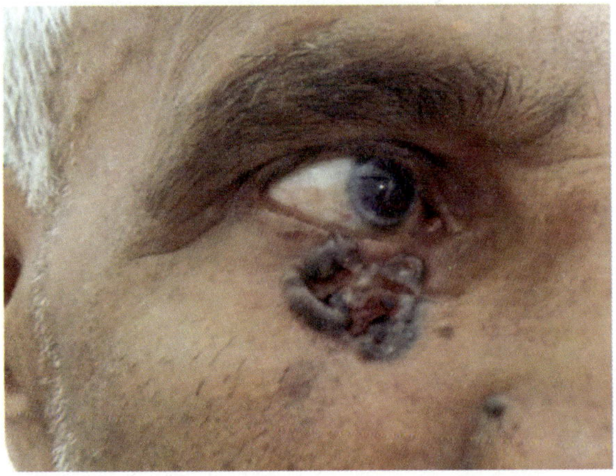

Fig. 2.69: Rodent ulcer (basal cell carcinoma) over the face

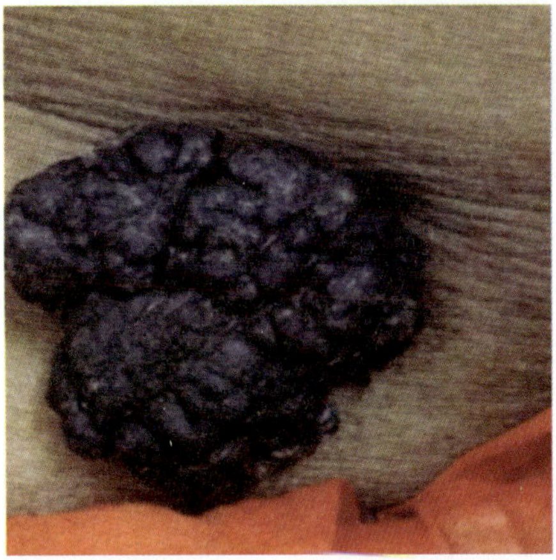

Fig. 2.70: Malignant melanoma—most dangerous skin carcinoma (a neoplasm of melanocytes)

• Occipital	Scalp infection (e.g., louse, dandruff), rubella, secondary syphilis
• Axillary	Breast carcinoma, infection of ipsilateral upper extremity, ALL or CLL, tuberculosis, lymphoma, melanoma (Fig. 2.70)
• Epitrochlear	Ipsilateral hand infection, lymphoma (especially, NHL), sarcoidosis, ALL or CLL, secondary syphilis, cat-scratch disease, HIV infection
• Mediastinal and hilar	Metastases from lung (commonest)/breast/stomach/colon, lymphoma (commonly HD), sarcoidosis (hilar glands +), tuberculosis and fungal diseases
• Abdominal	Lymphoma, intestinal tuberculosis, carcinoma of stomach/pancreas/ colon
• Inguinal	Infection/trauma of lower limb, plague, filariasis, metastases from genital/ uterus/rectal malignancy, genital herpes, tuberculosis, lymphoma, chancroid, lymphogranuloma venereum
• Popliteal	Local skin/muscle infection, melanoma

*Cervical lymphadenopathy may be confused with lipoma, thyroid nodule, branchial cyst, thyroglossal cyst and parotid gland. Similarly, inguinal lymphadenopathy may be misguided by femoral hernia.

Q. What are matted nodes?

Matted (periadenitis) means that the lymph nodes are adhered to form a mass, and are common in tuberculosis, and rarely seen in chronic lymphadenitis and NHL.

Q. What is Waldeyer's ring?

It is the ring of lymphoid tissue within the oral cavity, and is commonly involved in NHL. It is composed of:

- Adenoids,
- Faucal tonsils, and
- Lingual tonsils.

Q. What is Sister Marie Joseph's nodule?

It is the metastatic nodule around umbilicus developing out of adenocarcinoma of stomach.

Q. Why do you examine oral cavity in a case of lymphadenopathy?

It is done in the search of:

- Waldeyer's ring/tonsillar enlargement (Fig. 2.71)/peritonsillar abscess
- Carcinoma of lip/cheek/tongue (Fig. 2.72)
- Petechiae at junction of hard and soft palate (e.g., in infectious mononucleosis)
- Pharyngeal infection
- Any ulcer within oral cavity.

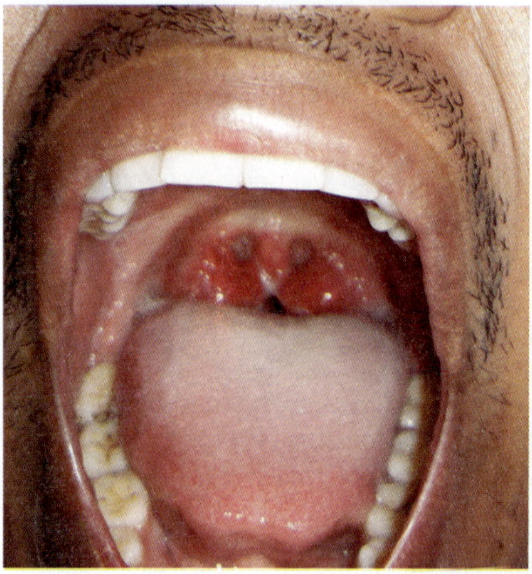

Fig. 2.71: Acute follicular tonsillitis

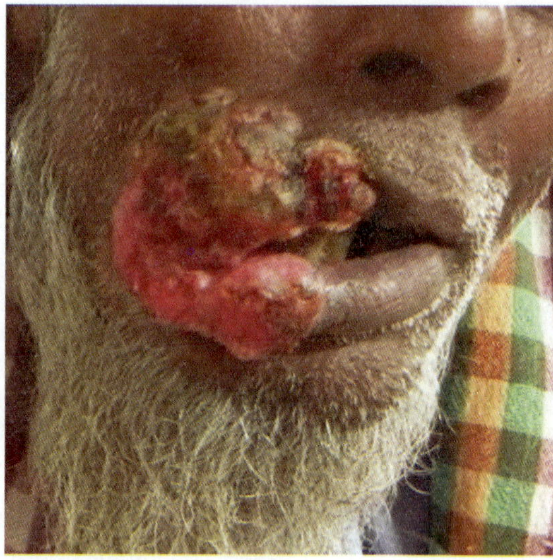

Fig. 2.72: Squamous cell carcinoma (also known as epidermoid carcinoma)

Q. What are the causes of fixed/painful/or nodes with sinus formation?

Nodes in different situations	*Clinical abnormality*
• Nodes fixed to surrounding structures	Metastatic nodes, tuberculosis
• Painful and tender nodes	Pyogenic/fungal/viral/parasitic infection, diphtheria, infectious mononucleosis, malignant nodes (may be non-tender)
• Lymphadenopathy with sinus formation	Tuberculosis, actinomycosis

Q. Describe characteristics of lymphadenopathy in lymphoma and tuberculosis.

Lymphoma is of two types: Hodgkin's disease (HD) and non-Hodgkin's lymphoma (NHL).

- *Hodgkin's disease:* Enlarged, non-tender, smooth surface, with *India-rubbery feel*, neither fixed to skin nor to deeper structures, discrete, no sinus, no rise of temperature in the overlying skin, and without any softening or suppuration. Commonly, cervical nodes are initially affected.
- *Non-Hodgkin's lymphoma:* Enlarged, non-tender (rarely tender), smooth or nodular surface with *firm or variegated feel*, may fix to deeper structures, discrete, without

any sinus formation, may be with elevated local skin temperature, and there is neither softening nor any suppuration. Any area of body may be affected initially.

- *Tuberculosis:* Enlarged, *matted*, usually painless but may be painful, firm and without any rise in local temperature. Rarely, there may be sinus formation in overlying skin or cold abscess formation underneath. Discrete nodes are found in early diseases; hard and craggy nodes are common in healed and calcified tuberculosis. Commonly affected area is upper deep cervical lymph nodes.

THYROID GLAND

Q. How to confirm the neck swelling as thyroid gland?

Thyroid swelling is confirmed by:

- Ask the patient to swallow (or, may give a glass of water to swallow) and observe that *thyroid swelling moves upwards with swallowing* because of its laryngeal attachment.
- Other swellings in neck which moves upwards with deglutition are thyroglossal cyst (moreover, it also moves upwards with protrusion of tongue), subhyoid bursitis, and pretracheal and prelaryngeal lymph nodes fixed to trachea and larynx respectively. Other than these, no other swelling in front of the neck moves upwards with deglutition (Fig. 2.73).

Q. Outline of examination of the thyroid gland.

The thyroid gland is a butterfly-shaped endocrine gland lying in front of the neck below the thyroid cartilage. It has two symmetrical lobes connected by the isthmus in the middle; the isthmus covers the second and third tracheal rings. The thyroid may extend into superior mediastinum, or may be purely retrosternal. In health, the normal gland is not palpable, and weighs 20–25 g. The method of examination of thyroid gland goes like this:

- *Inspection:* With the neck slightly extended, from the front, observe for position, extent, shape and contour, size, symmetry, overlying skin (thyroidectomy scar, dilated veins, or signs of inflammation), localised or diffuse nature of swelling; look for the lower border as soon as the gland moves up with deglutition.

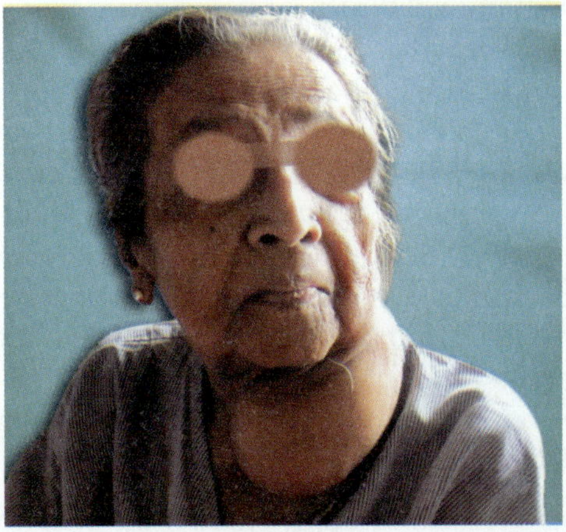

Fig. 2.73: A cystic swelling in front of the neck (not a thyroid swelling)

- *Palpation:*
  - *From behind: At the first step, palpation of thyroid should always be done from behind.* Stand behind the seated patient; slightly flex the neck to relax the sternomastoids and encircle the neck by both hands with the fingers slightly flexed, and continue palpation for size, shape, consistency, mobility, etc. Both the lobes and isthmus should be palpated.
  - *From front:* Each lobe is better palpated from front i.e., for palpation of the left lobe, the gland is pushed to the left from the right side; when the left lobe becomes prominent, it is palpated by the right hand and so on (Lahey's method). Now look for:
    - Size (small, medium, large)
    - Shape (localised or diffuse)
    - Surface (smooth or irregular)
    - Consistency (soft—Graves' disease, firm—simple goitre, hard—carcinoma of thyroid; remember, a cystic thyroid swelling may feel solid and a solid one cystic)
    - Mobility (lost in carcinoma of thyroid)—Gland is moved vertically as well as horizontally
    - To get below the swelling (observe while swallowing)
    - Temperature (warm in Graves' disease)
    - Tenderness (tender in thyroiditis/carcinoma) or non-tender
    - Relation with neighbouring structures (pressure effects, fixity, etc.) like:
      - ❖ Trachea: Deviated or not
      - ❖ Oesophagus: C/o dysphagia
      - ❖ Carotid sheath: No pulsation in carcinoma of thyroid (increased pulsation in Graves' disease)
      - ❖ Recurrent laryngeal nerve: C/o hoarseness of voice
      - ❖ Sympathetic trunk: Produces Horner's syndrome
      - ❖ Sternomastoid muscle: Malignancy may infiltrate the muscle with its loss of function
      - ❖ Skin and subcutaneous tissue
    - Thrill (felt over thyroid gland in Graves' disease due to increased vascularity)
    - Cervical lymph nodes are palpated from behind for lymphadenopathy, if there are any.
- *Percussion:* Sternum is normally resonant on percussion; if the note of percussion becomes dull, it may be presumed that retrosternal extension may be present.
- *Auscultation:* Ask the patient to hold breath, and now auscultate for systolic bruit over the lobes. Systolic bruit is present over thyroid gland in Graves' disease because of increased vascularity. Thyroid bruit may be confused with carotid bruit or venous hum present in the neck.
- *Measurement (mensuration):* Circumference of the neck is measured by a tape at the most prominent part.

NB: Hard consistency of thyroid, rapid growth, male sex, no movement of the gland on swallowing, Horner's syndrome, enlarged and hard cervical lymphadenopathy, and past H/o irradiation in the neck increase the chance of malignancy of the thyroid gland.

Q. What is goitre?

Goitre refers to an enlargement of the thyroid gland. Most of the patients with goitre are euthyroid (i.e., no thyroid dysfunction) (Fig. 2.74).

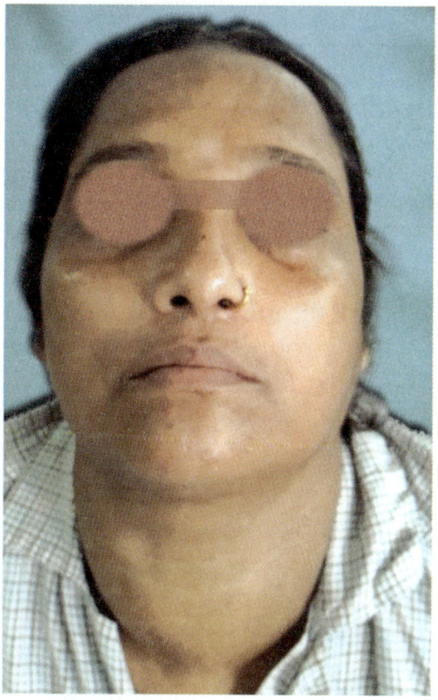

Fig. 2.74: Goitre (i.e., thyroid swelling) in front of the neck

Q. What are the common causes of thyromegaly?

- Goitre
  - Diffuse (e.g., Graves' disease)
  - Nodular
    - Single (Fig. 2.75)
    - Multiple
- Thyroiditis (e.g., Hashimoto's thyroiditis)
- Autoimmunity
- Neoplastic
  - Benign
  - Malignant.

Q. Give short notes on hypothyroidism and hyperthyroidism.

Hypofunction of thyroid gland at birth is cretinism, and that after puberty is myxoedema. Excess function of thyroid gland is hyperthyroidism. Vide the chapter on 'Endocrine system' for details.

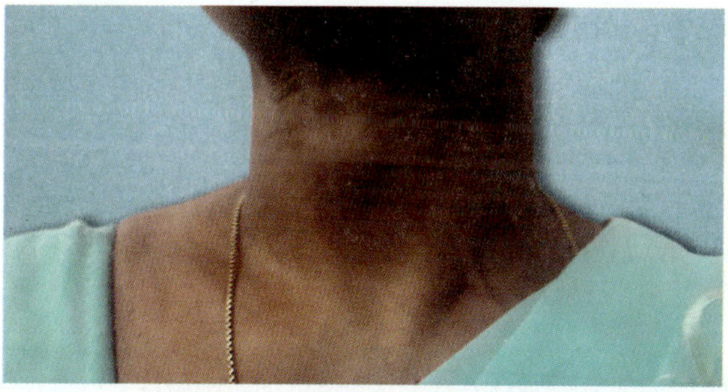

Fig. 2.75: Solitary thyroid nodule

OEDEMA

Q. Can you define oedema?

Oedema is the accumulation of excess interstitial fluid resulting in swelling of the tissue, or in other words, it is the clinically apparent increase in extracellular fluid volume. A weight gain of several kilograms often precedes overt manifestation of oedema. The older name of oedema was dropsy.

Q. What is the examination sequence to demonstrate oedema?

1. First inspect the leg for any swelling.
2. Apply firm pressure for at least 15 seconds (up to maximally 30 seconds) by tip of your right thumb sequentially over medial malleolus, above medial malleolus, lower end of medial surface of tibia and the upper part of shin bone (i.e., press over a bony background). Now, *watch for any pitting or dimple*; one can press dorsum of the swollen foot now. Repeat the same manoeuvre on the opposite side.
3. Now make the patient in prone position and press over the sacrum by tip of your right thumb to demonstrate 'sacral oedema'. In *bed-bound patients*, oedema is confined to sacrum. However, sacrum must be examined in all patients with oedema.
4. Examine for 'parietal oedema': Press the tip of your five fingers of right hand, over the abdominal parietis or thigh for a few seconds, and look for signs of pitting or dimpling (Fig. 2.76).

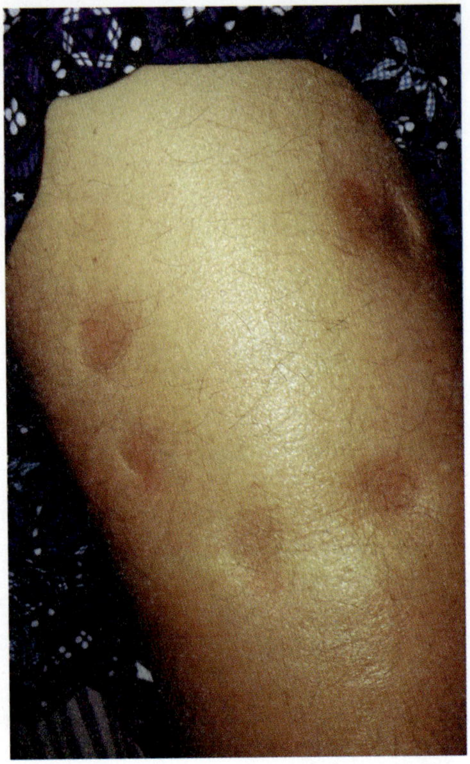

Fig. 2.76: Demonstrating parietal oedema over thigh

NB: Oedema may be restricted to limited region like pedal/sacral/genital/facial, or becomes generalised (anasarca). Other than peripheral oedema (the chapter in discussion) there are pulmonary oedema, cerebral oedema and macular oedema in eye in internal medicine.

Q. Some essential facts about oedema: Do you know?

1. In *ambulatory patients*, oedema develops in the dependent part i.e., the ankle. *Pitting* (i.e., skin indentation) is the cardinal sign of subcutaneous oedema. Pitting oedema is due to increased interstitial fluid while non-pitting oedema reflects protein deposition.
2. If upper part of body seems swollen, press sequentially over wrist, lateral epicondyle at elbow, sternum, vertebra and forehead.
3. Grades of oedema (according to some clinicians): Grade 1 (oedema below ankle), grade 2 (oedema below knee), grade 3 (oedema of thighs), and grade 4 (generalised oedema).
4. *Non-pitting oedema*: It is difficult to recognise at the bedside. Look for the pallid and glossy appearance of skin with less prominent superficial veins, and at times its doughy feel gives a clue.
5. At least 10–15% increase in body weight, and/or 10% of increase in circumference of the limb is necessary for demonstration of pitting oedema. In a case of anasarca,

search carefully for bilateral hydrothorax, ascites, hydrocele (± scrotal oedema) and pericardial effusion.

6. Oedema may be *postural* (e.g., prolonged bus journey), which may result from failure of muscular movement.

NB: Ambulant patient: Pedal oedema, and **bed-bound patient**—sacral oedema.

Q. How oedema is classified in clinical medicine?

- Whether pits on pressure or not:
  - *Pitting oedema:*
    - Congestive cardiac failure (CCF) (Fig. 2.77)
    - Nephrotic syndrome
    - Cirrhosis of liver
    - Hypoproteinaemia with severe anaemia (nutritional oedema): Protein-losing enteropathy (Crohn's disease), kwashiorkor
    - Pericardial effusion
    - Constrictive pericarditis
    - Others: Venous obstruction, beriberi, drug-induced (amlodipine, corticosteroids, oestrogens, NSAIDs, fludrocortisone), cyclical oedema.
  - Non-pitting or 'solid' oedema:
    - Myxoedema (due to deposition of mucinous material)
    - Lymphatic oedema (late stage) e.g., filariasis (Fig. 2.78)
    - Angioneurotic oedema
    - Early phage of scleroderma.
- In relation to distribution of oedema:
  - Generalised (**anasarca**):
    - Includes first 4 causes under *pitting oedema*; may add cause 5 and 6
  - Localised (i.e., localised to one region or limb):
    - Venous obstruction: Deep vein thrombosis (DVT), SVC syndrome, pregnancy, varicose veins
    - Lymphatic obstruction (lymphoedema): Filariasis, carcinoma of breast, post-radical mastectomy, Milroy's disease (Fig. 2.79)

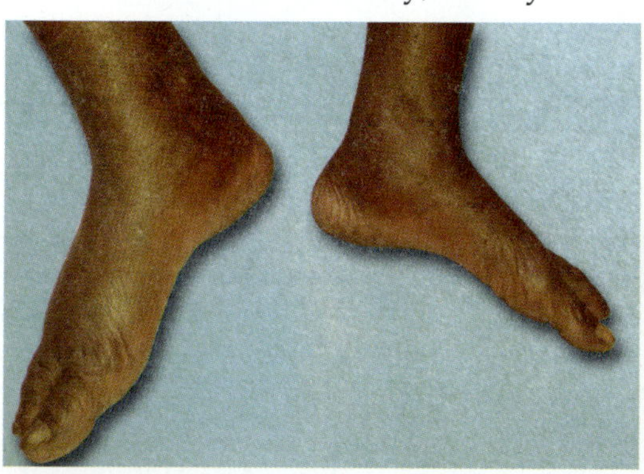

Fig. 2.77: Dependent bipedal pitting oedema from congestive cardiac failure

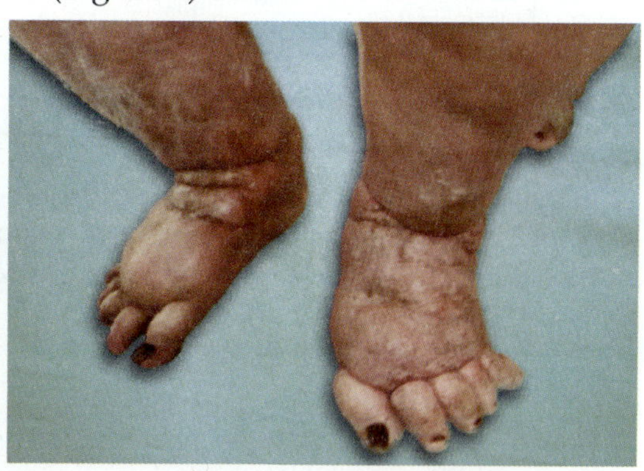

Fig. 2.78: Acquired lymphoedema (with non-pitting oedema)—filariasis

- Inflammatory: Insect/snake bite, severe septicaemia (increased capillary permeability due to liberation of histamine), vasculitis
- Allergic: Angioneurotic oedema, acute anaphylaxis
- Others: Bruises, gout, cellulitis, sprains, fracture.

NB: Low protein extracellular fluid (CCF, nephrotic syndrome): Pits easily and recover quickly on release of pressure.

High protein extracellular fluid (lymphoedema, angioneurotic oedema): Resist pitting and recovers slowly on release of pressure.

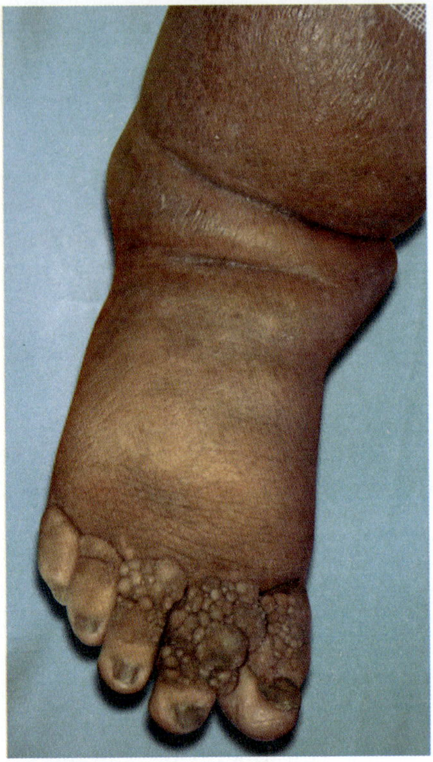

Fig. 2.79: Congenital lymphoedema (with non-pitting oedema)—Milroy's disease

Q. Five basic facts of oedema.

1. *Oedema may be due to:*
   - Low plasma oncotic pressure: Nephrotic syndrome, cirrhosis of liver
   - Increased hydrostatic pressure: DVT, pregnancy, CCF, excess IV fluid
   - Increased capillary permeability: Amlodipine, acute allergy, severe septicaemia
   - Lymphatic obstruction: Elephantiasis (filariasis), malignant infiltration.
2. Presence of oedema always makes the clinician suspicious of underlying serious diseases.
3. In early stage, lymphoedema is soft and pits on pressure. In late stages, the skin feels thickened and indurated (brawny) due to increased protein concentration in the interstitial fluid, which makes the oedema intractable and non-pitting.
4. Periorbital and scrotal loose subcutaneous tissue favour collection of fluid there because of low tissue tension (with reference to renal oedema).
5. Idiopathic cyclical oedema occurs in females in child bearing age group, which has temporal relationship with menstrual cycle.

Q. What is slow-pitting and rapid-pitting oedema?

They are:

- *Slow oedema:* Slow return (>40 seconds) of displaced fluid after pitting in CCF
- *Rapid oedema:* Rapid return (<40 seconds) of displaced fluid after pitting in hypoalbuminaemic states e.g., nephrotic syndrome.

Q. What is angioneurotic oedema?

Features of angioneurotic oedema are:

- It is a solid oedema from hypersensitivity, which commonly affects tongue, lips, face, eyelids; usually patchy involvement; pale or pink swelling develops rapidly with itching.

- *Two types:* Congenital and acquired (e.g., ACE-inhibitor induced). Hereditary variety is due to C_1 esterase inhibitor deficiency; if larynx or trachea is involved, it may threaten life by suffocation.

Q. Do you know the evolution of oedema in a case of anasarca?

Diseases with anasarca	*Evolution of oedema*
• CCF	Legs → face → ascites
• Nephrotic syndrome	Face (periorbital swelling) → legs → ascites (with scrotal swelling)
• Cirrhosis of liver	Ascites → legs → face (rarely involved)
• Nutritional oedema	Oedema of feet with facial puffiness → ascites

Q. Can you enumerate common causes of pedal and facial oedema?

- *Pedal oedema:*
  - Causes mentioned in 'pitting oedema'
  - *Others:* DVT, varicose veins, abdominal mass pressing IVC, filariasis, cyclical oedema (females during menstrual cycle), postural oedema, prolonged immobility (e.g., paraplegia), irradiation, ruptured Baker's cyst (from rheumatoid arthritis), fluid overload.
- *Facial oedema (puffiness)*
  - Acute glomerulonephritis, nephrotic syndrome
  - CCF, SVC syndrome (oedema restricted to upper half of body)
  - *Others:* Angioneurotic oedema, Cushing's syndrome, pericardial effusion, constrictive pericarditis, myxoedema, hypoproteinaemia (severe anaemia, PEM).

Q. Do you know causes of 'unilateral' pedal oedema?

The causes are:

- DVT or varicose veins
- Cellulitis
- Trauma, sprain or fracture
- Filariasis
- Ruptured Baker's cyst
- Arthritis (e.g., gout)
- *Others:* Diabetic foot, hemiplegic side, angioneurotic oedema.

Q. Can you enumerate the causes of 'unilateral' swelling of leg?

Unilateral swelling of leg is due to:

- Causes of 'unilateral' pedal oedema (question above)
- Calf muscle strain or haematoma (muscle is tender to lateral compression)
- Postphlebitis syndrome (leg pain with chronic unilateral leg swelling which was previously affected by DVT)
- Lymphatic obstruction
- Calf muscle infarction (the muscle becomes swollen, tender and tense due to bleeding within the compartment or embolism within the artery supplying the muscle).

Q. What are special of cardiac, renal and hepatic oedema?

Special features of oedema due to involvement of different systems are:

- *Cardiac oedema (e.g., CCF):* Oedema (pitting) starts at dependent part and then ascends progressively. Oedema is usually noticed at the end of day's work. Bed-bound patients have sacral oedema too. The patient may be dyspnoeic.
- *Renal oedema (e.g., nephrotic syndrome):* Oedema (pitting) starts in face (chiefly periorbital), arms and then descends. Oedema is usually noticed in the early morning while getting up from bed. Swelling of scrotal sacs and lower eyelids are characteristic. Non-ambulatory patients may have sacral oedema too.
- *Hepatic oedema (e.g., cirrhosis of liver):* Abdominal distension with symptoms and signs of ascites is the first manifestation (due to hepatocellular failure plus portal hypertension), which is followed by bipedal pitting oedema.

SKELETON

Height/weight/arm-span/upper segment–lower segment ratio (anthropometry).

Q. What is arm-span?

Arm-span is the distance between fingertips when hands are stretched parallel to the ground. Normally arm-span is equal to height.

- Arm-span > height: Seen when lower segment of body > upper segment (Fig. 2.80).
- Arm-span < height: Hyperpituitarism, precocious puberty, adrenal cortical tumour.

*Read the section on 'Build' for arm-span, height, and upper and lower segment.

** Read the section on 'Nutrition' for weight-related queries.

Q. What is kyphoscoliosis?

Description of kyphoscoliosis goes like this:

- Kyphosis means exaggerated anterior curvature of the spine with an increased convexity posteriorly. It is examined from sides of the patient with a tangential view.

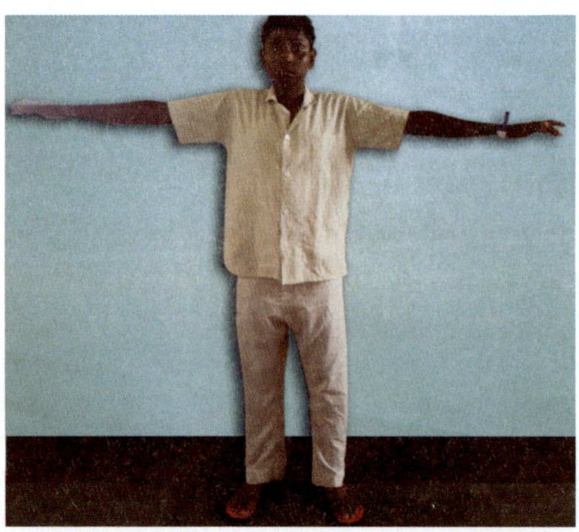

Fig. 2.80: Demonstrating arm-span > height in Klinefelter's syndrome

- Scoliosis is the lateral bending of the vertebral column. It should be examined from patient's back.
- The common causes of kyphoscoliosis are:
  - Congenital or developmental
  - Neurological causes like neurofibromatosis (Fig. 2.81), poliomyelitis, Friedreich's ataxia, syringomyelia
  - Ankylosing spondylitis, caries spine (with 'gibbus' i.e., acute angulation in the spine), senile osteoporosis, rickets, osteoarthritis
  - *Others:* Occupational (e.g., porters carrying weight in back), Marfan's syndrome, Turner's syndrome, Paget's disease, acromegaly, traumatic, postural.

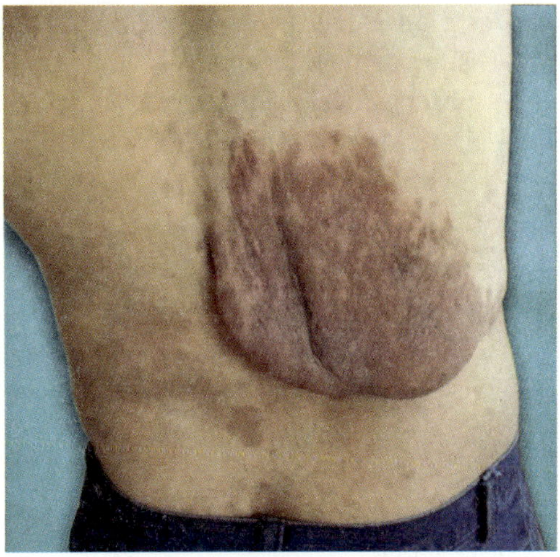

Fig. 2.81: Plexiform neurofibroma (an uncommon variant of neurofibroma)

Q. What is lordosis?

It is the exaggerated inward curvature of spine i.e., lumbar spine is more convexed anteriorly. Exaggerated lumbar lordosis (hyperlordosis) is common in advanced pregnancy, muscular dystrophy, disorders of hip joints, massive ascites/large abdominal tumour.

Q. Do you know the causes of pes cavus and pes planus?

- *Pes cavus (high-arched foot)* (Fig. 2.82): An important window in clinical medicine:
  - Friedreich's ataxia (pes cavus with hammer toes called Friedreich's foot)
  - Syringomyelia
  - Poliomyelitis (Fig. 2.83)
  - Peroneal muscular atrophy (Charcot-Marie-Tooth disease)
  - Others: Congenital, cerebral palsy, spina bifida, Refsum's disease, trauma.

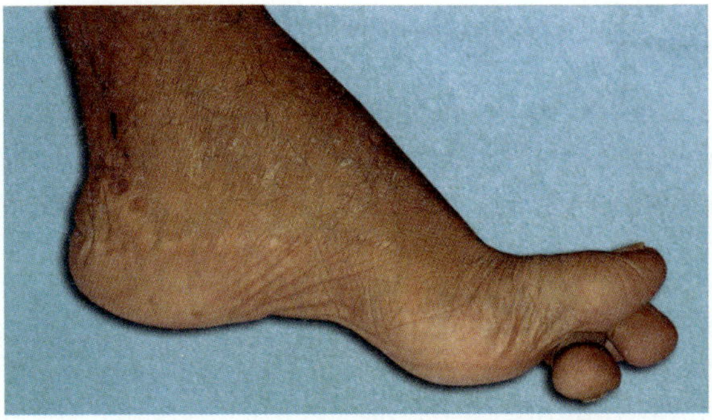

Fig. 2.82: High-arched foot or pes cavus

- Pes planus (flatfoot) (Fig. 2.84):
  - Marfan's syndrome
  - Ehlers-Danlos syndrome
  - Osteogenesis imperfecta
  - Dysfunction of posterior tibial tendon.

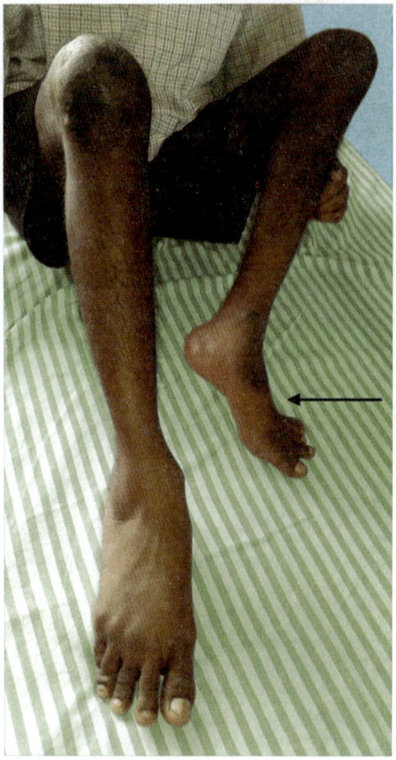

Fig. 2.83: Poliomyelitis with gross wasting of muscles along with contracture at knee; pes cavus is noted in left foot

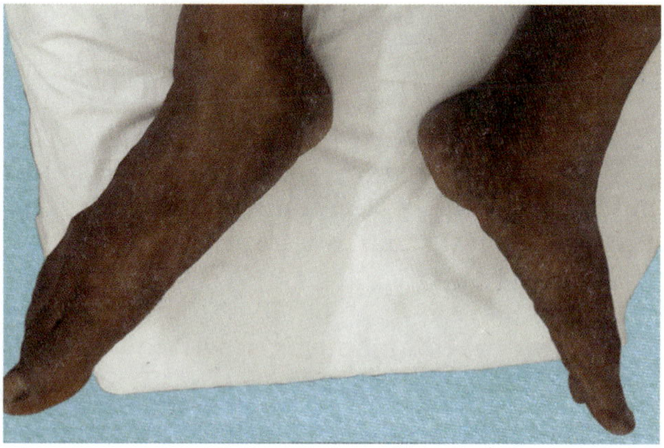

Fig. 2.84: Flatfoot or pes planus

Q. Do you know the common skeletal abnormalities in neurology?

Skeletal abnormalities observed in neurology are:

- Kyphoscoliosis (a combination of kyphosis and scoliosis)
- Pes cavus
- Short neck (e.g., in cranio-vertebral anomaly)
- Gibbus (i.e., from caries spine, metastasis, or trauma to spine) (Fig. 2.85)
- Various skull deformities: Microcephaly (e.g., cerebral palsy), macrocephaly (hydrocephalus, Paget's disease), dolichocephaly (long narrow skull, seen in Marfan's syndrome), brachycephaly (slightly flattened head, seen in Down's syndrome), turricephaly (tower-like peaked appearance of skull, seen in Apert's syndrome), oxycephally (cone-shaped and pointed head)
- Spina bifida occulta (diagnosed by observing presence of tuft of hair, fibrofatty tumour, dimpling, nevus or cicatricial thickening of skin over the sacrum).

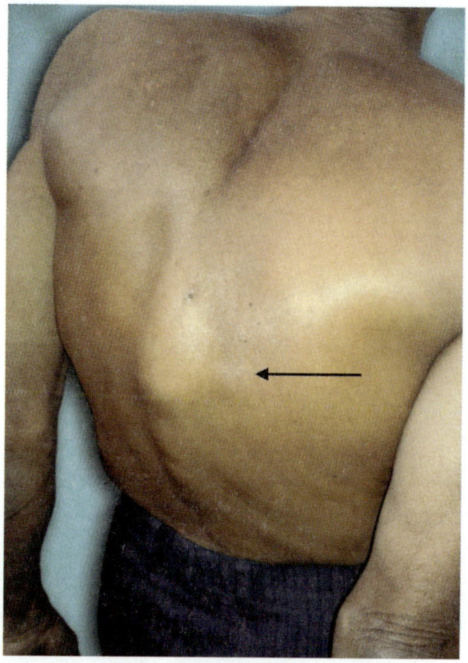

Fig. 2.85: Severe kyphosis with gibbus (acute angulation in the spine) formation

Q. Describe the causes of the following entities.

Physical abnormalities	*Diseases associated with*
• Frontal bossing (prominence) of skull	Thalassaemia, rickets, acromegaly, achondroplasia, hydrocephalus, congenital syphilis
• Quadrate skull	Rickets, osteopetrosis (marble bone disease)
• Prominent supraorbital ridges	Racial, acromegaly, Paget's disease, achondroplasia
• Depressed bridge of the nose (Fig. 2.86)	Racial, traumatic, cretinism, thalassaemia, lepromatous leprosy, ectodermal dysplasia, Wegener's granulomatosis, congenital syphilis, Down's syndrome, achondroplasia
• Saddle nose (Fig. 2.87)	Lepromatous leprosy, ectodermal dysplasia, achondroplasia, congenital syphilis, fractured nasal bone (i.e., trauma)
• High arched palate*	Marfan's syndrome, Turner's syndrome, Down's syndrome, achondroplasia, cyanotic congenital heart disease
• Perforation of palate	Congenital, leprosy, tuberculosis, irradiation, syphilis
• Perforation of nasal septum	Leprosy, Wegener's granulomatosis, tuberculosis, syphilis, trauma
• Polydactyly (extra finger) (Figs 2.88 and 2.89)	Congenital, Laurence-Moon-Biedl syndrome, associated with retinal degeneration/mental retardation/genital hypoplasia
• Syndactyly (fused fingers)	Poland syndrome, Apert's syndrome, Holt-Oram syndrome
• Arachnodactyly (long, slender fingers)	Marfan's syndrome, hypogonadism

*If the roof of the palate is not visible when the examiner's eyes are kept at the level of patient's upper incisor teeth (keep the patient's mouth wide open), it is known as high arched palate.

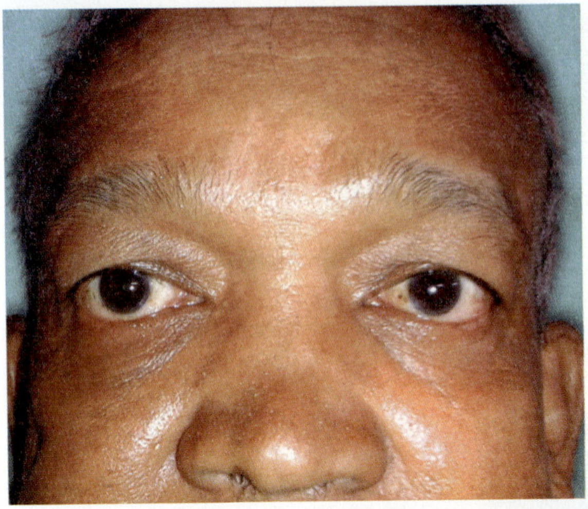

Fig. 2.86: Depressed bridge of the nose

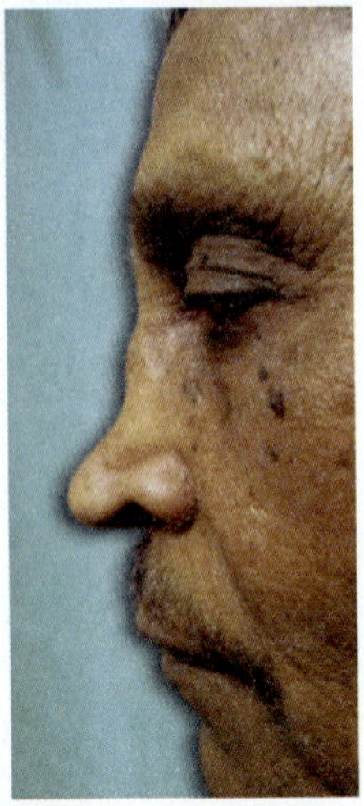

Fig. 2.87: Saddle nose as a result of nasal trauma

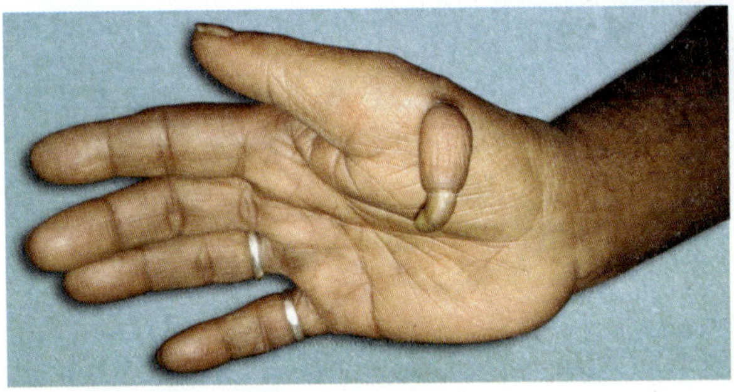

Fig. 2.88: Polydactyly of right hand

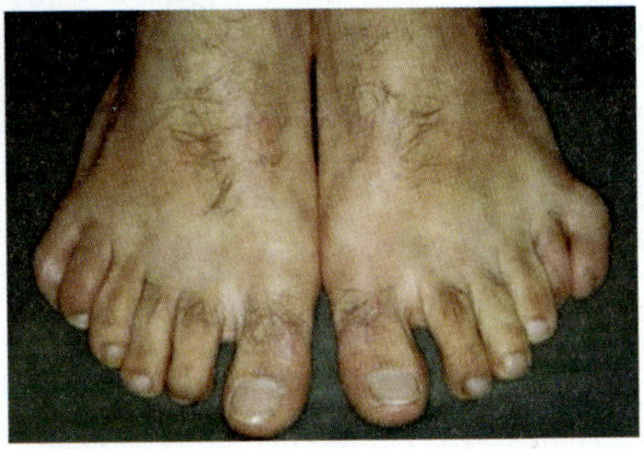

Fig. 2.89: Polydactyly of both feet having six toes in each

Q. Do you know these physical stigmata which immensely help in clinical diagnosis?

Physical stigmata	*Clinical abnormality*
• Hypertelorism (widely set eyes)* (Fig. 2.90)	Racial, Down's syndrome, cretinism, thalassaemia, Turner's syndrome, craniostenosis
• Hypotelorism (decreased distance between orbits)	Patau's syndrome, ethmocephaly, cebocephalia
• Upwards-slanting (mongoloid) of eyes	Racial, Down's syndrome, ectodermal dysplasia
• Anti-mongoloid slant of eyes	Noonan's syndrome, Turner's syndrome
• Blue sclera (Fig. 2.91)	Osteogenesis imperfecta, Marfan's syndrome, Ehlers-Danlos syndrome, newborn baby, hypophosphatasia, pseudoxanthoma elasticum
• Low set ears**	Down's syndrome, Patau's syndrome (trisomy 13), Edwards syndrome (trisomy 18)
• Diagonal ear lobe crease	An independent risk factor for coronary heart disease
• Short neck***	Cranio-vertebral anomaly, cretinism, Turner's syndrome, Down's syndrome

Contd.

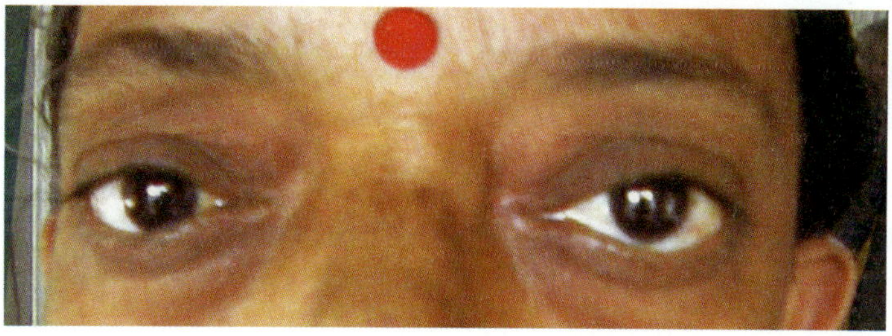

Fig. 2.90: Hypertelorism—increased distance between two eyeballs

Fig. 2.91: Blue sclera

Contd.

• Webbed neck	Turner's syndrome, pseudoxanthoma elasticum, Noonan's syndrome, Klippel-Feil anomaly
• Low hair line (below C_4 vertebra)	Klippel-Feil anomaly, Turner's syndrome, pseudohypoparathyroidism, Noonan's syndrome
• Brachycephaly	Head is unusually short in diameter from front to back (e.g., Down's syndrome)
• Dolichocephaly	Head is longer than would be expected, relative to its width (e.g., Marfan's syndrome)
• Hutchinson's triad (in congenital syphilis)	Hutchinson's teeth, interstitial keratitis, deafness (VIIIth cranial nerve involvement)
• Small chin (micrognathia)	Turner's syndrome, Treacher Collins syndrome, Foetal alcohol syndrome, Pierre Robin syndrome
• Prognathism (bull-dog jaw)	Acromegaly, osteopetrosis, fragile-X syndrome
• Big lips	Cretinism, acromegaly, myxoedema, hamangioma or lymphangioma of the lip
• Teeth present at birth (natal teeth)	Ellis-van Creveld syndrome
• Short 4th metacarpal/metatarsals	Turner's syndrome, pseudohypoparathyroidism, Down's syndrome, trauma
• Sabre tibia (anterior tibial bowing)	Rickets, Paget's disease, osteogenesis imperfecta, osteopetrosis, congenital syphilis

*Hypertelorism literally means an increased distance between two organs, usually referring to an increased distance between the eyes. When the inter inner-canthal distance between two eyes is more than half of inter-pupillary distance, hypertelorism is said to be present.

**Low set ears: When less than one-third of pinna is present above the arbitrary horizontal line drawn from the outer canthus of ipsilateral eye.

***Short neck is usually associated with low hair line.

NB: High arched palate, hypertelorism and low set ears are frequently associated with different congenital anomalies of heart.

VITAL SIGNS

PULSE

Q. What are the 'vital signs' of a patient?

The 4 main vital signs routinely monitored by health care providers (doctors, nurses, social workers, etc.) are:
- Pulse
- Blood pressure (BP)
- Respiration
- Temperature.

NB: A few clinicians believe that 'level of consciousness' can be added with those four signs. In many countries, 'O_2 saturation in peripheral capillaries or SpO_2' (usually which is 94–98% in health, and 88–92% in COPD patients) is regarded as 5th vital sign in clinical medicine.

Q. How pulse is defined?

It is the expansion and elongation of the arterial wall (transmitted pressure wave) conveyed by the column of blood, and is passively produced by the pressure changes during ventricular systole and diastole.

Q. What are the points in examination of pulse to be taken into account?

Pulse should always be examined considering these 8 points:
1. Rate
2. Rhythm
3. Volume
4. Condition of the arterial wall (i.e., vessel wall thickening present or not)
5. Comparison between two radial pulses (i.e., radio-radial delay)
6. Radio-femoral delay
7. Special character, if any
8. Palpation of other peripheral pulses.

* 'Tension' is the indirect measurement of BP; estimation of tension by palpation of pulse is unreliable, and should be accurately measured by sphygmomanometer.
** Commonly, the right radial artery is examined for pulse.
*** The rate and rhythm are better palpated in radial artery, while volume and character of pulse should be examined in big arteries like carotid, brachial or femoral artery. Collapsing pulse of aortic regurgitation (AR) and pulsus alternans of LVF are better palpated in radial artery. Palpation of brachial artery is needed to record BP.

Q. What is the normal pulse rate?

The method of assessing pulse rate is:
- Count the pulse for 15 seconds and multiply by 4; in arrhythmia, count the pulse for full 1 minute. Normal pulse rate is 60–100 beats/minute (average 72/min). At birth, the rate remains 120–160/min, averaging 140/min.

- Use the middle three fingers (index, middle and ring) to palpate the radial pulse of the patient at right wrist; the patient's forearm should be semipronated and the wrist slightly flexed (it is the 'method of trisection' where the examiner applies pressure by his three fingers over patient's radial pulse until the pulse is maximal) (Fig. 2.92).

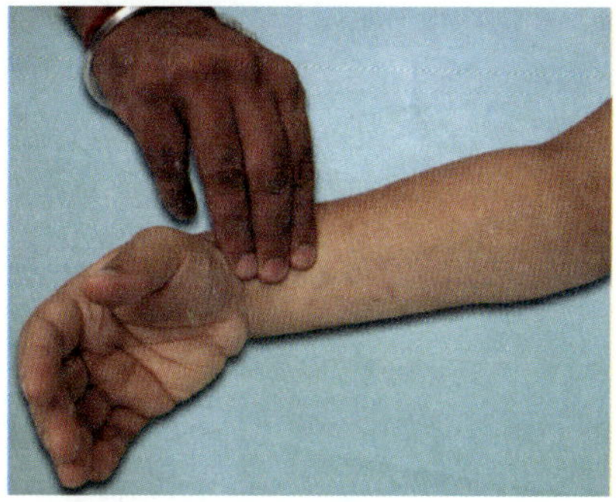

Fig. 2.92: Palpation of radial artery (the 'pulse')

Q. What are the variations in pulse rate?

Variations	*Causes*
• Tachycardia (pulse rate > 100 / min)	Exercise, emotion, fear, anxiety, heart failure, fever, severe anaemia, thyrotoxicosis, myocarditis, shock (e.g., AMI), hypoxia, pregnancy, acute haemorrhage, drugs (salbutamol, atropine, nifedipine)
• Bradycardia (pulse rate < 60 / min)	Trained athletes, meditation, yoga, during deep sleep, myxoedema, obstructive jaundice, increased intracranial tension, complete heart block (CHB), sick sinus syndrome, vasovagal attack, hypersensitive carotid sinus, hypothermia, viral myocarditis, drugs (β-blockers, digitalis, verapramil), organophosphorus poisoning

Q. What is the pulse–temperature relationship?

Remember, with per degree (°F) rise of temperature in an adult, the pulse rate is increased by 10 beats/minute. Undermentioned relative tachycardia and bradycardia (pulse–temperature relationship) often helps the clinician to solve the puzzle of fever.

Variations	*Causes*
• Relative tachycardia [increase in pulse rate >10 beats/minute with per degree (°F) rise of temperature]	Acute rheumatic carditis, tuberculosis, myocarditis (viral, diphtheritic), polyarteritis nodosa
• Relative bradycardia [increase in pulse rate <10 beats/minute with per degree (°F) rise of temperature]	Any viral fever (e.g., yellow fever, dengue), first week of enteric fever, brucellosis, Weil's disease, Lyme disease, drug fever

Q. Do you know any pulse-respiration ratio?

The ratio goes like this:

- *Normal* pulse: respiration = 4 : 1 (72 : 18)
- *Increased* pulse: respiration e.g., 13 : 1 (78 : 6) is seen in narcotic poisoning
- *Decreased* pulse: respiration e.g., 2 : 1 (100 : 50) is seen in acute lobar pneumonia.

NB: Normal respiratory rate in a relaxed adult is 14–18 breaths/minute. In narcotic overdose, respiratory rate becomes low, while respiratory rate is grossly increased in pneumonia; in pneumonia, pulse rate is also increased as a result of infective aetiology and resultant pyrexia.

Q. What is sinus tachycardia and sinus bradycardia?

These are defined as:

- *Sinus tachycardia:* Pulse rate is >100/min, and the impulse has been originated from SA node. The heart rate usually varies between 100 and 160/min.
- *Sinus brachycardia:* Pulse rate is <60/min, and the impulse has been originated from SA node.

NB: Paroxysmal tachycardia: Pulse rate is >160/min, and it is of two types: 1. Supraventricular (PSVT), and 2. Ventricular (VT); the causes are rheumatic carditis, ischaemic heart disease (IHD), hypertensive heart disease, thyrotoxicosis, cardiomyopathy and WPW (Wolff-Parkinson-White) syndrome.

Q. What are the causes of increased sleeping pulse rate?

Increased sleeping pulse rate is found in:

- Thyrotoxicosis
- Rheumatic carditis
- Atropinised patient
- Fever due to any cause
- Tuberculosis.

*In anxiety neurosis, the diurnal pulse rate is high (e.g., tachycardia) but the sleeping pulse rate remains normal.

Q. What is 'pulse deficit'?

Pulse deficit is common in different arrhythmias (i.e., rhythm disturbances).

It is the difference between heart rate and pulse rate. First count the heart rate for 1 minute and then count the pulse rate for 1 minute—if the rate is not same, then it is said that pulse deficit is present (it is better to count the pulse rate by one examiner, and heart rate by other examiner simultaneously for full one minute). It is due to the fact that some weak heartbeats cannot reach radial artery, and pulse deficit develops. Usually it is >10/min in *atrial fibrillation*, and <10/min in *multiple ectopics*.

Q. What is sinus rhythm, nodal rhythm and idioventricular rhythm?

These definitions go like this:

- *Sinus rhythm:* SA node is the natural pacemaker of the heart. Normal cardiac rhythm ranges between 60 and 100/min (average 72/min), and is known as sinus rhythm as the heart beat is generated from SA node.
- *Nodal rhythm:* If SA node fails, AV node takes the charge to originate impulse at the rate of 40–60/min, and the pulse rate becomes 40–60/min; it is nodal rhythm.
- *Idioventricular rhythm:* In this rhythm, the cardiac impulse originates from the walls of ventricles at a rate of 30–40/min (average 36/min), and the pulse rate becomes 30–40/min; its ideal example is complete heart block (CHB).

Q. What is an ectopic beat?

- Ectopic beat is synonymous with extrasystole and premature beat.

- In ectopic rhythm, the impulse arises from atrial wall, AV node or ventricular wall instead of SA node. The ectopic beat is small, occurs a bit earlier and is followed by a compensatory pause. The compensatory pause mimics a 'missing' beat in pulse.
- Pulse feels like (**classical cadence**): Small pause followed by small beat, then big pause comes which is followed by a big beat.
- Common causes: Overindulgence of tea, coffee, cigarettes, alcohol; anxiety; rheumatic, hypertensive, ischaemic, thyrotoxic and cardiomyopathic heart diseases.
- Vagotonic procedures (e.g., carotid sinus massage, self-induced vomiting, Valsalva manoeuvre, stretching of arms and body) abolish ectopics, while vagolytic procedures (exercise, atropine, amyl nitrite) increase the ectopics.

Remember, vagotonic procedures have no effect on ventricular ectopics.

Q. What is rhythm of pulse?

- It is the spacing of successive pulse waves in time. Normal pulse is regular in rhythm and is known as sinus rhythm. Irregularities in rhythm are of two types:
  - Regularly irregular (i.e., irregularity comes in a regular interval e.g., a worker is punctually late by ten minutes everyday, in arrival at office)—ectopics, 2° heart block, pulsus bigeminus, pulsus trigeminus, *sinus arrhythmia* (pulse rate increases with inspiration and decreases with expiration; itself a physiological phenomenon, and is commonly seen in children and athletes).
  - Irregularly irregular (irregularity between two pulse beats in every aspect like rate, rhythm, volume etc. i.e., extremely chaotic with no discernible pattern)—*atrial fibrillation, multiple ventricular ectopics*, atrial flutter with varying degree of heart block.

Q. What is volume of the pulse?

It is the amplitude of the pulse wave (i.e., uplift felt at the wrist), and reflects the *pulse pressure* (systolic BP minus diastolic BP). Normal pulse pressure is 30–60 mm of Hg. Volume of a pulse depends on stroke volume and compliance of the arteries. It is of two types: High volume and low volume.

Type of volume	*Causes*
1. High volume pulse (pulse pr. >60 mm of Hg)	a. *Hyperkinetic circulatory states* like post-exercise, pyrexia, severe anaemia, pregnancy, thyrotoxicosis, aortic incompetence, PDA, arteriovenous shunts, chronic cor pulmonale (hypercarbia), hepatocellular failure
	b. Atherosclerosis (i.e., rigid arteries), systemic hypertension, complete heart block (slow, bounding pulse) or bradycardia due to any cause
2. Low volume pulse (pulse pr. <30 mm of Hg)	a. Shock due to any cause (e.g., AMI, septicaemia), CCF
	b. Severe AS, tight MS, pericardial effusion, constrictive pericarditis

Q. What do you mean by condition of the arterial wall?

In health, arterial wall is impalpable and may be palpable due to arteriosclerosis (in old age), when the artery becomes tortuous and feels like a cord (known as "Monckeberg's medial sclerosis" i.e., calcification of medial coat of large arteries). The condition of the arterial wall is clinically assessed by rolling the radial artery over the radius bone. Remember, atherosclerosis occurs in intimal coat, and the artery is neither palpable nor tortuous.

Q. Causes of radio-radial and radio-femoral delay.

Inequality	*Causes*
• Radio-radial delay	Normal anatomic variation, thoracic inlet syndrome, pre-subclavian coarctation, supravalvular AS, atherosclerosis, peripheral embolism, aneurysm of the arch of aorta, aortic dissection, Takayasu's disease
• Radio-femoral delay	Coarctation of the aorta (important bedside clue in a young hypertensive), atherosclerosis of aorta, thrombosis or embolism of aorta

**Normally, there is no radio-radial delay*. Similarly, *there is no radio-femoral delay in health* but pulsation of arteria dorsalis pedis comes 0.02 to 0.03 second later than radial artery. To diagnose radio-femoral delay, palpate both radial and femoral artery simultaneously to find out any perceptible delay in the arrival of femoral beat compared to radial pulse.

Q. How to palpate different peripheral pulses?

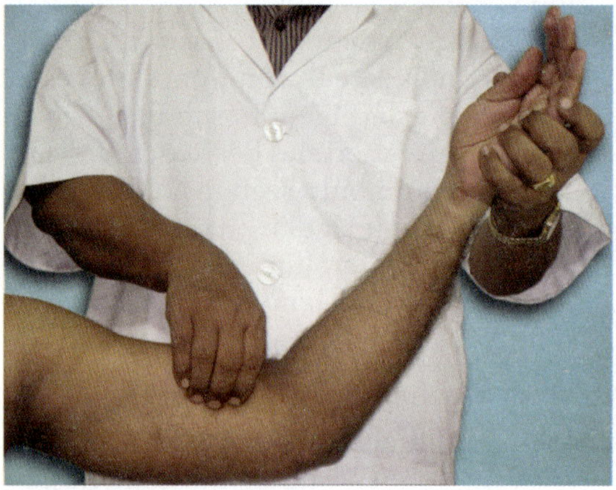

Fig. 2.93: Palpation of brachial artery

Remembering the surface marking of each artery, try to palpate them in the following way:

1. *Subclavian artery:* Felt above the middle of clavicle, while standing behind the patient.
2. *Brachial artery:* Felt at or above the elbow, just medial to the tendon of biceps brachii (Fig. 2.93).
3. *Carotid artery:* Palpate right carotid with left thumb and left carotid with right thumb, medial to strenomastoid at or just below the thyroid cartilage (some clinicians palpate the right carotid with his/her middle three fingers of right hand, and vice-versa for the left) (Figs 2.94 and 2.95).
4. *Radial artery:* Patient's forearm should be slightly pronated and wrist slightly flexed. It is palpated (present lateral to flexor carpi radialis tendon) with pulp of three fingers i.e., index, middle and ring fingers by compressing the artery against head of the radius (Fig. 2.92).
5. *Superficial temporal artery:* Felt just in front of tragus of the ear.
6. *Femoral artery:* Felt at the level of inguinal ligament, midway between anterior superior iliac spine and pubic tubercle; femoral artery lies lateral to femoral vein.
7. *Popliteal artery:* Patient lies supine with slightly flexed knee. The fingertips of both hands are pressed in the popliteal fossa against the posterior aspect of tibial condyle.
8. *Posterior tibial artery:* Felt behind the medial malleolus, midway between it and the heel (Fig. 2.96).
9. *Arteria dorsalis pedis:* Felt lateral to tendon of extensor hallucis longus in the 'proximal' part of dorsum of foot; may be absent in 10% of normal subjects (Fig. 2.97).

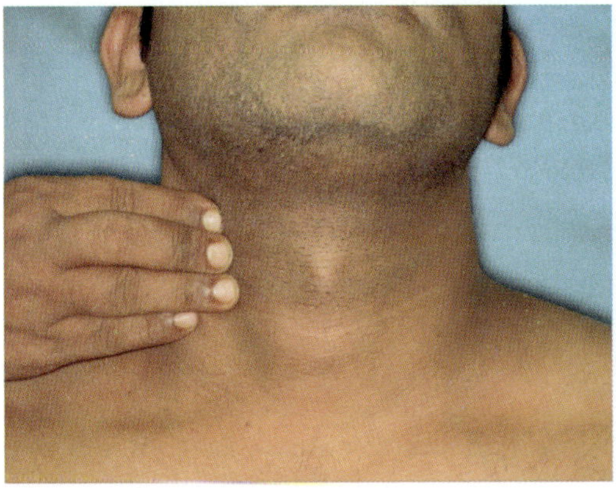

Fig. 2.94: Palpation of right carotid artery (right carotid pulse)

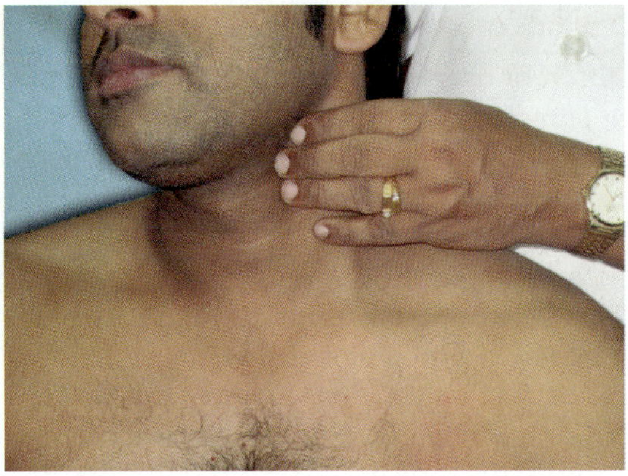

Fig. 2.95: Palpation of left carotid artery (left carotid pulse)

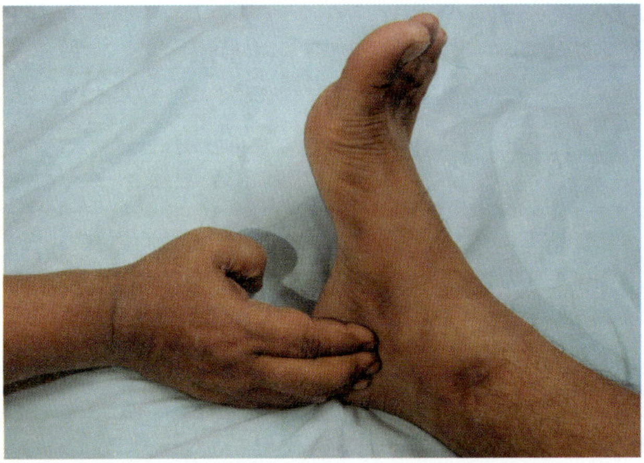

Fig. 2.96: Palpation of posterior tibial artery

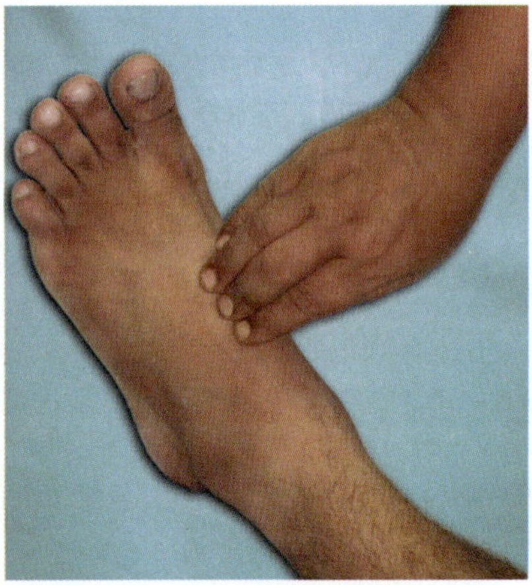

Fig. 2.97: Palpation of arteria dorsalis pedis (the 'pedal pulse')

Q. What are complaints of patients experiencing bradycardia?

It is light-headedness, weakness, dizziness, fainting (syncope), or palpitations. In very slow pulse rate, patient may experience confusion or seizures.

Q. Do you know the causes of absent radial pulse?

Absent radial pulse is seen in:

- Anatomical abnormality
- Severe atherosclerosis
- Takayasu's disease (pulseless disease)
- Embolism into radial artery (from atrial fibrillation, SBE)
- Death (i.e., the end of the life).

Q. What are thready pulse, bounding pulse, jerky pulse and collapsing pulse?

Different characters of pulse are analysed by:

- *Thready pulse:* It is a low volume (feeble) pulse with rapid pulse rate e.g., peripheral circulatory failure, severe LVF, intense vasoconstriction.
- *Bounding pulse:* The pulse volume is high with increased blood flow e.g., hyperkinetic circulatory states.
- *Jerky pulse:* Pulse may feel a rapid upstroke due to vigorous contraction of hypertrophic left ventricle but pulse wave recedes quickly due to sudden obstruction of left ventricular outflow, and is known as jerky pulse. It is found in hypertrophic obstructive cardiomyopathy (HOCM).
- *Collapsing pulse:* It is a high volume pulse with collapsing nature, that means the pulse disappears fast from palpating hand. Remember, all collapsing pulses are of high volume but all high volume pulses are not of collapsing in character.
- *Asymmetric pulse:* Pulse in both hands looses symmetry in subclavian artery atherosclerosis, thoracic inlet syndrome or dissection of aorta.

Q. What are the significances of absent upper or lower limb pulse?

Situation	*Possibilities*
• Upper limb pulse weak/absent but lower limb pulse felt	Takayasu's disease, aortoarteritis
• Upper limb pulse felt but lower limb pulse weak/absent	Coarctation of aorta, Leriche's syndrome (saddle-shaped thrombosis at bifurcation of aorta)
• Absence of peripheral pulse here and there (randomly)	Atherosclerosis, embolism, vasculitis

Q. How will you differentiate atrial fibrillation (AF) from multiple ectopics at bedside?

Clinically, these rhythm disturbances are differentiated by:

1. Pulse of AF is totally chaotic **(irregularly irregular)** though ectopics may follow the classical cadence (see question above in ectopic beat).
2. Count the pulse: If >100/min, it is usually AF; if <100/min, it is probably multiple ectopics.
3. Count the pulse deficit: If >10/min, it is AF; if <10/min, it is ectopics.
4. Now ask the patient to perform mild exercise (patient will sit and touch the toes with his/her hands, and will lie down again to repeat it for 5–6 times), if his/her condition permits. The heart of AF becomes more irregular after exercise, and thus if pulse deficit (post-exercise) becomes >10/min, it is AF, and if remains same or goes <10/min, it is ectopics.

Q. Findings after examining a patient of atrial fibrillation (AF).

Characteristics of AF are:

1. Ventricular rate is usually 100–140/minute. Pulse is irregularly irregular with pulse deficit >10/min. Pulse is irregular in rate, rhythm and volume i.e., totally chaotic.
2. Variable intensity of S_1.

3. Absent *a*-wave in JVP.
4. Embolic manifestations may be evident e.g., CVA, intermittent claudication.

NB: In atrial fibrillation, atria usually fire impulses at a rate of 350–600/minute while the ventricle responds at a rate of 100–140/minute, and the pulse rate is usually 100–120/minute. It is the most common arrhythmia in clinical practice.

Aetiology of atrial fibrillation is rheumatic (commonly mitral stenosis), ischaemic, hypertensive, thyrotoxicosis, myocarditis, cardiomyopathy, pericarditis, following cardiothoracic surgery and 'lone' atrial fibrillation (commonly in elderly persons where no cause can be found).

Q. What is catacrotic pulse?

It is the normal pulse found in health. It has three waves chronologically like P, T and D representing Percussion (P, on top of ascending limb), Tidal (T, near top of descending limb) and Dicrotic waves (D, on descending limb). The wavy pattern is not felt in health since it is obliterated by normal vascular tone.

Q. What is complete heart block (CHB)?

In CHB, all supraventricular impulses are blocked to traverse downwards to ventricles due to coronary artery disease, cardiac surgery, degenerative disease of conducting system, etc. The ventricle runs by ventricular pacemaker i.e., by idioventricular rhythm at a rate of 30–40/min (averaging 36/min); atrial chamber beats of its own by impulses originated from SA node with a rate of 72/min which may be reflected in neck veins. The pulse of CHB is of low rate at 36/min (i.e., bradycardia) with a high volume. The patient may be unconscious during ventricular asystole period (Stokes-Adams syndrome).

Q. Can you focus on different well-known characters of pulse?

Character	*Terminologies*	*Description*
• Double-beating pulse	Anacrotic pulse	Low volume, twice beating, systolic peak observed in ascending limb. Found in severe AS
	Dicrotic pulse	Low volume. Upstroke felt in descending limb; first wave is 'P', and second is 'D'. It is due to hypotonia of vessel wall. Found in 2nd week of typhoid, endotoxic shock
	Pulsus bisferiens (bifid pulse)	High volume. Percussion (P) and tidal (T) waves both are felt. Common in isolated AR, AS with AR, and HOCM
• Changing amplitude of pulse	Pulsus parvus	Parvus means low volume, and is found in tight MS, severe AS
	Pulsus 'parvus et tardus'	Pulsus tardus means slow or late. Pulse of severe AS will have slow rising upstroke, small volume and sustained peak. A 'carotid shudder' may be felt at neck

	Water-hammer pulse	High volume collapsing pulse which will have sharp rise, ill-sustained and sharp fall. Found in all causes of 'high volume pulse' (AR should come first in list). It is appreciated clinically by raising the hand upwards (Fig. 2.98)
• Pulse of specific characters	Pulsus alternans	Low volume, and alternate pulse waves are weak (rhythm is regular in contrast to ectopics). Common in severe LVF
	Pulsus bigeminus	Coupling of pulse waves in pairs and a pause thereafter recur in a regular fashion; the second beat is ectopic, and thus the pause. Found in digitalis toxicity, 3:2 heart block
	Pulsus paradoxus	Appreciable reduction in volume of pulse in inspiration and increase in expiration (due to exaggerated inspiratory fall in systolic BP >10 mm of Hg). Seen in acute severe asthma, cardiac tamponade, SVC syndrome, pulmonary embolism, constrictive pericarditis (rare)

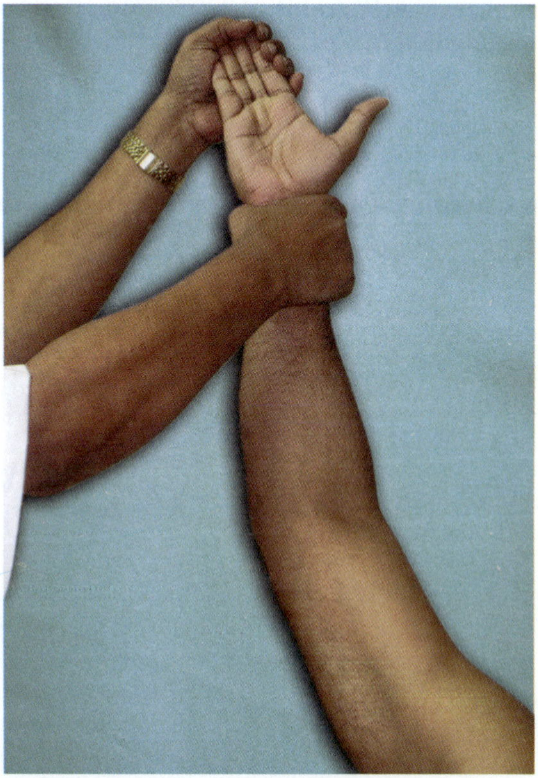

Fig. 2.98: Demonstration of water-hammer pulse (collapsing radial pulse)

BLOOD PRESSURE (BP)

Q. What is blood pressure?

It is the:

- Lateral pressure exerted by the column of blood on the vessel walls while flowing through it. From minute to minute, BP varies with activity, emotion, exercise, respiration, pain, temperature, diet, posture, tobacco or alcohol consumption, or medications.
- Persistent rise of BP above the normal is known as *hypertension.*

Q. Do you know systolic pressure, diastolic pressure, pulse pressure and mean arterial pressure?

These are defined as:

- *Systolic pressure (SP):* It reflects the cardiac output
- *Diastolic pressure (DP):* It reflects the peripheral resistance
- *Pulse pressure (PP):* It is SP minus DP; normal PP is 30–60 mm of Hg
- *Mean arterial pressure (MAP):* It is the average BP in an individual, and is usually calculated by DP + 1/3rd of PP. Normal MAP is approximately 100 mm of Hg, which is required to perfuse brain, coronary arteries, kidneys and other vital organs.

Q. What are the sounds you heard during measurement of BP manually?

These are known as 'Korotkoff sounds' (after Nikolai Korotkoff described the sounds in 1905), and they are:

- *Phase I:* Sudden appearance of tapping sound (indicates SP)
- *Phase II:* Tapping sound is replaced by soft murmur-like sounds
- *Phase III:* Gong sounds replace murmur
- *Phase IV:* The loud sounds suddenly becomes muffled
- *Phase V:* All sounds cease (indicates DP).

Q. Some basic facts in BP to be known.

1. Korotkoff sounds may be audible up to 0 mm of Hg in aortic regurgitation, arteriovenous (AV) fistula and pregnancy.
2. Multiple BP recording with averaging is advised in atrial fibrillation.
3. DP is more important in persons <50 years, while SP is important in persons >50 years of age. SP continuously increases with age.
4. SP in lower limbs are higher by up to 20 mm of Hg than SP in upper limbs, while DP remains same. Lower limb BP is higher (e.g., >20 mm of Hg) than upper limb BP in aortic regurgitation, and lower limb BP is lower than upper limb BP in coarctation of aorta and occlusive arterial disease.
5. BP difference in right and left arm may be up to 10 mm of Hg; if more, think of Takayasu's disease, thoracic inlet syndrome, pre-subclavian coarctation, atherosclerosis of aorta, etc. On standing, systolic BP falls though diastolic BP rises.
6. BP should be measured in both upper and lower limbs (to diagnose above entities), and in supine and erect posture (to diagnose postural hypotension). BP should be

measured in the unparalysed upper limb in a patient of hemiplegia. Night time BP is 10–20% lower than daytime BP.

Q. Do you know different types of BP machine?

Two common types used are:
- Mercury column type (sphygmomanometer) (Fig. 2.99)
- Aneroid type or spring dial type (less accurate) (Fig. 2.100).

NB: Digital (electronic) BP machine is used by lay people at home.

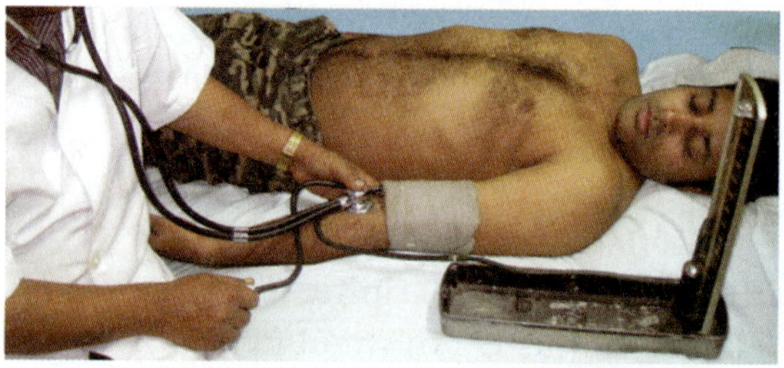

Fig. 2.99: Recording of blood pressure by sphygmomanometer (mercury column type)

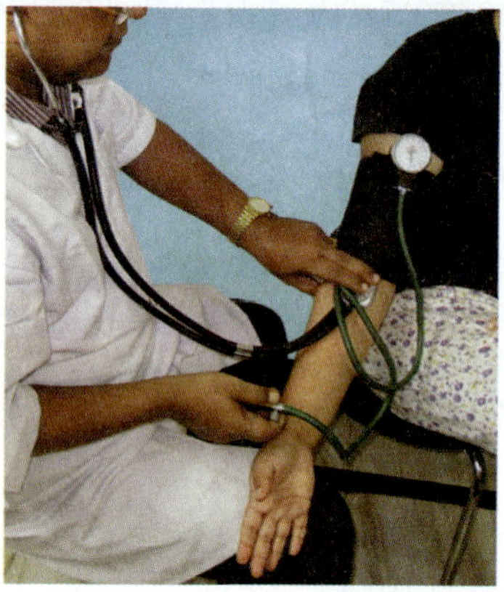

Fig. 2.100: Recording of blood pressure by aneroid machine (spring dial type)

Q. Do you have any idea about measurement of sphygmomanometer cuff?

The sphygmomanometer cuff should be:
- *Length:* Should not be <10 inches
- *Width:*
  - *Adults:* 5 inches
  - *Young children:* 3 inches
  - *Infants:* 1 inch.

NB: If adult-sized cuff is used in a child, it will falsely record low BP, and similarly a falsely high BP is recoded if infant-sized cuff is used in an adult. An adult ideally requires 8 inches wide cuff for recording lower limb BP (to wrap in thigh); an obese adult require a more wider cuff for arm i.e., 6 inches.

Q. Use of sphygmomanometer in clinical practice.

The sphygmomanometer can be used for:

1. To measure the BP
2. To demonstrate and confirm: Pulsus paradoxus, pulsus alternans, water-hammer pulse
3. To demonstrate Hill's sign in aortic regurgitation
4. To look for Hess' capillary fragility test or 'Tourniquet test' (e.g., in dengue)
5. To elicit latent tetany (Trousseau's sign)
6. To demonstrate orthostatic (postural) hypotension
7. To draw venous blood (e.g., for blood biochemistry or in blood donation camp).

Q. What is auscultatory gap?

This is also known as silent gap. In some patients with hypertension, there is a period of silence that may occur between phase I and phase II, and this silent period is known as auscultatory gap. If the clinician misses the phase I, he/she will record the phase II as systolic BP, which is lower than the actual systolic BP. Thus, mercury column should be raised up to 200 mm of Hg or more at the initial part of BP recording. It is due to venous distension or diminished flow velocity in arteries.

Q. Indications of ambulatory BP recording for 24 hours.

The indications are:

- To rule out white-coat hypertension (see below)
- Unusual variability in BP recording.

Q. Do you know aetiological classification of hypertension?

Systemic hypertension is of two types: *Primary* (essential or idiopathic; 80–90%) and *secondary* hypertension. Secondary hypertension occurs as a result of specific disease or abnormality, and thus it is often treatable though it is a severe hypertension. The cause of primary hypertension is unknown.

Causes of secondary hypertension

1. Renal diseases	Acute and chronic glomerulonephritis, polycystic kidney disease, renal artery stenosis, chronic pyelonephritis, chronic renal failure, renal involvement from diabetes or SLE
2. Endocrine disorders	Cushing's syndrome, pheochromocytoma, primary hyperaldosteronism (Conn's syndrome), acromegaly, myxoedema, hyperparathyroidism, congenital adrenal hyperplasia, Liddle's syndrome
3. Drugs	Corticosteroids, oral contraceptive pills, oestrogens, carbenexolone, sympathomimetics, anabolic steroids
4. Vascular	Coarctation of aorta, non-specific aortoarteritis
5. Others	Obesity, pre-eclampsia/eclampsia, obstructive sleep apnoea, alcohol, porphyria

NB: Commonest cause of hypertension is idiopathic, and the second common causes are renal disorders.

Q. Do you know orthostatic hypotension or postural hypotension?

If a person stands from lying down position and BP is measured within 3 minutes, systolic BP may fall up to 20 mm of Hg while diastolic BP may decrease up to 10 mm of Hg. Anything more than this is orthostatic hypotension. This 'postural drop' is commonly observed in blood loss, fluid loss (e.g., acute gastroenteritis), autonomic neuropathy (e.g., diabetes mellitus), shock, and patients on antihypertensive drugs. It is an important 'cause of fall' in the geriatric (i.e., old age) population.

Q. What is the summary of recommendations of JNC VIII (Joint National Committee, 2014) guidelines of treatment of hypertension?

The basic recommendations are:

1. Encourage lifestyle changes even in patients with pre-hypertension (120–139/80–89 mm of Hg).
2. Patients <60 years, or with diabetes or chronic kidney disease: Start pharmacotherapy at 140/90 mm of Hg.
3. Patients 60 years or older, start pharmacotherapy at 150/90 mm of Hg.

NB: So, it seems that normal BP should be 120/80 mm of Hg. Hypertension is defined as BP >140/90 mm of Hg.

Q. Have you heard about white-coat hypertension?

This is the high BP recorded in some patients by physicians in his/her chamber, outdoor or indoor of a hospital, while the BP is otherwise normal. Thus, it is often called office or clinic hypertension, which is a well-known cause of refractory hypertension. Recent studies have shown that patients may be associated with target organ damage (LVH, carotid atherosclerosis). Accurate diagnosis needs 24-hour ambulatory monitoring of BP. These patients should be under regular follow-up by physician or cardiologist.

Evidence of anxiety-induced sympathetic drive like perspiration, cold hands, tremor or tachycardia may be associated with.

Q. How to measure BP in a case with atrial fibrillation?

A rough assessment of BP is done after measuring BP for several times due to variability of cardiac output.

Q. Describe the undermentioned terminologies.

Terminologies	*Description*
• Accelerated hypertension	Recent and rapid increase in BP level with evidence of vascular damage on fundoscopic examination but without papilloedema
• Malignant hypertension	Severe accelerated hypertension with diastolic BP >140 mm of Hg along with haemorrhages, exudates and papilloedema in optic fundi, and is often associated with either deteriorating renal function, or cardiac decompromise (e.g., LVF), or hypertensive encephalopathy
• Hypertensive emergency	Severe elevation of BP with impending or accompanying target organ damage, demanding prompt and rapid control of BP within 1 hour by parenteral therapy e.g., hypertensive encephalopathy, dissection of aorta

• Hypertensive urgency	Markedly elevated BP without any target organ damage, demanding control of BP within hours by oral therapy e.g., asymptomatic severe hypertension
• Labile hypertension	Patients having high BP for sometime of the day, but not always (fluctuating BP, which requires constant monitoring periodically)
• Pseudo hypertension	Recording of falsely elevated high BP in old age due to stiff and non-compliant arterial wall (Osler's sign)
• Paroxysmal hypertension (episodic hypertension)	Sudden shooting of BP, and is classically seen in pheochromocytoma
• Paradoxical hypertension	Elevation of BP after initiation of antihypertensive drugs e.g., ACE-inhibitors in treating renal artery stenosis
• Transient hypertension	Hypertension may be seen for a short period of time in pregnancy, acute glomerulonephritis, CVA or AMI, which may be stress-induced or disease-induced
• Isolated systolic hypertension (ISH)	Commonly found in old age, where systolic BP ≥140 mm of Hg and DP <90 mm of Hg
• Decapitated hypertension	Sudden lowering of systolic BP in a hypertensive patient as a result of LVF due to varying aetiology (systolic decapitation of normal BP occurs in aortic stenosis)
• Refractory hypertension	If in spite of full compliance and with three or more antihypertensives, BP cannot be reduced to 140/90 mm of Hg, it is called refractory or resistant hypertension. It is due to non-compliance of drug therapy (commonest), inadequate treatment or failure to recognise secondary hypertension
• Gestational hypertension	High BP during pregnancy or first 24 hours postpartum in absence of previous H/o persistent high BP or proteinuria

Q. What are the target organs which are commonly damaged by hypertension?

The target organs commonly jeopardised by long-continued hypertension are:

- *Heart and vessels* e.g., LVF, AMI, peripheral vascular disease
- *Cerebrovascular* e.g., CVA (transient ischaemic attacks, cerebral thrombosis, hypertensive encephalopathy, subarachnoid haemorrhage)
- *Renal:* Leads to impaired renal functions terminating in renal failure
- *Eye:* Associated with retinal haemorrhages and exudates, and papilloedema
- *Nose:* Complicated by epistaxis.

RESPIRATION

Q. What are the points to be noted clinically in 'Respiration'?

Respiration is described by these 5 points:

- Rate
- Rhythm
- Type
- Depth
- Breathing pattern

Q. Can you analyse each point of 'Respiration'?

A. ***Rate:*** Normal respiratory rate in a relaxed adult is 14–18 breaths/minute. At the time of birth, the rate is 40/minute.

Rate of respiration is counted surreptitiously (i.e., without attracting patient's attention), by placing the right hand in the patient's epigastrium while observing the anterior chest movements for a full minute. A wide variation in rate may occur in health, and they are:

1. *Tachypnoea (polypnoea):* Rate >20/minute is tachypnoea, and is commonly found in anxiety, exertion, pyrexia, acute lobar pneumonia, bronchial asthma, COPD (chronic obstructive pulmonary disease), shock, metabolic acidosis, and hysteria. Very high respiratory rate is found in pneumonia. Many a time, tachypnoea is the only clue to a respiratory disease.
2. *Bradypnoea:* Low respiratory rate <10/minute is bradypnoea, and is common in narcotic poisoning (opium or morphine), increased intracranial tension, metabolic alkalosis, myxoedema coma, hypothermia, and respiratory centre abnormality.

B. ***Rhythm:*** Alterations in rhythm are diagnosed by inspecting the anterior movement of the chest. Wide variations may be noted in rhythm like:

1. *Irregularly irregular or Biot's breathing:* Here, the rhythm of respiration is just like atrial fibrillation as reflected in pulse. The respiration is sometimes slow, sometimes rapid, sometimes superficial, and sometimes deep without any constant relationship between two types; respiration starts abruptly and stops with longer periods of apnoea. It is seen in pontine lesion, and meningitis (especially in children).
2. *Regularly irregular or Cheyne-Stokes respiration:* This is a form of periodic respiration where periods of apnoea rhythmically alternate with hyperpnoea, each phase lasting for about 30 seconds, and the whole cycle is usually completed in less than 2 minutes. The hypercapnoea (retention of CO_2) resulting out of apnoea stimulates brainstem respiratory centres which gives rise to hyperventilation drive, and ultimately washes out CO_2 which henceforth produces depression of respiratory centre leading to apnoea. This is commonly seen in healthy infants, deep sleep in adults, severe LVF, uraemia, increased intracranial tension (e.g., CVA), narcotic poisoning, and severe cardio-respiratory embarrassment.
3. *Miscellaneous:* Kussmaul's breathing, stertorous breathing, prolonged inspiration or prolonged expiration.

C. ***Type:*** Easily diagnosed by observing the movement of anterior chest wall and abdomen. The common types are:

1. *Abdominal:* Adult males (as diaphragm plays more in respiration), young children.
2. *Thoracic:* Adult females (as intercostal muscles play more in respiration).
3. *Abdomino-thoracic:* Young children, sometimes in adult males.

NB: Abdominal type of respiration is also seen in conditions like painful conditions in chest (e.g., pleurisy, chest injury), ankylosing spondylitis, intercostal muscles paralysis.

Similarly, thoracic type of respiration is also prevalent in anxiety, huge ascites, painful conditions in abdomen (e.g., peritonitis), diaphragmatic palsy, hysteria.

D. ***Depth:*** Inspect the excursion of chest, which easily gives the clue to depth of respiration, and they are:

1. *Shallow:* Narcotic poisoning (usually associated with bradypnoea)
2. *Deep:* Hyperpnoea, hyperventilation (e.g., metabolic acidosis).

E. ***Breathing pattern:*** Wheezing or stridor, air hunger, sighing, shallow breathing, mouth-breathing, purse-lip respiration or gasping. One may comment on movement of accessory muscles of respiration or intercostals suction, if present.

Q. What are the different alterations of breathing?

Types	*Description*	*Example*
• Dyspnoea	Abnormally uncomfortable subjective awareness of breathing	Bronchial asthma, LVF, pneumothorax, severe anaemia
• Orthopnoea	Breathlessness in lying down position and is of such a degree as to make the patient sit upright for relief	COPD, LVF, pericardial effusion, massive ascites
• Tachypnoea	Increased respiratory rate of respiration i.e., >20/min	Exertion, pneumonia, bronchial asthma, pyrexia, metabolic acidosis
• Bradypnoea	Low respiratory rate of respiration i.e., <10/min	Narcotic overdose, hypothermia, myxoedema coma, respiratory depression
• Hyperpnoea	Increased rate and depth of respiration	Metabolic acidosis
• Hyperventilation	Increased depth of respiration	Metabolic acidosis, salicylate poisoning, hysteria
• Trepopnoea	Breathlessness only in left or right lateral decubitus	CCF, pleural effusion, pneumothorax
• Platypnoea (orthodeoxia)	Respiratory distress only on assuming upright posture (i.e., opposite to orthopnoea)	Hepato-pulmonary syndrome, left axial myxoma, pulmonary thromboembolism
• Cheyne-Stokes respiration	Periods of apnoea alternate with hyperpnoea	Severe LVF, uraemia, narcotic poisoning
• Kussmaul's breathing (air hunger)	Deep sighing, rapid breathing with a hissing sound (laboured breathing pattern)	Diabetic ketoacidosis, lactic acidosis, uraemia
• Sighing respiration	Shallow nervous breathing with intermittent deep inspiration	Anxiety, depression, hysteria
• Paradoxical respiration	Depression of abdomen with inspiration, and bulging with expiration	Diaphragmatic palsy, high spinal cord lesion
• Gasping respiration	Deep, irregular, intermittent inspirations mimicking 'fish out of water'	In dying patients, which is the terminal respiratory pattern of lower brainstem damage
• Cogwheel breathing	From time to time interruption in normal breathing pattern	Nervous, anxious or weeping individuals

• Stertorous breathing	Respiration with a noisy sound coming from throat; or cheeks puff in and out in a comatose patient	Due to fall-back of tongue, or coming from pharyngeal secretions (e.g., 'death rattle' in pulmonary oedema)
• Purse-lip respiration	Breathing consists of exhaling through tightly pressed lips and inhaling through nose with mouth closed	COPD (i.e., chronic bronchitis, emphysema and chronic bronchiolitis)
• Apneustic breathing	Breath is held at end-inspiration mimicking bradypnoea	Pontine haemorrhage, anoxia, hypoglycaemia, severe meningitis
• Biot's breathing	Irregular breathing in time and depth	Meningitis (especially in children), brainstem damage
• Sleep apnoea	Loud snoring with periods of apnoea terminating in a gasping snore, usually noticed by bed-partner	Usually in obese persons (in contrast to regular snoring, sleep apnoea is associated with excess daytime somnolence)
• Paroxysmal nocturnal dyspnoea (PND)	Sudden (paroxysmal), severe and dramatic development of acute breathlessness (dyspnoea) in early hours of night (nocturnal)	Acute left-sided heart failure (e.g., left atrial failure from MS, or acute LVF from hypertension)
• Ataxic respiration	Rhythm of respiration is chaotic, varying in rate and depth	Lesion in medulla of brainstem

Q. What do you mean by wheezing and stridor?

Clinical conditions	*Features*	*Examples*
• Wheezing	High-pitched continuous musical sound *heard from a distance*. It is better audible in *expiratory phase* and indicates *smaller airway obstruction*; rhonchi in the chest is audible by stethoscope	Bronchial asthma (classical), COPD, tropical eosinophilia, cardiac asthma (e.g., acute LVF), GERD with aspiration, toxic gas inhalation, carcinoid syndrome
• Stridor	Low-pitched crowing sound *heard from a distance*. It is better heard in *inspiratory phase* and indicates partial *obstruction of larger airways* like larynx, trachea and major bronchus. It is an ominous sign with impending complete airway closure (*a medical emergency*), which demands urgent respiratory support. Stridor is more common in children	Aspirated foreign body, laryngeal oedema (angioedema), diphtheria, acute epiglottitis (severe sore throat with thick muffled voice), recurrent laryngeal nerve palsy, tetany (laryngismus stridulus), croup, mucus plug

* Reversible wheezing: Bronchial asthma, and irreversible wheezing: COPD

** Nocturnal wheezing: Acute LVF (giving rise to PND), and GERD with aspiration

Q. What is intercostal suction?

It is the drawing-in of the intercostal spaces with inspiration; in health, intercostal spaces expand and draw-out with inspiration. Intercostal suction is prognostically worse for the patient.

When air entry in the respiratory tract is compromised, the positive atmospheric pressure presses the lower chest wall in the face of negative intrathoracic pressure. The common conditions, which are associated with:

- Foreign body in respiratory tract
- Oedema of the glottis (e.g., in anaphylaxis)
- COPD
- Bronchiolitis in infants and children
- Diphtheria
- Diaphragmatic palsy (bilateral).

Q. What are the 'accessory muscles of respiration'?

In health, normal muscles of respiration are intercostals (external and internal) and diaphragm. Accessory muscles of respiration assist breathing in respiratory embarrassment (e.g., acute severe asthma, COPD), and becomes active and prominent. The muscles are:

- Alae nasi (nasal flare)
- Sternomastoid
- Scalenii
- Latissimus dorsi
- Trapezius
- Pectoralis major
- Serratus anterior
- Anterior abdominal muscles.

Q. How do you assess 'respiratory depression' at the bedside?

Respiratory depression is hypoventilation (i.e., inadequate ventilation) to a clinician. It may develop as a result of different pulmonary diseases (e.g., bronchial asthma, bronchiectasis, emphysema, etc), head injury, anaesthesia, diaphragmatic palsy, poliomyelitis, Guillain-Barré (GB) syndrome, narcotic overdose, metabolic abnormality, morbid obesity or chest injury. Respiratory depression is assessed by:

1. Features of hypoxia (see below). As the patient worsens, there is difficulty in speaking; he/she will speak only one or two words at a time and is not being able to complete a sentence.
2. Central cyanosis.
3. Bradypnoea (low respiratory rate).
4. Shallow respiration (chest expansion will be reduced).
5. Diminished air entry in lungs (clinically diagnosed by auscultation). Even, the clinician may experience with abnormal sounds like wheezes (bronchial asthma), crepitations (pneumonia), or even decreased breath sounds (emphysema).
   Ultimately, mechanical ventilation is required to salvage the moribund patient.

Q. How to diagnose 'upper airway obstruction' clinically?

Obstruction of upper airways like larynx, trachea or major bronchus is a medical emergency. It is easily diagnosed by *proper history* and features like:

1. Restless patient with prominent accessory muscles of respiration
2. Dyspnoea which may lead to orthopnoea
3. Cough
4. Stridor
5. Central cyanosis
6. Intercostal suction.

Q. What is meant by 'respiratory failure'?

It is a condition when normal arterial gases are no longer maintained and the lung function is inadequate for the metabolic needs of the individual, and is characterised by abnormality in blood gases (PaO_2 <60 mm of Hg and/or $PaCO_2$ >50 mm of Hg). Respiratory failure is of four types (mainly type I and II):

1. ***Type I*** (hypoxic features are more prominent): Low PaO_2 with normal or low $PaCO_2$; it is common in pneumonia, acute asthma, ARDS, pulmonary oedema, pulmonary thromboembolism (PTE), hysterical hyperventilation. Usually the patient becomes restless.

   Here, high concentration of O_2 therapy is required i.e., >35%, usually 60%, with high-flow (6–8 L/min).
2. ***Type II*** (hypercapnoeic features are more prominent): High $PaCO_2$ with low PaO_2; it is common in chronic bronchitis, emphysema, acute exacerbation of bronchial asthma or COPD, ankylosing spondylitis, respiratory depression by narcotics or anaesthetics, end-stage type I failure. Usually the patient becomes drowsy.

   Here, low concentration (24–28%), low-flow (1–2 L/min) O_2 therapy by Ventury mask is employed because a few patients are dependent on 'hypoxic drive' to breathe.
3. ***Type III*** (peri-operative) e.g., lung atelectasis.
4. ***Type IV*** (shock): Secondary to cardiovascular instability.

Commonest cause of respiratory failure is chronic bronchitis

Q. Clinical manifestations of hypoxia and hypercapnoea at the bedside.

Features of hypoxia	*Features of hypercapnoea*
1. *Restlessness*, tachypnoea, orthopnoea	1. *Drowsiness*, reduced psychomotor activity, confusion, or even coma
2. Confusion, impaired judgement	2. Headache
3. Central cyanosis	3. Asterixis (flapping tremor)
4. Tachycardia, hypotension	4. Flushed and warm extremities (i.e., hands)
5. Arrhythmias	5. Water-hammer pulse, capillary pulsation, hypertension
6. Damage to vital organs like kidney, liver	6. Chemosis of the conjunctiva
7. Convulsions	7. Fasciculation (twitching of muscles)
8. Even coma may supervene	8. Papilloedema

TEMPERATURE

Q. What is fever or pyrexia?

It is the rise in body temperature commonly caused by cellular response to infection, immunological aberration or malignancy.

Fever is both a symptom and sign. It should always be recorded as part of clinical examination.

Q. What are the methods of recording body temperature?

1. *Oral:* Thermometer is *placed under the tongue* with mouth closed, while the patient breathes through nose. Before putting the thermometer in mouth, wash it with antiseptic solution and gently shake it, so that the mercury column goes below normal temperature. Do not take any oral feed before putting the thermometer in mouth. Always try to record oral temperature, if no contraindication prevails.
2. *Axillary:* Before putting the thermometer *in armpit*, wipe off the sweat present there. Axilla, groin (thigh folded over abdomen) and natal cleft are avoided in adults, and may be practised in children and unconscious patients.
3. *Rectal:* Most reliable and accurate, though not routinely practised (*introduced through rectum*). It is a special 'low-reading' thermometer with a rounded bulb to reduce risk of injury, and is graduated up to 90°F.

Oral, rectal and ear (tympanic membrane electronic thermometer used in ear) temperature record core temperature of body. In health, the temperature in rectal and aural > oral > axillary temperature by 0.5–1°F. Thermometer should be placed in all the sites for at least 2 minutes.

Axilla is an unreliable site to record temperature. Electronic thermometer, which is more safe and accurate, is gradually replacing age-old mercury thermometer. Try to assess the temperature by using your dorsum of hand, which is more sensitive than palmar aspect.

In diagnosing 'fever in ICU', many a time intravascular, intravesical (i.e., urinary bladder), and rectal temperature is recorded in a desperate situation.

Q. Condition when recording of rectal temperature is preferred.

Rectal temperature is recorded in:

- Hypothermia
- Cholera patients, or in algid malaria
- In collapsed, comatosed, or invalid patients.

Q. What are the normal body temperature and its variations in clinical practice?

Variations	*Degree (Celsius/Centegrade/ 'C')*	*Degree (Fahrenheit/ 'F')*
Normal	36.6–37.2	98–99
Subnormal	36.6	<98
Pyrexia or febrile	>37.2	>99
Hypothermia	<35	<95
Hyperpyrexia	>41.5	>106.7

Fever or pyrexia: Oral temperature >99°F; axillary temperature > 98.6°F (i.e., 98.6°F or 37°C, where the arrow in thermometer indicates cut off point of normal temperature).

Recent studies reveal that oral AM temperature of > 98.9°F or an oral PM temperature >99.9°F would define fever. The conversion formula (C versus F) is C/5 = F–32/9.

There is a 'diurnal variation' of body temperature, when temperature is recorded lowest in early morning and reaches maximum between 6 and 10 PM. Remember, ovulation in females increases body temperature by 1°F. Absence of diurnal variation points towards a central source (e.g., encephalitis). Reversal of diurnal pattern can be seen in disseminated tuberculosis, polyarteritis nodosa and salicylate toxicity.

In hypothermia, at 82.4–89.6°F patient becomes drowsy, comatose at 82.4°F and cardiac asystole and death occurs at 68°F. *Hyperthermia* is an increase in body temperature over the body's thermoregulatory set-point, and thus it is not regarded as fever.

Q. What are the different types of fever?

There are basically three types of fever, namely:

A. *Intermittent:* Fever is present only for several hours and **always touches the baseline** sometimes during the day. It is divided into three subtypes:
   1. *Quotidian:* When fever occurs daily i.e., daily rise and daily fall, it is quotidian temperature. The examples are: Malaria (i.e., double infection of *P. vivax*), urinary tract infection (UTI), tuberculosis, septicaemia, pent-up pus anywhere in body (e.g., lung abscess), or amoebic liver abscess.
   2. *Tertian:* When the paroxysm of fever occurs on alternate days (i.e., once in every 48 hours), it is tertian temperature. The examples are: Benign tertian malaria (commonly by *P. vivax* and rarely by *P. ovale*), malignant tertian malaria (*P. falciparum*).
   3. *Quartan:* When two days intervene between two paroxysmal attacks (i.e., once in every 72 hours), it is quartan temperature. The example is quartan malaria (*P. malariae*), which is rare in India.

B. *Continued (continuous or sustained):* Fluctuation of temperature not more than 1°C (1.5°F) during the 24-hours, and it **does not touches the baseline**. The common examples are: Second week of enteric fever, lobar pneumonia, acute rheumatic fever, miliary tuberculosis, meningitis, collagen vascular diseases (e.g., SLE).

C. *Remittent:* Daily fluctuation of fever is more than 2°C (3°F) and it **does not touches the baseline**. The classical examples are: Third week of enteric fever, acute bronchopneumonia, acute tonsillitis, amoebic liver abscess, bacteraemia, pyaemia.

Q. Situations where you cannot record oral temperature?

Recording of oral temperature is avoided in:

- Infants and children
- Mentally dull patients (e.g., low IQ in cretinism or Down's syndrome)
- During severe respiratory distress or mouth breathers
- During repeated convulsions, tetanus or protracted sneezing
- Immediately after taking hot tea or coffee, smoking or chewing tobacco

- Ulcers within the mouth, paralysis of the tongue, Bell's palsy
- Comatose or restless patient.

Q. Enumerate major causes of hyperpyrexia, hypothermia, and fever with chill and rigor.

Hyperpyrexia	*Hypothermia*	*Fever with chill and rigor*
• Cerebral malaria • Encephalitis, meningitis • Septicaemia • Lobar pneumonia • Pontine haemorrhage • Heat stroke • Thyrotoxic crisis • Neuroleptic malignant syndrome • Malignant hyperthermia • Drug-induced (e.g., barbiturates) • Hypothalamic dysfunction	• Myxoedema coma • Prolonged exposure to cold/immersion in cold water (e.g., beggars, mountaineering, with alcohol intoxication) • Hypoglycaemia • Adrenal insufficiency • Near-drowning • Artificial hypothermia (e.g., in open heart surgery) • Autonomic dysfunction • Panhypopituitarism • Peripheral circulatory failure	• Malaria • UTI • Pent-up pus in body (e.g., subdiaphragmatic abscess) • Ascending cholangitis • Thrombophlebitis • Acute pyelonephritis • Septicaemia/pyaemia • SBE • Pyrogen reaction after fluid infusion or blood transfusion • Filariasis

NB: Fever is due to elevated set-point of the thermostat while hyperpyrexia results from inadequate heat dissipation.

Heat-related illnesses are heat cramps, heat syncope, heat exhaustion and heat stroke.

Q. Do you know the mechanism of chill and rigor associated with fever?

In health, normal temperature is maintained by regulating a balance between heat gain and heat loss, governed by the hypothalamus. If the thermostat situated in hypothalamus is suddenly reset to a higher temperature (e.g., due to presence of pyrogen), the patient feels a sensation of cold. When the temperature is rising to a higher level, body tries to conserve heat by cutaneous vasoconstriction and involuntary contraction of skeletal muscles, experienced as **chill**. If the patient **shivers** violently, it is called **rigor**. Many a time, a profound chill with piloerection (goose flesh) is associated with severe shivering, rigor and chattering of the teeth (a classical example is malaria). When the higher temperature is reached, heat loss starts by heat dissipation through dilatation of cutaneous vessels; the patient feels hot and sweating starts (sweating assists heat loss mechanism).

Q. Enumerate causes of 'evening rise' of temperature.

Though, in health, body temperature is increased in the evening, it is not felt by a healthy person. Classically, evening rise of temperature is recorded in (probably, cortisol secretion is decreased in the evening):

- Tuberculosis
- Lymphoma

- Leukaemias
- Autoimmune disease (e.g., rheumatoid arthritis).

Q. Describe hectic temperature and periodic fever.

Hectic temperature: There is a big swing in temperature pattern, which rises with chill and rigor, persists for a few hours and suddenly falls with profuse perspiration. The causes are:

- Pent-up pus anywhere in the body (liver abscess, lung abscess, subdiaphragmatic abscess, empyema thoracis)
- Septicaemia or pyaemia
- Advanced tuberculosis, hypernephroma, lymphoma
- Ascending cholangitis, pyelonephritis, drug reactions
- Periodic fever syndrome (e.g., familial Mediterranean fever).

Periodic fever: Periodic attacks of fever alternating with an afebrile period, and is seen in:

- Relapsing fever (arthropod-borne infection)
- Hodgkin's disease (Pel-Ebstein fever)
- Brucellosis
- Malaria
- Rat bite fever
- Dengue.

Q. What is PUO (pyrexia of unknown origin) or FUO (fever of unknown origin)?

- PUO/FUO is defined as (most recent):
  - Fever lasting for ≥3 weeks
  - Fever >101°F on at least two occasions
  - No cause can be found despite thorough history taking, proper clinical examination and related basic investigations.
- Examples of PUO are infections (tuberculosis, toxoplasmosis, brucellosis, HIV), occult abscess anywhere in the body, collagen vascular diseases (e.g., SLE), carcinoma (e.g., hypernephroma), lymphoma, factitious fever, drug fever.
- PUO is commonly caused by an uncommon presentation of a common disease. Diagnosis rests on intelligent interviewing of the patient, 'repeated' physical examination and specific investigations. Hidden and deeper sites like retroperitoneum, subdiaphragm, sinus, teeth (Fig. 2.101), prosthesis, prostate, kidney, ovary and spleen should be looked for meticulously.

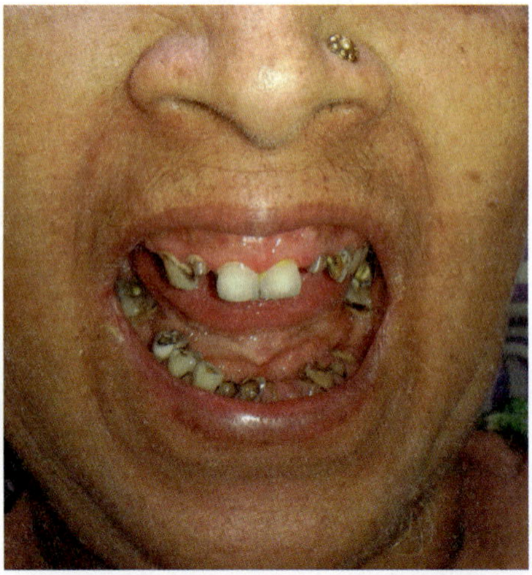

Fig. 2.101: Unhealthy teeth—a source of many diseases

- PUO in India or in any developing country are commonly due to tuberculosis, enteric fever, amoebic liver abscess, malaria, kala-azar, filariasis, brucellosis and AIDS.
- Known immunocompromised states have been excluded from PUO in recent classification.

Q. Common causes of fever.

Fever is due to:

1. Different infections (e.g., tuberculosis, staphylococcal infection)
2. Non-infective causes
   - Autoimmune diseases (e.g., SLE, rheumatoid arthritis, vasculitis)
   - Autoinflammatory disorders (e.g., familial Mediterranean fever)
3. Malignant conditions (e.g., hypernephroma)
4. *Miscellaneous:* Drug fever (e.g., rifampicin), factitious fever, habitual hyperthermia
5. Undiagnosed fever (in spite of repeated and judicious investigations, the aetiology is not revealed).

Q. Can fever occur without infection?

Yes, *aseptic fever* (i.e., no role of antibiotics) is due to:

1. Collagen vascular diseases e.g., SLE
2. Pontine haemorrhage
3. Heat stroke
4. Lymphomas, leukaemias, disseminated malignancy
5. Thyroid storm (i.e., thyrotoxic crisis)
6. Drug fever e.g., rifampicin-induced
7. Acute myocardial infarction (AMI)
8. Gout
9. Crush injury
10. Radiation sickness.

Q. How remission of a fever occurs?

Most of the raised temperature falls by lysis, while antipyretics (e.g., paracetamol) may precipitate fall by crisis.

- *Fall by 'crisis':* Here, the elevated temperature falls to normal or subnormal level very quickly within 6–12 hours and is associated with severe sweating, which is commonly seen in acute lobar pneumonia, enteric fever complicated by perforation or haemorrhage, septicaemia and adrenal crisis.
- *Fall by 'lysis':* Here, the temperature falls gradually in steps over several days, and is commonly seen in uncomplicated enteric fever, acute rheumatic fever and acute bronchopneumonia.

Q. What is factitious fever?

Patients occasionally purposefully show false elevation of temperature, which are often self-induced like falsely registering higher temperature (e.g., by immersing the thermometer in hot water), or ingesting thyroxine tablets. Usually, they are young women, many a time attached to health sectors. The puzzled diagnosis is reached by:

- History of (H/o) personality disorder
- Dissociation between pulse and temperature; records very high temperature (e.g., 106°F)
- Absence of chills, sweating, tachycardia, or even tachypnoea
- Absence of normal diurnal variation in temperature.

Q. Signs and symptoms associated with pyrexia or fever.

- *Constitutional symptoms:* Headache (due to vasodilatation), anorexia, lassitude, myalgia, constipation, shivering, chill and rigor, furring of tongue, outbreak of miliaria, sudaminal rash (sweat-retention rash) in body in high fever, herpes labialis ('fever blisters') (Fig. 2.102), rash of exanthematous fever (e.g., measles), febrile convulsions (children in the age group of 6 months to 5 years), confusion and/or delirium.
- *Signs:* Fever, flushing of face, tachycardia or relative bradycardia, tachypnoea, dehydration.

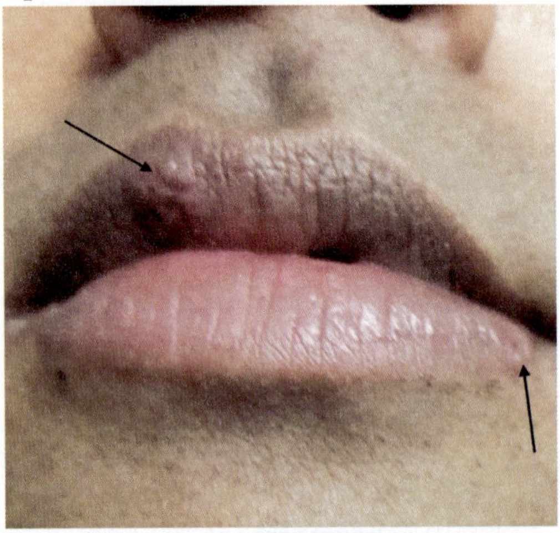

Fig. 2.102: Herpes simplex infection in lips after viral fever (known as 'herpes labialis' of 'fever blisters')

Q. Do you know these different types of fever?

- Step-ladder pattern pyrexia (temperature of today exceeds that of previous day): Enteric fever.
- Double quotidian fever (or 'camel hump fever' or 'rabbit-ear pattern' pyrexia, where there is double fever spikes in a single day): Kala-azar (classical example), gonococcal perihepatitis.
- Saddle-back pyrexia (pyrexia continues from 1 to 10 days where there is a fall of temperature for 2 to 3 days in the middle): Dengue.
- Pel-Ebstein temperature (days or weeks of fever alternates with afebrile period for few days): Hodgkin's disease (classical), brucellosis and hypernephroma.
- Black water fever (intravascular haemolysis and haemoglobinuria from *P. falciparum* infection, turning urine dark reddish in nature along with renal failure): Malaria.
- Black fever (skin turns black due to hyperpigmentation, especially of the face): Kala-azar.

Q. Clinical clues in solving the diagnosis of fever.

1. *Toxic look:* high pyrexia, enteric fever, typhus (Fig. 2.103), septicaemia.
2. *Marked sweating:* Septicaemia (Fig. 2.104), rheumatic fever, amoebic liver abscess.
3. *Petechiae or purpuric eruptions:* Acute leukaemias, meningococcaemia, Rocky Mountain spotted fever, septicaemia.

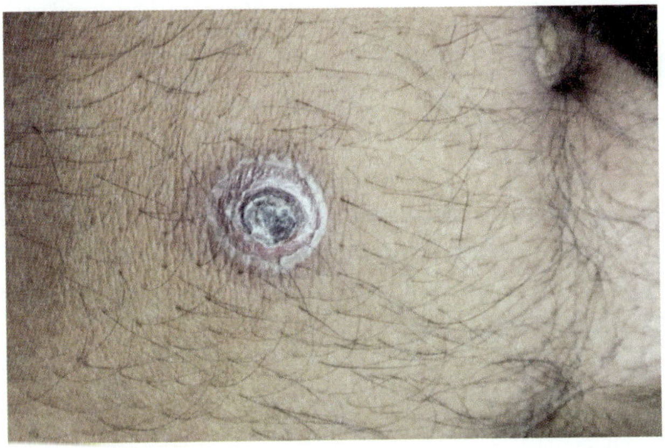

Fig. 2.103: Typical eschar formation in scrub typhus which is a valuable bedside clue to the diagnosis

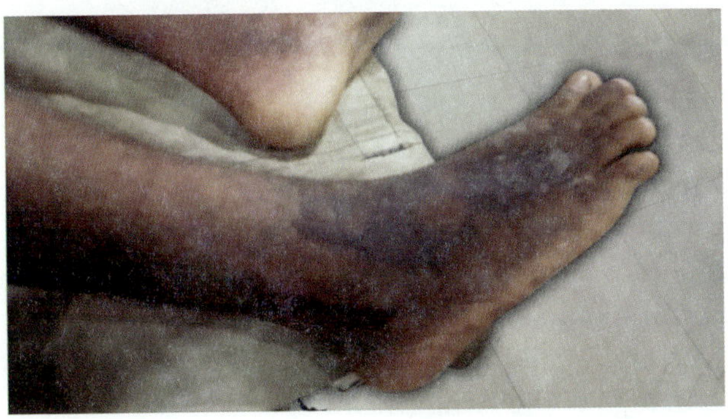

Fig. 2.104: Big ecchymosis in septicaemia

4. *Severe myalgia:* Influenza, dengue, chikungunya, leptospirosis, or any viral illness.
5. *Lymphadenopathy:* Tuberculosis, lymphoma, leukaemia, secondary syphilis, SLE, AIDS.
6. *Hepatosplenomegaly:* Malaria, kala-azar, miliary tuberculosis, SLE, leukaemias or lymphomas, Still's disease, brucellosis.
7. *Convulsions:* Febile (in children), meningoencephalitis, tuberculoma, cerebral abscess.
8. *Pustular lesions in skin:* Gonococcaemia, staphylococcal sepsis.
9. *Scalp tenderness or jaw claudication:* Giant cell arteritis (or, temporal arteritis).
10. *Choroidal tubercle on fundoscopy:* Miliary tuberculosis.

Q. Common 'factors' responsible for development of fever.

1. Infection (bacteria, virus, fungus)
2. Immune-mediated (e.g., SLE)
3. Tissue necrosis (AMI)
4. Malignancy (hypernephroma, lymphoma)
5. Drug fever (may have eosinophilia) e.g., sulphonamides, iodides/bromides, rifampicin ('flu syndrome'), barbiturates, penicillin, ecstasy (recreational drug), phenytoin.

6. Neurological disorders (pontine haemorrhage, hypothalamic dysfunction)
7. Factitious fever.

Q. Should you treat all kinds if fever?

Fever has some beneficial effects in the body. It increases the bactericidal and phagocytic activity of neutrophils; cytotoxic effects of lymphocytes are also increased. So, always think before initiating the treatment of fever. However, the following conditions associated with fever should always be treated as soon as possible e.g.,

- In infants and children
- In pregnant women
- With co-morbidities like diabetes mellitus, hepatic or renal dysfunction
- Prolonged fever for >7 days
- High rise of temperature (e.g., >102° F).

ANY OBVIOUS DEFORMITY OR OUTSTANDING FEATURES

Q. Points to be noted.

Be careful to note these points:

- Halitosis (pyorrhoea alveolaris, bronchiectasis, hepatic encephalopathy)
- Shaking hands (static tremor in parkinsonism)
- Continuous crying (i.e., from pain anywhere in body, fear, or emotional upset)
- Instability on standing (ataxia)
- Asymmetry in face while talking or smiling (Bell's palsy)
- Sudden bending of legs while lying (flexor spasm in a paraplegie patient)
- Restlessness (akathisia in thyrotoxicosis)
- Head nodding (tics, mental retardation, cerebellar disorder, parkinsonism)
- Deformity of skull (macrocephaly in hydrocephalus, or microcephaly in cerebral palsy), or severe kyphoscoliosis
- Semi-purposive, rapid, jerky movements of upper limb (chorea)
- Breathlessness (e.g., pleural effusion, pneumothorax, pericardial effusion, pulmonary hypertension, huge ascites or hysteria)
- Squatting (indicating cyanotic congenital heart diseases)
- Wheezing (smaller airways obstruction e.g., bronchial asthma)
- Huge swelling of abdomen (ascites)
- Stooped posture (parkinsonism, ankylosing spondylitis, osteoporosis of spine with vertebral collapse).

GENERAL OBSERVATION: ANY ACUTE DISTRESS PRESENT OR NOT

Q. Points to be taken care of.

Following acute conditions should be taken care of immediately:

- Breathlessness
- Acute chest pain

- Ongoing haematemesis, haemoptysis, haematuria, haematochezia, melaena, epistaxis or bleeding from any part of the body
- Acute abdominal pain
- Incessant vomiting, continuous hiccough
- High rise of temperature with or without rigor
- Severe headache
- Convulsions
- Delirious (with acutely disturbed state of mind and shouting relentlessly)
- Psychosis (e.g., with abnormal behaviour)
- Blue tongue and periphery (e.g., central cyanosis)
- Functional overlay (e.g., hysterical personality).

NB: A proper history cannot be elicited in comatose, drowsy, dysphasic, deaf, delirious, psychotic, severely dementic, or mentally retarded patient. In this setting, history should be obtained from the relatives or accompanying persons.

HANDEDNESS WITH LEVEL OF INTELLIGENCE

Handedness of a person is important to localise their 'speech area'. In general, 90–95% people are right-handed and their speech area is located in the left cerebral hemisphere. Moreover, in left-handed and ambidextrous persons (who use right and left hand equally well) too, the left hemisphere is the dominant one. The speech areas are distributed in motor or Broca's area (area 44 and 45), and sensory or Wernicke's area (area 22) in the dominant hemisphere.

So, a person with left-sided cerebral haemorrhage or infarction (i.e., CVA) will have right-sided hemiplegia *with* dysphasia or aphasia. While a person with right-sided cerebral haemorrhage or infarction will have left-sided hemiplegia but *may not* suffer from dysphasia or aphasia.

Intelligence is a total assessment of judgement, reasoning, arithmetic ability, abstract thinking, attention, insight, etc. During communication with the patient, you can have a rough idea about the intelligence of the patient. Try to get an idea about the IQ (intelligence quotient) of the patient, which is: Mental age/chronological age, multiplied by 100. Mini-mental state examination (MMSE) in neurology assesses intelligence in a better way.

BREAST, HYDRATION AND BONY TENDERNESS

A. ***Breast:*** It is a part of routine clinical examination, especially during examination of the chest and respiratory system. Male doctor must call a female attendant, and will examine the female breast giving dignity to the patient's self-respect and sensitivity. Ask her to undress up to the waist and sit upright on a stool.

- *Ask her to hang the arms relaxed by the sides:* Observe the size, symmetry, contour and colour of the breast; look for peau d'orange (orange peel skin) colour and texture of the skin commonly found in breast carcinoma (Fig. 2.105). Look for any asymmetry or inversion (especially of recent origin) of the nipple, or retraction of the areola; nipple should be examined by index finger and thumb, while the colour and consistency of the discharge from the nipple is noted, if there is any. Dimpling on overlying skin should be noted.

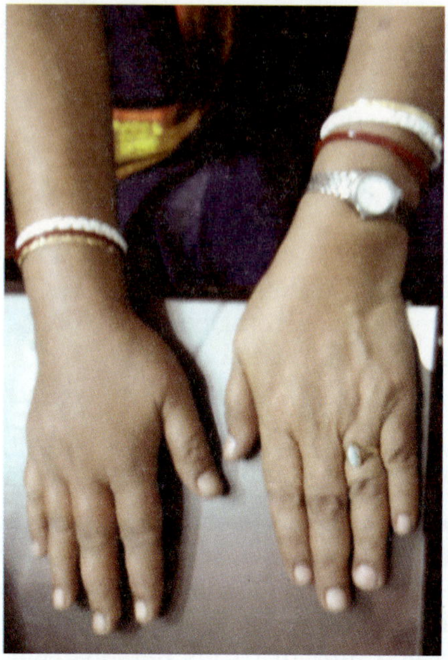

Fig. 2.105: Early swelling of right hand due to lymphoedema from right-sided breast carcinoma

- *Ask her to raise her arms above her head:* It may reveal very minor contour abnormality.
  Ask her to lie supine and to rest one arm above her head: Now examine all the four quadrants of relaxed and widespread breast tissue with holding your hand flat over the breast tissue, especially using the pads of your middle three fingers. In a larger breast, other hand of yours may support the breast tissue during examination. Compare the texture of one breast with the other one. Palpate all quadrants very meticulously and systematically in the search of a nodule (note the size, shape, consistency, mobility, tenderness, or any tethering or ulceration present on the overlying skin) or tumour; use rotatory movements of your hands with compression of the breast tissue on the chest wall. Palpate the axillary tail present in the upper outer quadrant, and the areola.
  Normal breast tissue is variable in feel ranging from smooth to granular.
- *Now ask her to press her hands against her hips:* Again examine the nodule or lump for mobility; it will be less mobile, if attached to pectoral muscles. Assess the fixity of skin overlying the lump.
- According to some clinical surgeons, *inspection* of the breast is done in a standing patient adopting the following position by: (a) hands resting on thighs, (b) hands pressed on to hips, (c) both the arms rest above head, and (d) leaning forward while the breasts become pendulous. *Palpation* of one-sided breast is better done on a supine patient with her head on a pillow and her hand placed under her head on the side of examination.
- Male breast is also examined for gynaecomastia or for any tumour (rare). Lipomastia (no breast tissue, only fat deposition due to obesity) (Fig. 2.106) is better palpated by flat of the hand while gynaecomastia is best appreciated by fingers.

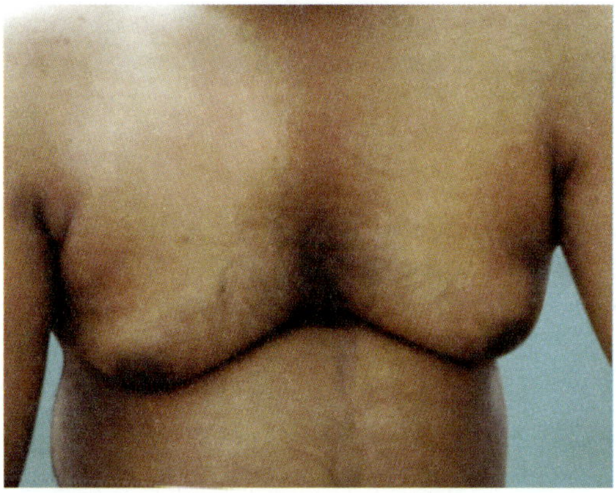

Fig. 2.106: Lipomastia mimics gynaecomastia

B. ***Hydration:*** To assess the **hydration status**, look for the following sites and facts. *Signs of dehydration* are dry tongue, shrunken eyes, loss of skin turgor, presence of postural hypotension, low intraocular tension (i.e., soft eyeballs), low jugular venous pressure in supine position of the patient, and oliguria. Facies in dehydration (facies Hippocraticus) has been described in the section of 'Facies'.

   Some pathological conditions may cause *overhydration*, which need early diagnosis like congestive cardiac failure (CCF), nephrotic syndrome, chronic renal failure, cirrhosis of liver, uncontrolled diabetes mellitus and as a side effect of NSAID (non-steroidal anti-inflammatory drug) use.

C. ***Bony tenderness:*** It may be present in primary malignancy of bone, metastases in bone, infection (osteomyelitis), trauma, osteomalacia, multiple myeloma, leukaemias (acute leukaemias and chronic myeloid leukaemia), osteoporosis, or in overuse.

   Bony tenderness may be tested over sternum (the so-called *sternal tenderness* is elicited by pressing the ball of the thumb over the upper part of the body of sternum for 2–3 seconds, when the patient winces with pain if it is present), pelvic bones, ribs, upper part of shin bone, spine (i.e. vertebrae), and frontal bone.

HAND EXAMINATION IN CLINICAL MEDICINE

Q. Hand examination in systemic diseases.

Handshake with the patient may clinch some clinical diagnosis:

- Warm and moist hand—thyrotoxicosis, type II respiratory failure
- Cold and moist hand—anxiety neurosis
- Cold and dry hand—myxoedema
- Cold and clammy hand—shock (may be with peripheral cyanosis)
- Patient not releasing (slow relaxation) examiner's hand—myotonia
- Painful shaking hand—rheumatoid arthritis, hand injury, gout.

Others:

- Palmar erythema—cirrhosis of liver, chronic alcoholics, thyrotoxicosis, pregnancy, high pyrexia.

- Colour changes (in palm)—yellow in jaundice, pale in anaemia (especially palmar creases), orange-yellow in carotenaemia, blue in cyanosis (especially tips of fingers and nail-beds), or triphasic colour response in Raynaud's phenomenon (e.g., scleroderma).
- Clubbing—vide the section on 'Clubbing'.
- Both clubbing and cyanosis—cyanotic congenital heart disease, fibrosing alveolitis, bilateral extensive bronchiectasis, cystic fibrosis.
- Wasting of small muscles of hand—leprosy (Fig. 2.107), motor neuron disease (MND), syringomyelia, long-continued rheumatoid arthritis.
- Capillary pulsation and digital artery pulsations—aortic iregurgitation, hyperkinetic circulatory states (severe anaemia, thyrotoxicosis).
- Tremor—different types like static, action, intention, or flapping tremor.
- Swellings—Osler's node (e.g., SBE), Heberden's and Bouchard's node over dorsal aspect of distal interphalangeal (DIP) and proximal interphalangeal (PIP) joints respectively in osteoarthritis, gouty tophi or calcinosis (e.g., scleroderma), Gottron's papules (lilac-coloured papules over knuckles seen in dermatomyositis); oedema over dorsum of hands is seen after IV drip inserted over veins in dorsum of hand, or as a part of anasarca; a large finger may be due to local arteriovenous malformations (Fig. 2.108).

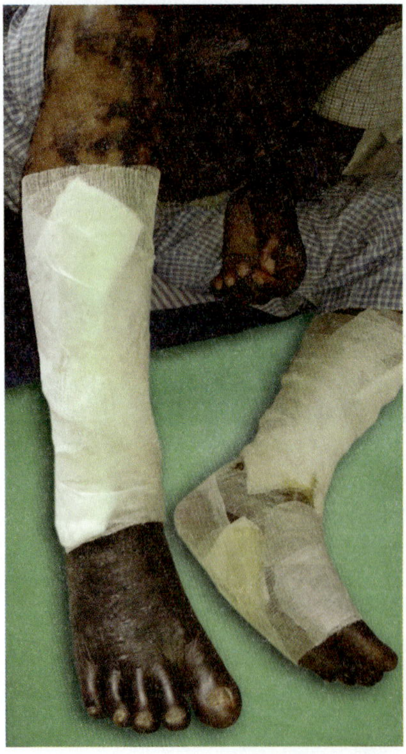

Fig. 2.107: Lepromatous leprosy (Hansen's disease) with ulcers (dressed) affecting lower limbs along with wasting of small muscles of hands

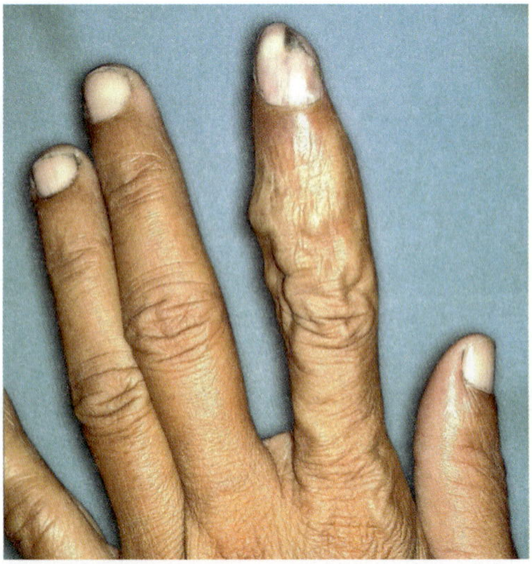

Fig. 2.108: Swelling of the left index finger due to arteriovenous malformations

- Deformities—they are swan-neck deformity, button-hole deformity or Z-deformity of thumbs are common in rheumatoid arthritis (Fig. 2.109), Dupuytren's contracture (painless flexion contracture of ring and little fingers may be due to alcoholic cirrhosis, diabetes, repeated trauma to palm or after phenytoin therapy) (Fig. 2.110), carpopedal spasm in tetany, short 4th metacarpal bone in pseudohypoparathyroidism and Turner's syndrome, polydactyly in Laurence-Moon-Biedl syndrome, fingerisation of thumb in Holt-Oram syndrome, arachnodactyly (long slender fingers) in Marfan's syndrome, sclerodactyly in scleroderma (Fig. 2.111), syndactyly (two or more fingers are fused together) in Apert syndrome, clinodactyly (incurved little finger) in Down's syndrome, and spade-shaped hand in acromegaly. Arteriovenous malformations may give rise to a larger hand than the normal side (Fig. 2.112).
- Claw hand—in claw hand, the martacarpophalangeal (MCP) joints are hyperextended, and PIP and DIP joints are flexed due to T_1 segment lesion or lesion

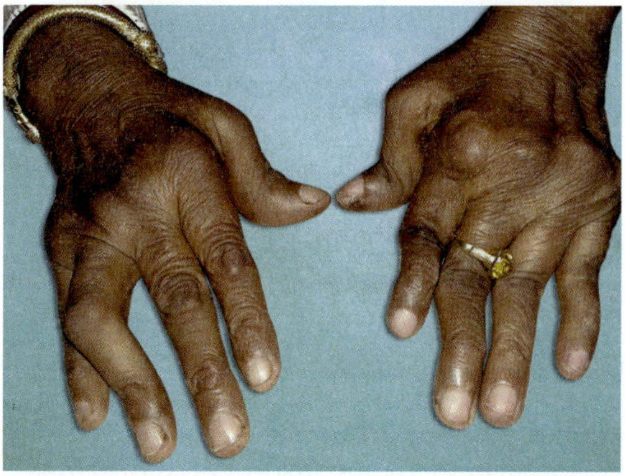

Fig. 2.109: Devastating deformities in hands—swan-neck deformity (lateral four fingers in left hand), button-hole deformity (right ring finger) and Z-deformity of both thumbs are evident

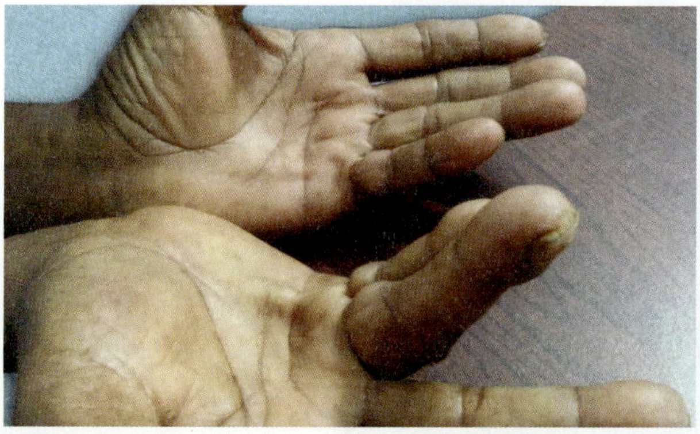

Fig. 2.110: Dupuytren's contracture in an alcoholic cirrhosis—the linear cord-like tissue (here, seen in right ring and left little finger) in palm contracts the fingers permanently

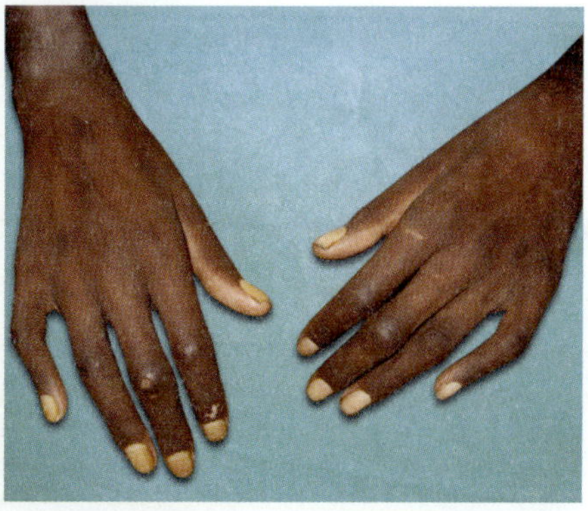

Fig. 2.111: Hands in scleroderma—skin over the fingers are taut (sclerodactyly) and thereby producing some deformity

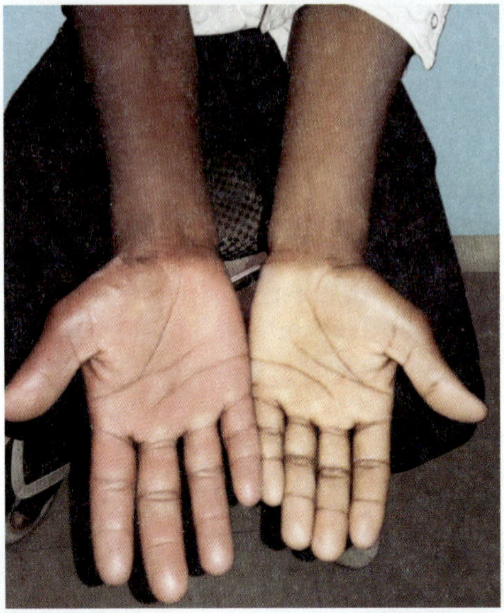

Fig. 2.112: A bit larger and reddish right hand due to local arteriovenous malformations

in both ulnar and median nerve. It is commonly seen in leprosy, MND, thoracic inlet syndrome, syringomyelia or cervical rib.

- Nail changes—vide the section on 'Skin, hairs and nails'.
- Pigmentary changes—vide the section on 'Skin, hairs and nails'.
- Miscellaneous—pulp atrophy, nail-fold thrombi, digital infarction/ulceration/ gangrene are features of vasculitis, e.g., in SLE, or scleroderma (Fig. 2.113), single palmar crease in Down's syndrome, nicotine staining in right index and middle finger in chronic smoker, palmar xanthoma in familial hyperlipidaemia, petechiae/ purpura/ecchymosis in haemorrhagic disorders, wrist drop in radial nerve palsy, or itchy drug rash over dorsum of hands.

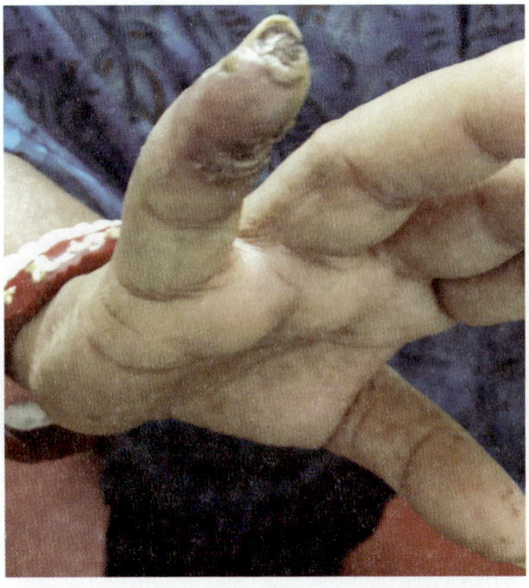

Fig. 2.113: Digital ulceration in scleroderma

Chapter

3

Systemic Examination

The present scenario: where do you stand?

- As of now, you are a bit knowledgeable and realised that what clinical medicine is!
- **Putting it all together:** Add the symptoms taken from 'history' with the clinical findings of 'general survey' to build-up an overall idea of the disease
- Take help of your teachers who are the ultimate saviour of the mass
- Match the outcome of clinical classes with the 'theory' classes going on simultaneously
- Maintain the habit of going medical wards everyday, what you have to develop from your initial days of training
- Now, proceed for different 'systemic examination' with the help of scheme of examination for respective system like:
  - Cardiovascular system (CVS)
  - Respiratory system
  - Gastrointestinal (GI) and hepatobiliary system
  - Genitourinary system
  - Nervous system
  - Endocrine system
  - Haemopoietic (lymphoreticular) system
  - Musculoskeletal (locomotor) system
  - *Others:* Dermatology, psychiatry, geriatric medicine, etc.

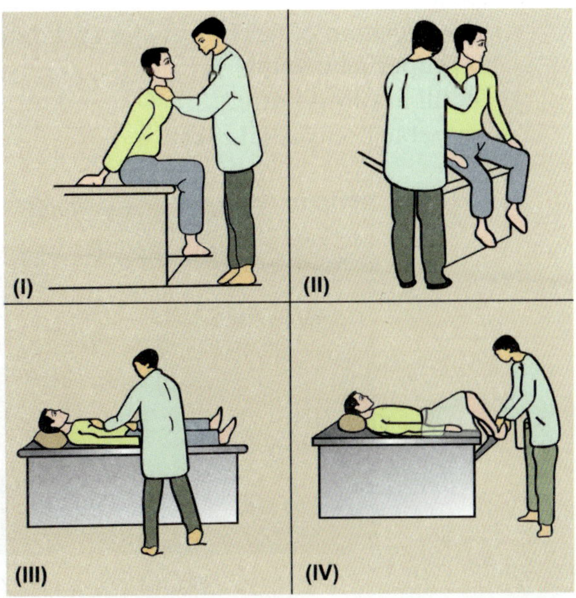

Chapter

4

Cardiovascular System

SCHEME OF SYSTEMIC EXAMINATION: AN OVERVIEW

I. *Examination of:* Pulse, blood pressure (BP), neck veins.

II. *Inspection:*

- Shape of precordium
- Position of apical impulse
- Pulsation
  - Over precordium (aortic, pulmonary, mitral, parasternal areas)
  - Neck (carotid pulsation), epigastrium
  - Suprasternal area, supraclavicular area, locomotor brachialis
- *Skin:* Engorged superficial veins, scar mark (e.g., for previous cardiac operation—Fig. 4.1), sinus, polythelia (additional nipple)
- Back (kyphoscoliosis, arterial or venous pulsations, skin condition).

III. *Palpation:*

- Appreciation of arterial pulses and determination of direction of venous flow (in superficial veins)
- Thrill in carotid artery
- Palpable pericardial rub

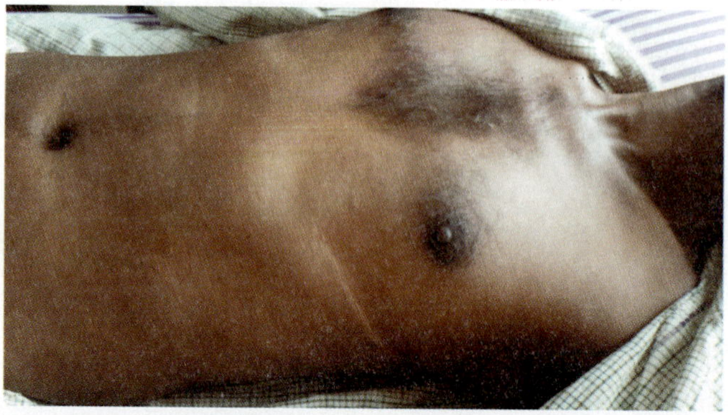

Fig. 4.1: Mitral valvotomy scar

- Mitral area: Apex beat (site and character), palpable heart sound (M_1), thrill
- Pulmonary area: Pulsation, palpable heart sound (P_2), thrill
- Aortic area: Pulsation, palpable heart sound (A_2), thrill
- Tricuspid area: Left parasternal heave, palpable heart sound (T_1), thrill.

IV. *Percussion:* Not done routinely (done in relevant cases like pericardial effusion, huge cardiomegaly, or aneurysm of the arch of aorta).

V. *Auscultation:*

- Cardiac rate (i.e., heart rate) and rhythm
- Mitral area: Heart sounds, murmur (in details), opening snap, ejection click, pericardial knock
- Pulmonary area: Similar to mitral area
- Aortic area: Similar to mitral area
- Tricuspid area: Similar to mitral area
- Neoaortic area (or, aortic II area): Similar to mitral area
- Auscultation for pericardial rub and over carotid arteries (i.e., for carotid bruit).

NB: *Left parasternal heave* is palpated by ulnar border of right hand placed in the lower left parasternum (Fig. 4.2). It denotes right ventricular hypertrophy (see below).

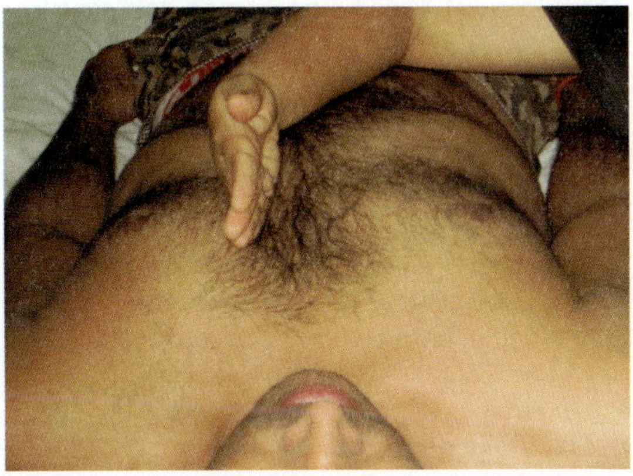

Fig. 4.2: Demonstration of left parasternal heave using ulnar border of right hand

Q. Mention the common presentations (chief complaints and H/o present illness) in cardiovascular system (CVS).

The patients having complaints of CVS commonly present with:

1. Chest pain (angina pectoris, acute myocardial infarction (AMI), pericarditis or aortic dissection).
2. Breathlessness (dyspnoea, orthopnoea, paroxysmal nocturnal dyspnoea or PND).
3. Palpitations (atrial fibrillation, paroxysmal tachyarrhythmias).
4. Recurrent respiratory tract infections (e.g., cough and expectoration).
5. Haemoptysis (i.e., 'expectoration of blood', seen in mitral stenosis or MS).
6. Syncope (aortic stenosis or AS, hypotension).
7. Swelling of feet or oedema, or facial puffiness (congestive cardiac failure or CCF).

8. Fatigue (whether present on exertion or not; seen in AS and β-blocker therapy. Fatigue is common in low output states like aortic stenosis (AS), tight MS or ischaemic heart disease (IHD).
9. Systemic hypertension (C/o occipital headache or symptoms related to target organ damage, e.g., oliguria in loss of renal function).
10. *Others:*
    a. Fever [subacute bacterial endocarditis (SBE), rheumatic activity, pericarditis, deep vein thrombosis or DVT, atrial myxoma, Dressler's syndrome].
    b. H/o squatting or cyanotic spells (indicating cyanotic congenital heart diseases like Fallot's tetralogy).
    c. Loss of appetite (from CCF), vomiting (digitalis toxicity) or loss of weight (cardiac cachexia).
    d. Fleeting joint pain (i.e., arthritis), subcutaneous nodules, erythema marginatum (i.e., markers of rheumatic fever).
    e. Convulsions or past H/o neurodeficit (i.e., paralysis)—MS with atrial fibrillation having a large clot in the left atrium may give rise to stroke.
    f. Pallor, pyrexia, Osler's node, Janeway's lesions, splinter haemorrhage, clubbing, Roth's spots in retina, and splenomegaly (i.e., markers of infective endocarditis).

Q. Describe points asked in past, family, personal and treatment history in CVS.

Past history	*Family history*	*Personal history*	*Treatment history*
1. Rheumatic fever 2. Recurrent respiratory tract infections 3. Cyanotic spells with H/o squatting 4. History suggestive of CCF 5. Hypertension, diabetes, IHD 6. Thyrotoxicosis	1. Hypertension, diabetes, dyslipid-aemia, obesity 2. Rheumatic or congenital heart disease, IHD 3. Whether born out of consanguineous marriage 4. H/o sudden cardiac death in the family	1. Smoking 2. Alcohol intake 3. Tobacco chewing 4. Drug addictions (especially, by IV route) 5. Occupation 6. Exercise 7. Diet	1. β-blockers (may aggravate heart block) 2. Antihypertensives (amlodipine may produce pedal oedema) 3. Thyroxine (increases angina) 4. Diuretics (may abolish gallop rhythm) 5. Oral contraceptives and corticosteroid (may increase BP)

Q. How to deliver a diagnosis in valvular heart diseases?

- *Anatomical:* Mitral, aortic, tricuspid, pulmonary
- *Structural:* Stenosis, regurgitation (or incompetence)
- *Aetiological:* Rheumatic, congenital, collagen vascular diseases
- *Complications:* Pulmonary hypertension, CCF, SBE
- *Rhythm:* Sinus rhythm or dysrhythmia (e.g., irregularly irregular pulse from atrial fibrillation)
- *Functional disability:* Mention the grading of dyspnoea according to New York Heart Association (NYHA) classification (see below).

Q. Some terminology you should know at the beginning.

- What is your diagnosis?
  Give the provisional diagnosis e.g., it is a case of aortic regurgitation (incompetence) of rheumatic origin without any evidence of congestive cardiac failure and the patient is in sinus rhythm at present with Grade II disability according to New York Heart Association (NYHA) classification.
- What is your case?
  Describe the summary of the case directly.
- Can you discuss over your diagnosis (also known as 'clinical reasoning')?
  Deliver the information gathered from history and relevant clinical features (physical findings), and discuss how you have arrived the diagnosis.
- What is differential diagnosis (D/D)?
  Those are different diseases mimicking the present diagnosis (e.g., murmur of mitral incompetence or MI can be mimicked by ventricular septal defect or VSD).

NB: Try to avoid abbreviations like CCF, rather say congestive cardiac failure.

Q. What are the common CVS diseases?

They are:

- Rheumatic (i.e., acute rheumatic fever): Valvular heart diseases
- Ischaemic heart disease (e.g., from atherosclerosis): Coronary artery diseases
- Hypertensive heart disease (LVH/LVF from hypertension)
- Thyrotoxic heart disease (atrial fibrillation from thyrotoxicosis)
- Cardiomyopathy (disorder of cardiac muscles), myocarditis, pericarditis
- Infective endocarditis
- Cardiac arrhythmias (e.g., atrial fibrillation)
- Pulmonary heart disease (i.e., cor pulmonale) e.g., pulmonary hypertension from chronic obstructive pulmonary disease (COPD) or pulmonary thromboembolism
- Congenital heart disease (acyanotic like bicuspid aortic valve, or cyanotic like Fallot's tetralogy)
- Peripheral vascular disease (e.g., limb ischaemia, aneurysmal disorder).

Q. How valvular heart diseases develop?

Initially, the patient gets sore throat from Group A β-haemolytic streptococci at the age of 5–15 years. The susceptible patient develops *acute rheumatic fever* after 2–4 weeks; with proper treatment, majority of the patients recover but without proper penicillin prophylaxis for a certain period, the affected person may develop organic valvular heart disease (e.g., MS, MI, AS, AI, etc.). If a patient develops acute rheumatic carditis (valvulitis) from acute rheumatic fever at the onset, he/she is more prone to get affected by organic valvular heart disease within a couple of years.

In India, the patients may suffer from organic heart disease by 12–13 years (i.e., MS occurs very early), while in temperate climates the patient develops the same around 20 years of age.

Rheumatic heart disease commonly affects left side of the heart than right side, and that is why mitral and aortic valves are more involved than tricuspid and pulmonary valves. Each valve may be stenosed or incompetent, and thus commonly left-sided valvular heart diseases are encountered with valvular stenosis or incompetence in the community (i.e., MS and MI from mitral valve, and AS and AI from aortic valve involvement. One must be clinically acquainted with every bit of these 4 valvular heart diseases); TS and TI from tricuspid valve, and PS and PI from pulmonary valve involvement (i.e., affection of right side of the heart) from acute rheumatic fever are rare.

Valvular heart diseases are diagnosed clinically and confirmed by echocardiography.

Q. What are the different positions of the heart?

- *Levocardia:* Cardiac apex on the left side
- *Mesocardia:* Cardiac apex on the centre of chest
- *Dextrocardia:* Cardiac apex on the right side of chest

*Dextroversion: Always acquired. Cardiac apex is on the right side due to extracardiac cause like left-sided pleural effusion/pneumothorax, or right-sided fibrosis/collapse of the lung. The trachea is shifted to right side too, while trachea remains central in dextrocardia.

**Situs inversus: Like the rotation of heart (e.g., dextrocardia), here abdominal or thoracic organs rotate to opposite side.

Q. How do you diagnose acute rheumatic fever?

It is diagnosed by revised Jones criteria. The presence of two or more major manifestations, or one major and two or more minor manifestations strongly suggest acute rheumatic fever if associated with one of the supporting evidence of preceding streptococcal infection like recent scarlet fever, raised ASO (antistreptolysin O) or other streptococcal antibodies titre, or positive throat culture.

Major criteria	*Minor criteria*
• Carditis	• Fever
• Polyarthritis	• Arthralgia
• Chorea	• Previous rheumatic fever
• Erythema marginatum	• High erythrocyte sedimentation rate (ESR) or C-reactive protein (CRP)
• Subcutaneous nodules (Fig. 4.3)	• Leucocytosis
	• Increased PR interval in electrocardiography (ECG)

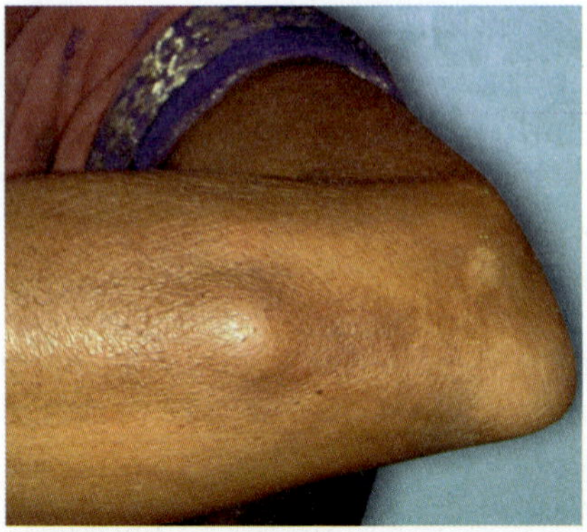

Fig. 4.3: Subcutaneous nodule along ulnar surface of forearm in acute rheumatic fever

Q. Do you know different causes of acute chest pain?

Acute chest pain may be of two types: Central and peripheral.

Central (retrosternal or behind the sternum):

- Cardiac: Angina pectoris, AMI, pericarditis
- Aortic: Dissecting aneurysm of aorta
- Pulmonary or mediastinal: Mediastinitis, pulmonary thromboembolism, acute tracheobronchitis
- Oesophageal: Diffuse oesophageal spasm, gastro-oesophageal reflux disease (GERD), oesophagitis
- Others: Musculoskeletal pain (e.g., osteoarthritis, trauma), anxiety neurosis.

Peripheral:

- Lung and pleura: Spontaneous pneumothorax, pleurisy, pulmonary thrombo-embolism
- Chest wall disorders: Myositis, fibrositis, trauma, rib fracture, intercostal myalgia (Bornholm disease), costochondritis (Tietze's syndrome), secondary deposits in ribs, osteomalacia, herpes zoster on the chest wall
- Anxiety neurosis.

NB: Abdominal disorders like hiatal hernia, acute pancreatitis, acute cholecystitis or perforated peptic ulcer may refer pain to the chest, which may be retrosternal (on the other hand, pain of AMI or basal pneumonia in the chest may refer to the abdomen.)

Sudden and severe chest pain may result from dissecting aortic aneurysm, tension pneumothorax, AMI and pulmonary thromboembolism.

Q. Describe chest pain of angina pectoris and acute myocardial infarction (AMI).

Coronary artery disease (CAD) or ischaemic heart disease (IHD) is commonly manifested as angina pectoris and acute myocardial infarction (AMI).

- Angina (ischaemic cardiac chest pain, which is commonly due to coronary atherosclerosis resulting in fixed stenosis)—retrosternal, constricting or chocking in nature (like a band around chest), typically radiates to the left upper extremity/ lower jaw/neck/back, commonly exertional, persists for 2–5 minutes (usually <10 minutes), relieved by rest or sublingual nitrates/nitroglycerine; may be associated with palpitation.
- AMI (acute ischaemic necrosis of an area of myocardium due to acute occlusion of a coronary artery resulting from plaque rupture and thrombosis)—the chest pain of AMI is more severe than angina (may be associated with shortness of breath), lasts longer (>20 minutes), evokes spontaneously, persists at rest, radiates like angina, not relieved by rest or nitrates/nitroglycerine, and is very often associated with nausea, vomiting, palpitation, pallor and profuse sweating.

NB: Angina pectoris is commonly of four types: Stable angina (described above), unstable angina (chest pain occurs at rest, or with exertion or stress), Prinzmetal's angina (vasospastic angina or variant angina), and nocturnal or decubitus angina (read 'Decubitus' in the section on 'general examination').

Q. Enumerate the 'risk factors' for coronary artery disease (CAD).

The recognised risk factors are:

- *Fixed*
  - Age
  - Male sex
  - Positive family history
- *Potentially changeable*
  - Smoking
  - Systemic hypertension
  - Diabetes mellitus
  - Hyperlipidaemia
  - Obesity
  - Homocysteinaemia
  - Sedentary lifestyle
  - *Others:* Elevated C-reactive protein (CRP), gout, drugs like oral contraceptive pills or rosiglitazone, excess alcohol consumption, high fibrinogen level.

Q. Physical stigmata and management of coronary artery disease (CAD)—an outline.

A. Physical stigmata of CAD:
- Xanthelasma (Fig. 4.4)
- Arcus senilis (Fig. 4.5)

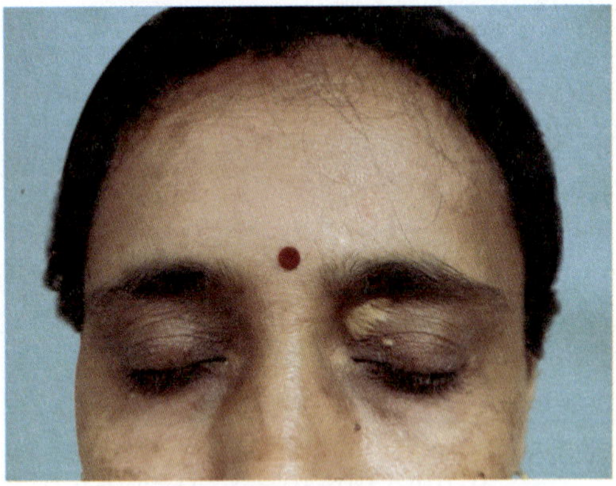

Fig. 4.4: Onset of xanthelasma

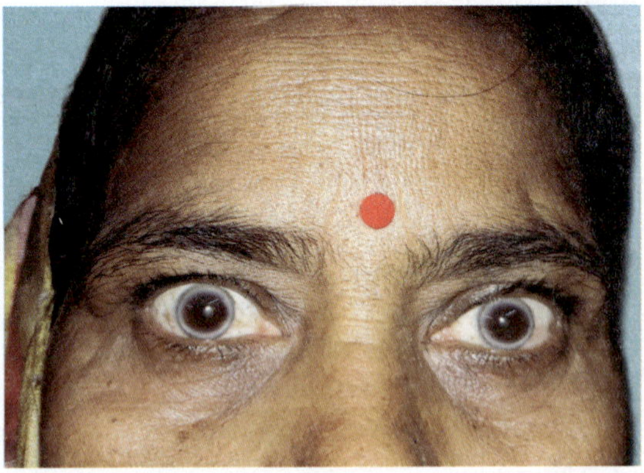

Fig. 4.5: Arcus senilis (with early cataract)—circular ring around cornea, commonly seen in older people due to deposition of phospholipid and cholesterol in corneal tissue

- Obesity
- Nicotine staining in fingers
- Diagonal ear lobe crease (Fig. 4.6)

B. Secondary prevention (Mnemonics: ABCDE)
- A: Aspirin and anti-anginal therapy
- B: Beta-blocker and BP control

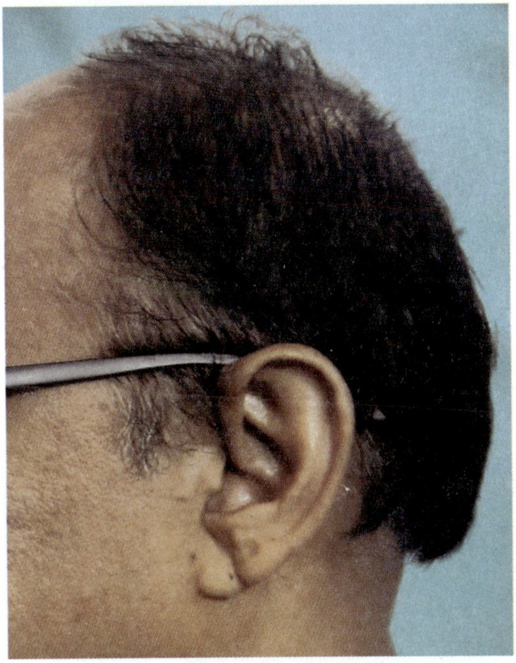

Fig. 4.6: Diagonal ear lobe crease—a physical sign for coronary artery disease

- C: Cessation of smoking and control of cholesterol
- D: Diet modification and control of diabetes
- E: Education of lifestyle modification and exercise

C. *Diagnosis:* The diagnosis of IHD depends on history and different investigations like rest ECG, stress ECG, thallium stress test, Holter monitoring (Fig. 4.7), echocardiography and Doppler study, and the most specific investigation coronary angiography.

D. *Definitive treatment:* If coronary angiography reveals blockage in coronary arteries, the patient is advised anti-anginal medications along with lifestyle modifications; the patient is then advised to undergo either:
- Coronary artery bypass grafting (CABG, Fig. 4.8), or
- Percutaneous transluminal coronary angioplasty (PTCA)

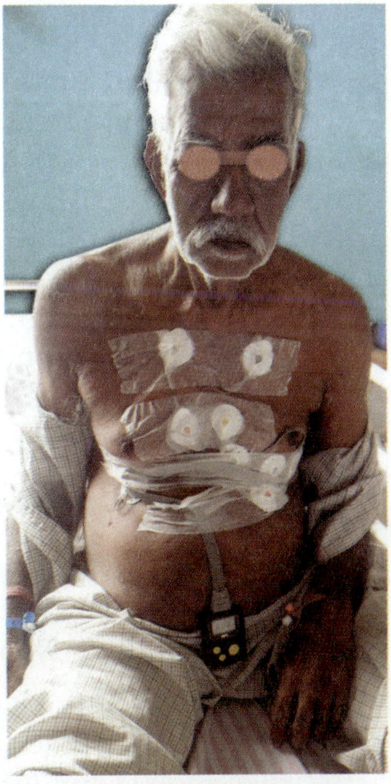

Fig. 4.7: An aged person on Holter monitoring who presented with bradycardia along with syncope

Q. What is dyspnoea?

It is the abnormally uncomfortable subjective awareness of breathing. Basically, diseases of CVS and respiratory system give rise to dyspnoea but dyspnoea may have its origin from involvement of other systems too. A

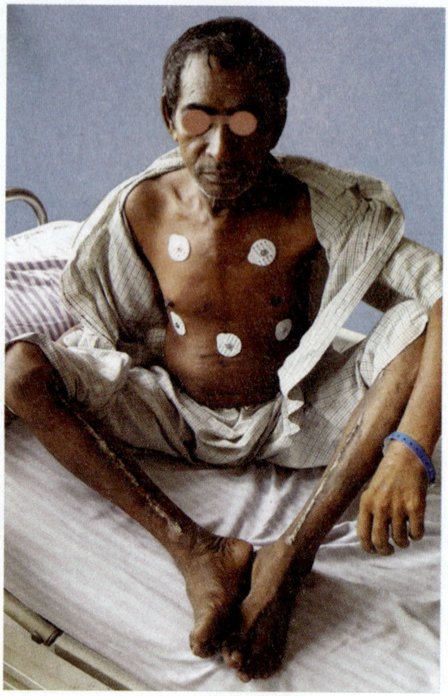

Fig. 4.8: Midline sternotomy incision mark with markings of saphenous venous grafts taken for coronary artery bypass grafting (CABG) performed for symptomatic ischaemic heart disease (IHD)

patient of dyspnoea needs emergency care and urgent aetiological evaluation. The major causes of dyspnoea are:

- *CVS:* Heart failure (left ventricular failure/LVF, or congestive cardiac failure/CCF), cyanotic congenital heart diseases, pericardial effusion, cardiac tamponade.
- *Respiratory:* Bronchial asthma, COPD, consolidation (i.e., pneumonia), pneumothorax, pleural effusion, fibrosing alveolitis (or interstitial lung disease/ILD), gross kyphoscoliosis, diffuse pulmonary tuberculosis, pulmonary thromboembolism, ARDS.
- *Neurological:* Diaphragmatic or respiratory muscle paralysis, myasthenia gravis, Guillain-Barré (GB) syndrome, depression of respiratory centre.
- *Gastrointestinal tract:* Massive (huge) ascites.
- *Miscellaneous:* High altitude, high pyrexia, unaccustomed exercise, severe anaemia, diabetic ketoacidosis, uraemia, hysterical hyperventilation.

NB: Dyspnoea with clear chest on auscultation: Severe anaemia, diaphragmatic palsy and hysterical hyperventilation.

Q. Queries related to dyspnoea while taking history.

Ask your patient for:

1. *Origin:* Acute or gradual? Does it occur at rest?
2. Paroxysmal (of sudden onset, or sudden increase in intensity) or exertional? Is it proportional to exertion?
3. Any H/o paroxysmal nocturnal dyspnoea (PND)? or, orthopnoea?

4. Any H/o seasonal variation?
5. Grading of dyspnoea [NYHA classification for cardiac dyspnoea and Medical Research Council (MRC) classification for dyspnoea of respiratory origin].
6. Presence of wheezing or stridor.
7. *Time of appearance:* Early night (PND or cardiac asthma), early morning (bronchial asthma), or irrespective of day and night (COPD, ILD).
8. Is it associated with pain chest (pneumothorax or acute myocardial infarction/AMI) or fever (consolidation)?
9. Is it progressive or not?
10. How is it relieved (by drugs, rest, adopting sitting posture, after expectoration of tenacious sputum, or squatting)?

NB: 'Dyspnoea threshold' means individual variation in tolerance to dyspnoea.

Q. What is paroxysmal nocturnal dyspnoea (PND)?

It is a paroxysmal (sudden onset) dyspnoea developing in early hours of night during sleep. During sleep, venous return increases to the heart which leads to pulmonary congestion and reduced compliance of the lungs; moreover, free diaphragmatic movement is hampered in lying down position due to liver and other viscera leading to dyspnoea in a susceptible patient (e.g., a patient of MS may not cope with increased venous return to the heart while lying). The patient gets relief of dyspnoea by adopting, sitting or standing position, which reduces the haemodynamic burden on heart.

As the left side of the heart cannot accommodate larger amount of blood, it fails and regurgitates blood to pulmonary veins leading to *pulmonary venous hypertension* → *acute interstitial oedema* (fluid collection in interstitial tissue of lungs leading to dry cough) → *acute pulmonary oedema* (fluid collection within alveoli of lungs, which is a fatal condition and a medical emergency; cough is now productive with profuse, watery, pinkish i.e., tinged with blood and frothy expectoration) → *cardiac asthma*.

PND is common in younger patient with MS and older patient with coronary artery disease (CAD) preceding impending left-sided heart failure. The patient is pale, anxious and becomes dyspnoeic (even orthopnoeic), with central cyanosis and tachycardia. Other prominent signs are raised JVP, S_3 gallop rhythm, scattered rhonchi and profuse crepitations in lungs.

PND or pulmonary oedema signifies acute left-sided heart failure (acute left ventricular or left atrial failure).

Q. What is 'Grading' of cardiovascular dyspnoea (of CVS) by New York Heart Association (NYHA)?

NYHA functional classification is actually a classification of cardiac disability (i.e., not only dyspnoea but it refers to symptoms like fatigue, palpitation and angina pectoris).

Grade I: No limitation of activities with ordinary physical work. There is shortness of breath on unaccustomed exertion.

Grade II: No limitation under resting condition but symptoms appear on ordinary activity.

Grade III: Comfortable at rest but limitation of activities on mild exertion or less than ordinary activity.

Grade IV: Limitation of activities at rest restricting the person to bed or chair.

Progression or regression of a disease is indicated by change in grade of dyspnoea.

Q. How to clinically differentiate cardiac dyspnoea e.g., acute heart failure, from respiratory dyspnoea e.g., acute exacerbation of bronchial asthma or COPD?

Cardiac dyspnoea	*Respiratory dyspnoea*
• Dyspnoea precedes cough and expectoration	Cough with expectoration precedes dyspnoea
• Seasonal variation: Absent	Seasonal variation: Common in winter
• Grade of dyspnoea: +++ (even with PND and orthopnoea)	Grade of dyspnoea: + / ++
• Cyanosis: Usually absent	Cyanosis: Present in late stage
• Polycythemia: Absent	Polycythemia: Present
• Associated features: Angina, syncope, palpitation, hypertension	Associated features: Wheezing or stridor
• Cardiomegaly: Usually present	Cardiomegaly: Absent
• Symptoms > signs, as a whole	Signs > symptoms, as a whole
• Heart: Murmurs may be present	Heart: Murmurs usually absent
• Lungs: Crepitations > rhonchi	Lungs: Rhonchi > crepitations

Q. What is precordium?

It is the anterior chest wall which overlies heart and great vessels. In health, precordium has a smooth convex contour.

Q. What are the different areas of heart?

Basically, there are four areas of heart; the fifth area is neoaortic area (Fig. 4.9).

1. *Mitral area (apical area):* Overlies apex beat (in health, it lies in the left 5th intercostal space, ½ inch inside the midclavicular line)
2. *Aortic area:* Right 2nd intercostal space close to the sternum
3. *Pulmonary area:* Left 2nd intercostal space close to the sternum
4. *Tricuspid area:* Left 4th intercostal space close to the sternum.

NB: *Neoaortic area* (Erb's point or aortic II area): Left 3rd intercostal space close to the sternum; the early diastolic murmur of aortic incompetence is often best audible here.

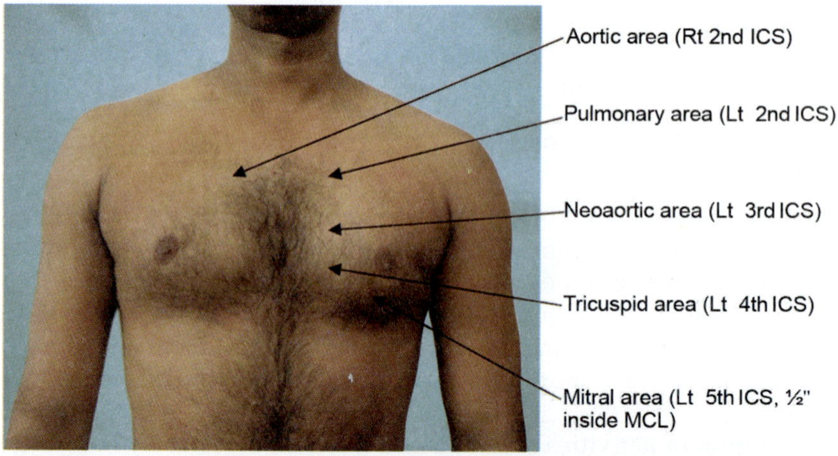

Fig. 4.9: Different areas of heart over the chest for examination in cardiovascular system

Different areas of heart mentioned above do not correspond to respective heart valve but point out the areas where cardiac events at these four valves are best appreciated by a clinician.

Q. How to auscultate different areas of heart?

During auscultation of each area, one has to be careful about position of the patient, phase of respiration and use of stethoscope (bell or diaphragm):

1. *Mitral area (apical area):* In left lateral position with the bell (for MS) or diaphragm (for MI) of stethoscope at the height of expiration (Fig. 4.10).
2. *Aortic area:* In sitting and leaning forward position with the diaphragm of stethoscope at the height of expiration (Fig. 4.11).
3. *Pulmonary area:* In sitting and leaning forward position with the diaphragm of stethoscope at the height of inspiration.
4. *Tricuspid area:* In supine or right lateral position with the diaphragm of stethoscope at the height of inspiration.
5. *Neoaortic area:* In sitting and leaning forward position with the diaphragm of stethoscope at the height of expiration.

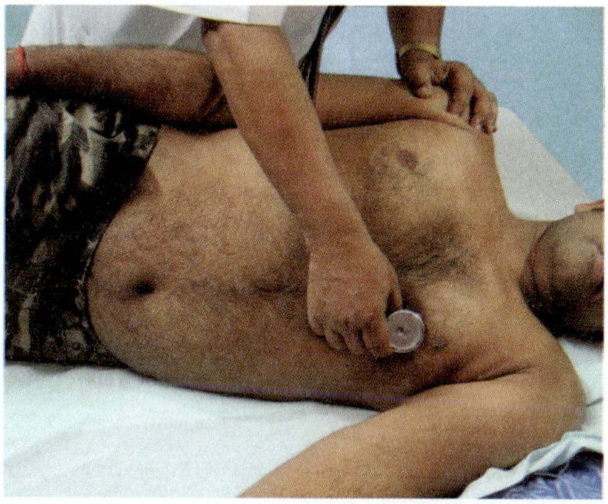

Fig. 4.10: Auscultation of the mitral area (for mitral stenosis) by bell of the stethoscope while the patient is in left lateral position (at the height of expiration)

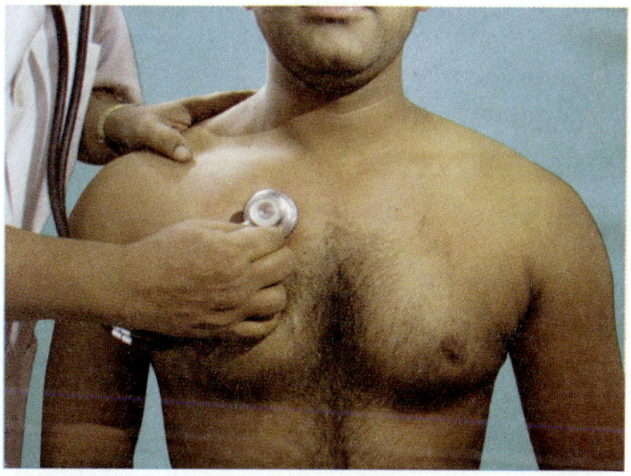

Fig. 4.11: Auscultation of aortic area by using diaphragm of the stethoscope while the patient is sitting and leaning forward (at the height of expiration)

NB: Position adopted during auscultation made murmurs more intense as the specific areas come closure to the chest wall. For auscultation of the *base of the heart* i.e., aortic and pulmonary area, it is customary to adopt a sitting and leaning forward position by the patient.

Due to more negative intrapleural pressure during inspiration, more blood comes to the right side of the heart, and thus right-sided events are more pronounced in inspiration and that of left-sided events are in expiration.

Low-pitched murmur of MS is best audible by bell, while others i.e., high-pitched murmurs are best audible by diaphragm of stethoscope.

Q. Heart sounds to be noted at bedside: A summary.

In health, one can listen two heart sounds (S_1 and S_2) among the four sounds (S_1, S_2, S_3, S_4). There are other sounds which are audible in a diseased heart.

Normally the S_1 is dull and prolonged (lubb in 'lubb-dup'), and is best audible over apex; it has two components like mitral (M_1) and tricuspid (T_1). S_1 may be soft (e.g., MI), loud (e.g., MS), or may be of varying intensity (e.g., atrial fibrillation).

In health, S_2 is short and high-pitched (dup in 'lubb-dup'). It has two components like A_2, which is best audible over aortic area, and P_2, which is best audible over pulmonary area. Normal physiological splitting of A_2 and P_2 is audible in children and adults in inspiration.

S_3 and S_4 are low-pitched sounds, which are usually not audible in health. S_3 and S_4 are found commonly in heart failure and IHD respectively, over the apical area.

NB: Normally, S_1 and S_2 are audible over precordium. If S_3 or S_4 is audible with S_1 or S_2, it is known as **triple rhythm**. Tripple rhythm with sinus tachycardia is called **gallop rhythm** (resembling the cadence produced by galloping horse). In one word, gallop rhythm indicates that the patient is in heart failure.

In different diseased states, other sounds audible over precordium are opening snap (MS), ejection click (AS), non-ejection click (MVPS), pericardial knock (constrictive pericarditis) and tumour plop (atrial myxoma).

Other than basic sounds in heart, one can hear murmur and pericardial rub (i.e., superficial, scratchy sound produced by rubbing of inflamed visceral and parietal pleura as a result of acute pericarditis).

Basics of heart sounds:

- S_1 (first heart sound): Produced as a result of closure of atrioventricular valves at the onset of ventricular systole.
- S_2 (second heart sound): Produced as a result of closure of semilunar valves at the beginning of ventricular diastole.
- S_3 (third heart sound): It is a ventricular filling sound which occurs in the first rapid filling phase of ventricular diastole.
- S_4 (fourth heart sound): It occurs during the last rapid filling phase of ventricular diastole which coincides with atrial systole.

NB: Clinically systole is the interval between S_1 and S_2, while diastole remains between the interval of S_2 and S_1. Systolic events occur with carotid pulsation (palpate right carotid artery of the lying patient with your left thumb) and diastolic events precede or follow carotid pulsation; in this way, timing of a murmur can be diagnosed (Fig. 4.12).

Q. What are thrill, murmur and bruit?

They are described as below:

- *Thrill:* It is the palpable low-frequency vibrations mimicking the sensation like 'purring of a cat'. This is always associated with a heart murmur, and is synonymous with 'palpable murmur'. A thrill is described by its site and timing (systolic, diastolic or continuous).

  In all areas, systolic thrill is commonly palpable, while diastolic thrill (e.g., thrill of MS) is more common in mitral area. A continuous thrill is palpable in PDA in left

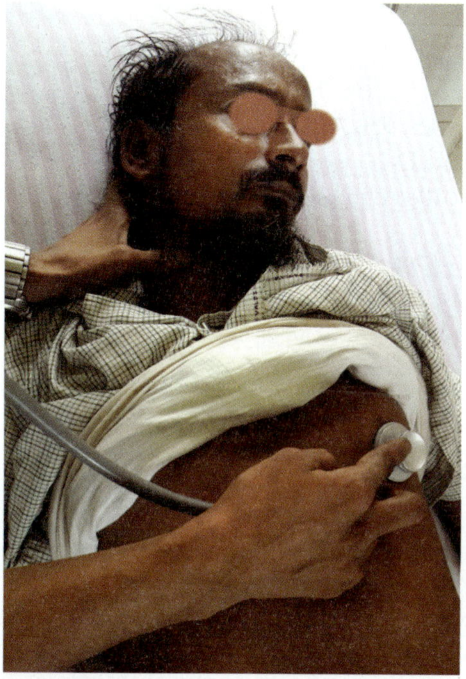

Fig. 4.12: Auscultation for murmur by stethoscope while palpating the right carotid artery simultaneously by the left thumb to ascertain the timing of murmur (i.e., systolic or diastolic)

infraclavicular area. A carotid thrill is not uncommon in root of the neck in AS (carotid shudder).

- *Murmur:* These are the unusual cardiac sounds produced by turbulent flow through the abnormal valves (e.g., MS, AS), normal valves (e.g., severe anaemia), great vessels (bruit from coarctation of aorta) or blood passing through an abnormal channel (e.g., ASD, VSD). Any murmur should be described by:
  - Where best audible (enumerate the specific area e.g., mitral area)
  - Timing (systolic, diastolic or continuous)
  - Character (rumbling, harsh, blowing), and pitch
  - Radiation or direction of selective propagation (do not say 'conduction')
  - Intensity (i.e., grading of murmur; if thrill is associated, the grade is IV or IV+ i.e., thrill is absent in grade I, II and III. Systolic murmurs are classified up to VI grades, where grade I is very faint murmur and grade VI is very loud murmur; diastolic murmurs are graded up to IV)
  - Change with respiration
  - Change with posture
  - Change after isometric exercise (MS murmur increases post-exercise; done only if the condition of the patient permits)
  - Whether best audible by diaphragm or bell of stethoscope (low-pitched murmur of MS and TS are best audible by bell; others are best audible by diaphragm).
- *Bruit:* Murmur which occurs at the site of arterial stenosis is known as bruit e.g., renal artery bruit in renal artery stenosis.

Q. Can you classify murmurs?

A. ***Organic murmurs***

- *Systolic:*
  - Ejection systolic: AS, PS, ASD
  - Pansystolic: MI, VSD
  - Late systolic: Papillary muscle dysfunction, MVPS
- *Diastolic:*
  - Early diastolic: AI, PI
  - Mid-diastolic: MS, TS, Carey Coombs murmur, Austin Flint murmur
  - Presystolic or late diastolic: MS
- *Continuous:*
  - PDA
  - Rupture of sinus of Valsalva
  - Pulmonary arteriovenous (AV) fistula.

B. ***Others***

- *Haemic murmur:* Ejection systolic murmur in aortic and pulmonary area resulting out of severe anaemia (so called **haemic**).
- *Innocent murmur:* Soft, systolic murmur, best heard over pulmonary area in supine position in children (Still's murmur) due to hyperkinetic circulation from increased heart rate. The murmur disappears as the child grows older.
- *Functional murmur:* Soft to medium grade systolic (may be diastolic) murmur, usually without a thrill, and is audible due to increased blood flow at the site of production (thus, often known as 'flow murmur'). Common examples are systolic murmur over pulmonary area in ASD and apical mid-diastolic murmur in severe AI (Austin Flint murmur).
- *Seagull murmur:* It is the murmur with a musical quality which is common in SBE (when developed over MI or AI), acute myocardial infarction or acute rheumatic fever.
- *Changing murmur:* Murmurs of atrial myxoma or infective endocarditis change their character from time to time.

**Organic murmur:* Increased pressure gradient across the abnormal valve.
Functional murmur: Increased flow of blood across the normal valve.

Q. What is apex beat?

It is the down most and outermost part of the precordium where a definite thrust can be felt. When the cardiac pulsation is seen, it is known as **'apical impulse'**. In an adult in health, normal position of the apex beat is in the left 5th intercostal space, ½ inch inside the midclavicular line. In lean and thin person, apex beat lies in left 6th intercostal space, while that of children lies in left 4th intercostal space.

Stand on the right side of the supine patient. First palpate the precordium with flat of the hand, and then localise it by pulp of index or middle finger (Fig. 4.13). If apex beat is not palpable in dorsal decubitus position, ask the patient to sit and lean forward, and try to locate it with outstretched fingers; if apex beat is still not palpable, try to palpate the right side of the chest (for dextrocardia or dextroversion). Never turn the

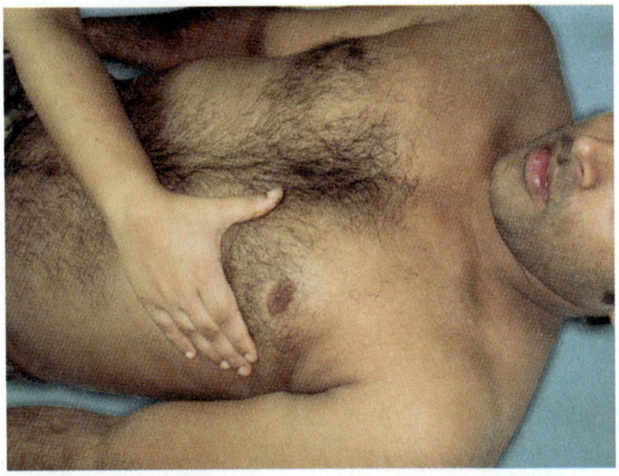

Fig. 4.13: Palpation of cardiac impulse and localisation of apex beat

patient to left lateral position to localise the apex beat because heart rotates 1–2 cm within the chest after adopting left lateral position; the character of apex beat is best palpable in left lateral position of the patient.

The five different *characters of apex beat* are:

- Normal (brief, non-sustained gentle tap which is palpable with certainty)
- Hyperdynamic (forceful and ill-sustained as in MI or AI)
- Heaving (forceful and well-sustained as in AS, systemic hypertension)
- Tapping (palpable first heart sound in MS)
- Hypokinetic (minimal thrust felt in AMI, pericardial effusion).

Q. Abnormalities of apical impulse/apex beat.

Different types	*Common examples*
1. Tapping (i.e., palpable S_1)	1. MS
2. Hyperdynamic	2. Left ventricular volume overload like MI, AI, VSD, PDA
3. Heaving	3. Left ventricular pressure overload like AS, systemic hypertension, coarctation of aorta
4. Hypokinetic	4. AMI, COPD, pericardial effusion
5. Diffuse	5. Left ventricular aneurysm
6. Double or triple	6. Hypertrophic obstructive cardiomyopathy (HOCM)
7. Retractile	7. Adherent pericarditis
8. Absent	8. Behind a rib, obesity, COPD (especially, emphysema), left-sided pleural effusion/pneumothorax, AMI, heart failure, remain elsewhere (i.e., dextrocardia)

Q. Features (signs at bedside) of LVH, RVH, LVF and RVF.

The clinical signs of ventricular hypertrophy and failure are as follows:

Clinical conditions	*Signs*
1. Left ventricular hypertrophy (LVH)	• Apex beat goes down and outwards
2. Right ventricular hypertrophy (RVH)	• Apex beat goes outwards • Left parasternal heave (pulsation at lower left side of sternum) • Epigastric pulsation

3. Left ventricular failure (LVF)	• Gallop rhythm • Fine crepitations at lung bases • Pulsus alternans **NB:** The patient may suffer from breathlessness, orthopnoea, central cyanosis, and nocturia
4. Right ventricular failure (RVF) or congestive cardiac failure (CCF)	• Engorged and pulsatile neck veins • Mildly enlarged, soft and tender liver • Dependent bipedal pitting oedema (Fig. 4.14) **NB:** The patient may complain of breathlessness, cough, oliguria, and may have peripheral cyanosis and pulsatile liver

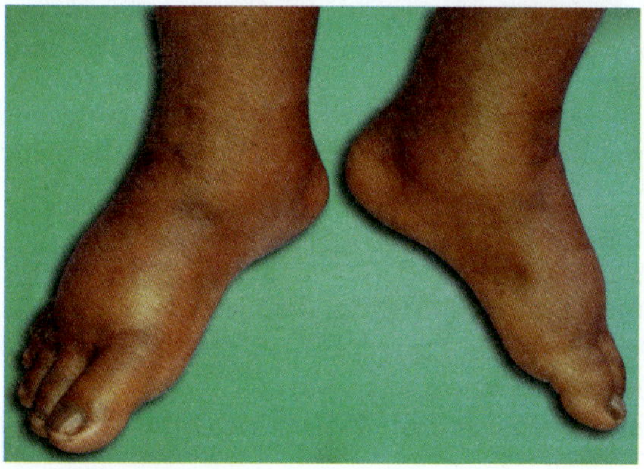

Fig. 4.14: Oedema of both feet in cardiac failure

Q. What is heart failure?

It is a clinical syndrome when there is inability of the heart to pump blood with normal efficiency and thus the heart cannot maintain an adequate cardiac output, or can do so at the expense of an elevated filling pressure.

Q. Do you know common causes of heart failure?

Different chambers of heart fail due to:

- LVF (acute pulmonary oedema): Systemic hypertension, ischaemic heart disease (IHD), AMI, AS, AI, MI, myocarditis, cardiomyopathy, severe anaemia, thyrotoxicosis, excess fluid overload.
- Left atrial failure (LAF): MS, left atrial myxoma, left atrial ball valve thrombus.
- RVF or CCF (congestive cardiac failure): Secondary to left-sided heart failure (e.g., MS), COPD, pulmonary hypertension due to any reason, ASD, VSD, PDA, PS, myocarditis, cardiomyopathy.
- Right atrial failure (RAF): TS, secondary to RVF.

Q. What are the precipitating factors for heart failure (CCF or LVF)?

The common precipitating factors are:

- Intercurrent illness e.g., infection or sepsis (e.g., respiratory tract infection or SBE)
- Increased metabolic demand e.g., anaemia, pregnancy, thyrotoxicosis

- Myocardial ischaemia or infarction
- Cardiac arrhythmias e.g., atrial fibrillation
- Pulmonary thromboembolism
- Myocarditis
- Infective endocarditis
- Administration of β-blockers (drug with negative inotropic properties)
- Ongoing rheumatic activity
- IV fluid overload or electrolyte disturbances.

Q. Can you define and enumerate causes of palpitations?

- *Definition:* Abnormal unpleasant subjective awareness of one's heartbeat.
- *Causes:*
  - *Cardiac:* Atrial fibrillation, ventricular ectopics, paroxysmal atrial tachycardia (PAT), AI, MI, ASD, VSD, PDA.
  - *Non-cardiac:* Hyperkinetic circulatory states like severe anaemia, thyrotoxicosis, anxiety, pyrexia, unaccustomed exertion; excessive smoking, hypoglycaemia, menopause, pheochromocytoma, sabutamol/nifedipine/atropine-induced hysteria.

Q. What is syncope (or black-out)?

It is the sudden and transient loss of consciousness with inability to stand upright due to reduced cerebral perfusion (i.e., postural collapse). The common causes are:

- Vasovagal attack (in an unpleasant sight, after prolonged standing).
- Stokes-Adams syndrome [recurrent unconsciousness due to ventricular asystole from complete atrioventricular (AV) block. Pulse is 36/minute, regular with large volume, with cannon waves in JVP and variable intensity of S_1].
- Postural hypotension (receiving antihypertensives).
- Micturition syncope (while voiding large volume of urine in standing position).
- Carotid sinus syncope (compression over neck by hand or tight collar).
- *Others:* Aortic stenosis (especially exertional), IHSS, sick sinus syndrome, hypoglycaemia, vertebro-basilar insufficiency, hyperventilation and hysterical fainting.

NB: Recovery from cardiovascular syncope is rapid, while recovery time from neurocardiogenic syncope (e.g., vasovagal attack) is slow with accompanying nausea and light-headedness.

Q. Which is the most common valvular heart disease?

Mitral valve is most commonly affected by acute rheumatic fever, and thus mitral stenosis (MS) is the commonest valvular heart disease.

Q. Do you know about infective endocarditis?

It is the microbial infection of a heart valve (e.g., mitral valve in MI, or prosthetic valve), the mural endocardium or a septal defect (e.g., VSD). The types are acute and subacute (i.e., subacute bacterial endocarditis or SBE). Its stigmata are given in 'common presentations in CVS'.

Q. Enumerate congenital heart diseases.

- *Cyanotic:* Tetralogy of Fallot (TOF), tricuspid atresia, transposition of great vessels, truncus arteriosus and total anomalous pulmonary venous connection (i.e., 5 'T').
- *Acyanotic:* ASD, VSD, PDA, coarctation of aorta, aortic stenosis, pulmonary stenosis.

Q. Which is the most common congenital heart disease?

Most common congenital cardiac anomaly is bicuspid aortic valve which remains asymptomatic until later life when the valve produces aortic stenosis or aortic incompetence.

VSD is the most common congenital heart disease.

Q. Can you tell the components of tetralogy of Fallot (TOF)?

The components of TOF are:

- Ventricular septal defect (VSD)
- Pulmonary stenosis (PS)
- Right ventricular hypertrophy (RVH)
- Overriding of aorta.

Q. What is a cyanotic or anoxic spell?

Cyanotic spells (Fallot's spells) occur between 2 months and 2 years of age. A child suffering from TOF suddenly becomes more cyanosed and starts hyperventilation, which ultimately leads to apnoea, syncope, seizures or sudden death, especially while crying, feeding, waking up, having pyrexia or doing exercise (these produce vasodilatation and thus blood goes by right-to-left shunt through VSD with less blood going to lungs, and maximum venous blood is being diverted to aorta resulting in cerebral hypoxia and unconsciousness). The child then adopt the squatting posture i.e., knee-chest position to reduce cyanotic spells. Squatting posture increases peripheral vascular resistance with reduction of right-to-left shunt; squatting also increases venous return to the heart with resultant increase in pulmonary blood flow.

Q. What is Eisenmenger's syndrome?

In course of time ASD, VSD and PDA (all are acyanotic congenital heart diseases) patients develop pulmonary hypertension. This phenomenon gives rise to right-to-left shunt within the heart from an initial left-to-right shunt in ASD, VSD, and PDA patients, which is known as Eisenmenger's syndrome. In this syndrome, the patients present with breathlessness, central cyanosis, clubbing, polycythemia, and features of RVH and RVF.

Q. Model description of murmurs and heart sounds in common valvular heart diseases.

1. ***Mitral stenosis (MS):*** Low-pitched, mid-diastolic rumbling murmur with presystolic accentuation of grade IV intensity (i.e., with a diastolic thrill), audible over mitral area without any radiation. The murmur is best audible at the apical area (i.e., mitral area), with the bell of stethoscope (placed lightly), in left lateral supine position, at

the height of expiration, and after doing mild isometric exercise (i.e., moderate exertion is done in doubtful cases if the condition of the patient permits). The presystolic murmur ends in a loud S_1 (short, sharp and accentuated), and the S_2 is audible. An opening snap is heard just after S_2.

2. ***Mitral incompetence (MI):*** High-pitched, soft blowing pansystolic murmur of grade III intensity (i.e., without a thrill), is present in the mitral area which is radiated towards the left axilla and inferior angle of left scapula (as commonly the anterior mitral leaflet is involved). The murmur is best audible with the diaphragm of stethoscope, in left lateral supine position and at the height of expiration. The S_1 is soft (muffled) and S_2 is audible.
   If the posterior mitral leaflet is involved, the pansystolic murmur of MI radiates to the anterior precordium and up to the pulmonary area (i.e., towards base of the heart). A pansystolic murmur starts immediately with the S_1 and continues through to the S_2, which always have a uniform intensity (thus known as 'holosystolic').
3. ***Aortic stenosis (AS):*** A harsh midsystolic ejection murmur of grade V intensity (i.e., with a systolic thrill) having a crescendo-decrescendo character with direction of selective propagation towards the carotids, is heard over the aortic area. The murmur is best audible with the diaphragm of stethoscope, in sitting and leaning forward position and at the height of expiration; occasionally the murmur is transmitted to the mitral area, and is known as Gallavardin's phenomenon. The S_1 is audible and S_2 (A_2) is soft (muffled). An ejection click may be present just after S_1 in mild valvular AS.
4. ***Aortic incompetence (AI):*** High-pitched, soft blowing, early diastolic decrescendo murmur of grade II intensity (i.e., without a thrill), is present over the aortic area with radiation towards the apex, and is often best heard in the neoaortic area. The murmur is best audible with the diaphragm of stethoscope, in sitting and leaning forward position and at the height of expiration. S_1 is audible and S_2 (A_2) is soft (muffled).

NB: Peripheral signs of aortic incompetence (AI) are due to 'wide pulse pressure' and hyperkinetic circulation, and they are:

- *Upper extremity:*
  - High-volume collapsing pulse or water hammer pulse
  - Visible capillary pulsation (Quincke's sign): Application of pressure over tip of fingers or nails gives rise to alternate flushing (redness) and pallor (blanching) of nail-bed
  - Blood pressure: High systolic and low diastolic pressure gives rise to wide pulse pressure
  - Locomotor brachialis: 'Tortuous and highly pulsatile' brachial artery (Fig. 4.15)
- *Lower extremity:*
  - 'Pistol shot' sound heard over the femoral artery (Traube's sign)
  - Systolic murmur on compression of the femoral artery proximally
  - Diastolic murmur on compression of the femoral artery distally (Duroziez's murmur)
  - Hill's sign: Femoral artery systolic BP is >20 mm of Hg than brachial artery systolic BP

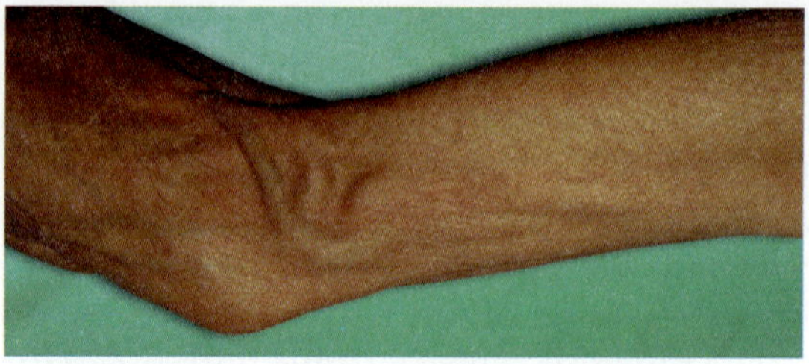

Fig. 4.15: Locomotor brachialis—tortuous and pulsatile brachial artery in aortic incompetence (AI)

- *Head, neck and adjacent area:*
  - de Musset's sign: Head-nodding synchronous with each carotid pulsation
  - Corrigan's sign: Dancing carotids in neck
  - Alternate redness and blanching are seen when a glass slide is pressed on the everted lower lip (i.e., visible capillary pulsation)
  - Visible pulsation in the jugular (suprasternal) notch.

Decoding Abbreviations

ECG	Electrocardiogram
MS	Mitral stenosis
MI/MR	Mitral incompetence/mitral regurgitation
AS	Aortic stenosis
AI/AR	Aortic incompetence/aortic regurgitation
PS/PI	Pulmonary stenosis/pulmonary incompetence
TS/TI	Tricuspid stenosis/tricuspid incompetence
ASD	Atrial septal defect
VSD	Ventricular septal defect
PDA	Patent ductus arteriosus
AMI	Acute myocardial infarction
CAD	Coronary artery disease
IHD	Ischaemic heart disease
RVH/RVF	Right ventricular hypertrophy/right ventricular failure
LVH/LVF	Left ventricular hypertrophy/left ventricular failure
CCF	Congestive cardiac failure
SBE	Subacute bacterial endocarditis
MVPS	Mitral valve prolapse syndrome
IHSS	Idiopathic hypertrophic subaortic stenosis
HOCM	Hypertrophic obstructive cardiomyopathy
ARDS	Acute respiratory distress syndrome.

Chapter

5

Respiratory System

SCHEME OF SYSTEMIC EXAMINATION: AN OVERVIEW

I. *Examination of the upper respiratory tract (URT):* Nose and alae nasi, nasal cavity, oral cavity, paranasal air sinuses, pharynx, mouth breathing, purse-lip respiration, larynx (cannot be examined clinically, examined by laryngoscope).

II. *Examination of the chest (lower respiratory tract or LRT).*

A. *Inspection:*

- Shape of chest (barrel-shaped in emphysema, pigeon-shaped in rickets, alar chest in tall-thin person, or funnel chest in cobblers, Fig. 5.1)
- Movement of the chest

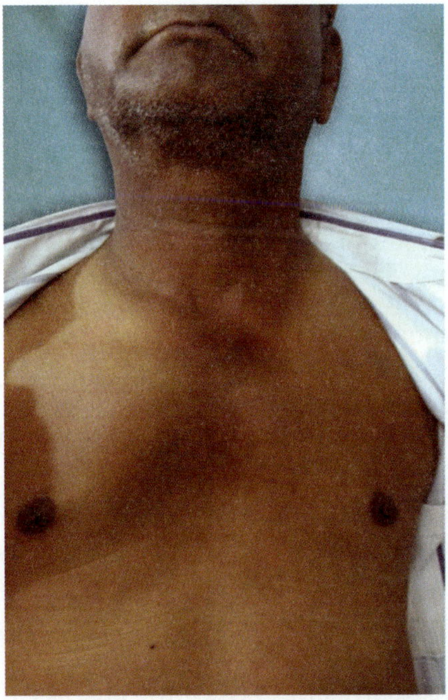

Fig. 5.1: Funnel chest (pectus excavatum)—depression seen in lower part of sternum

- Apical impulse, venous prominence (should be examined in standing or sitting position of the patient after a bout of cough)
- Respiration (vide section on 'General examination')
- Fullness or depression in the chest—unilateral or bilateral, localised or generalised
- Accessory muscles of respiration, intercostal suction, wheezing or stridor
- *Skin:* Gynaecomastia, ulcer, sinus, pigmentation, any swelling (i.e., cold abscess from tuberculosis), parietal oedema
- *Back:* Kyphoscoliosis, gibbus (acute angulation in the spine due to collapse of vertebrae from tuberculosis or malignant deposits), 'straight back', drooping of the shoulder, winging of the scapula, arterial or venous pulsations, skin conditions.

B. *Palpation:*
- Surface temperature and tenderness
- Corroboration of the findings of inspection, e.g., chest symmetry, spinal deformity, direction of venous flow, position of apical impulse, etc.
- Position of the trachea and apex beat
- Movement of the chest (to find out the symmetry of movement and expansion of the chest)—always measure the expansion of the chest by a measuring tape, in full inspiration and in full expiration
- Vocal fremitus and other tactile fremitus.

C. *Percussion:* Conventional percussion, shifting dullness, coin percussion, detection of hepatic and cardiac dullness, Traube's space percussion.

D. *Auscultation*:
- Breath sounds (vesicular or bronchial)
- Vocal resonance (increased or diminished, whispering pectoriloquy, aegophony)
- Adventitious sounds (wheezes or rhonchi, crackles or crepitations, pleural rub)
- *Others:* Succussion splash (splashing sound heard in hydropneumothorax), post-tussive suction, pneumothorax click, tinkling crepitations).

NB: Chest is a bilaterally symmetrical structure; thus, always compare the findings with the other side. Chest should be examined in sitting or standing position, if possible but avoid examining in recumbent position of the patient.

Q. Mention the common presentations (chief complaints and H/o present illness) in respiratory system.

The patients having complaints of respiratory system commonly present with:

1. Cough (pulmonary tuberculosis, bronchiectasis, lung abscess, lobar pneumonia, heavy smoker or bronchogenic carcinoma).
2. Expectoration or sputum production (bronchiectasis, lung abscess, resolution stage of pneumonia, chronic bronchitis).
3. Haemoptysis (tuberculosis, bronchiectasis, lung abscess, pneumonia, bronchogenic carcinoma).

4. Chest pain (pleurisy, spontaneous pneumothorax, acute tracheobronchitis, pulmonary thromboembolism).
5. Breathlessness or dyspnoea (bronchial asthma, COPD, consolidation, pneumothorax, pleural effusion, fibrosing alveolitis, ARDS).
6. Wheezing or stridor (bronchial asthma or COPD for wheezing, and laryngeal oedema or aspiration of foreign body for stridor).
7. *Others:*
   a. Heaviness in the chest (in pleural effusion, pneumothorax or hydropneumothorax, the affected side of chest feels heavy).
   b. Fever (tuberculosis, pleurisy, lung abscess, pneumonic consolidation, and lower respiratory tract infection/LRTI).
   c. Hoarseness of voice (laryngitis, diphtheria, angioedema, vocal abuse and especially, due to recurrent laryngeal nerve palsy from bronchogenic carcinoma).
   d. Loss of weight and/or loss of appetite (tuberculosis, lymphoma or bronchogenic carcinoma) or night sweats (tuberculosis or lymphoma).
   e. Swelling of feet or oedema (in chronic cor pulmonale, e.g., RVF from COPD).

Q. Points noted in past, family, personal and treatment history in respiratory system.

Past history	*Family history*	*Personal history*	*Treatment history*
1. Tuberculosis 2. Any allergic illness, especially nasobronchial allergy 3. Childhood illness like measles, tuberculosis, whooping cough 4. Exposure to STD 5. Occupation in coal mines, asbestos mines, silica factory, cotton dust, etc. 6. Any H/o unconsciousness which predisposes aspiration and lung abscess 7. Chest injury	1. Tuberculosis 2. Bronchial asthma 3. Any allergic illness 4. Eczema 5. Emphysema (due to α_1-antitrypsin deficiency)	1. Smoking* 2. Substance abuse (tobacco, betel nut chewing, alcohol** intake, or IV drug abuse) 3. Contacts with pets (e.g., pigeon), or exposure to allergen (e.g., pollen, feather) *Smoking may give rise to chronic bronchitis, COPD and bronchogenic carcinoma **Alcoholism may lead to aspiration and LRTI	1. Antituberculosis drugs; corticosteroids and immunosuppressants (i.e., increase susceptibility to different types of infections like bacterial, fungal or tubercular) 2. Bronchodilators (help assessing outcome of treatment) or cytotoxic drugs (e.g , busulphan-induced pulmonary fibrosis)

NB: 'Pack year' is the period of smoking in years multiplied by number of packets of cigarettes smoked per day. One packet of cigarette (containing 20 cigarettes) smoked per day for 10 years makes 10 pack years. If the pack year crosses 20 pack years, chance of COPD is quite increased while probability of bronchogenic carcinoma is much higher when pack year crosses 40.

Q. Some terminology you should know at the beginning.

- What is your diagnosis?
  Give the provisional diagnosis e.g., it is a case of pleural effusion of right side, probably of tuberculous in origin.
- What is your case?
  Describe the summary of the case directly.
- Can you discuss over your diagnosis (also known as 'clinical reasoning')?
  Deliver the information gathered from history and relevant clinical features (physical findings), and discuss how you have arrived the diagnosis.
- What is differential diagnosis?
  Those are different diseases mimicking the present diagnosis (e.g., D/D of pleural effusion are consolidation, thickened pleura or fibrosis/collapse of the lung).

Q. Applied anatomy of importance in respiratory system.

- Upper respiratory tract (URT) extends from external nares to the junction of larynx with trachea (i.e., up to lower border of cricoid cartilage), and includes nasal cavity, nasopharynx, paranasal air sinuses, oropharynx and larynx.
  Lower respiratory tract (LRT) includes trachea, lobar bronchus, segmental bronchi, generations of trachea-bronchial tree and alveolar air sacs.
- Right bronchus is more or less in the same line with trachea, and thus an aspirated material may directly go up to lower lobe of right lung resulting in aspiration pneumonia.
- Parietal pleura is pain sensitive, and is supplied by intercostal nerves and phrenic nerve. Visceral pleura is supplied by autonomic nervous system, and is pain-insensitive. Normally a small amount of pleural fluid (5–15 ml) may remain within each pleural cavity.

Q. Common diseases of respiratory system.

They are:

- Pneumonia (i.e., consolidation of the lung).
- Bronchial asthma.
- Tuberculosis.
- Chronic obstructive pulmonary disease or COPD (e.g., chronic bronchitis and emphysema).
- Bronchiectasis, lung abscess.
- Interstitial lung diseases (ILD, or fibrosing alveolitis).
- Bronchogenic carcinoma.
- Occupational lung diseases e.g., coal workers' pneumoconiosis.
- Pulmonary thromboembolism (PTE).
- *Pleural diseases:* Pleural effusion, pneumothorax, empyema thoracis, hydropneumothorax, pyopneumothorax, haemopneumothorax.
- Disorders of the diaphragm and mediastinal lesions (e.g., tumours).

Q. Chest pain due to respiratory system diseases.

Commonly they are due to pleurisy, spontaneous pneumothorax, acute tracheo-bronchitis, pulmonary thromboembolism and mediastinal diseases. The patterns are:

- *Retrosternal pain (central):* Pain of tracheitis and mediastinitis is felt behind the sternum mimicking cardiac pain (non-exertional). [Retrosternal pain may also be due to causes in other systems like angina pectoris, oesophagitis, acute pericarditis, dissecting aneurysm, or psychogenic].
- *Plerual pain (non-central or peripheral):* Sharp, stabbing and tearing in nature without any radiation, which increases with coughing, laughing, jolting, sneezing and deep inspiration. The pain is less with shallow breathing. The patient prefers to lie on the affected side to splint his/her chest wall with the bed. The cause is pleurisy as a result of tuberculosis, pneumonic consolidation, pleural infiltration by malignancy and pulmonary infarction (i.e., pulmonary thromboembolism); patients of pneomothorax may C/O severe pleural pain.
- *Musculoskeletal pain (non-central or peripheral):* Rib fracture, costochondritis, fibromyalgia, intercostal myalgia, trauma in the chest.

Q. Discuss causes of dyspnoea due to respiratory diseases, wheezing and stridor.

Read the section on CVS for dyspnoea, and 'General examination' for wheezing and stridor.

Q. Causes of chronic breathlessness, and sudden severe dyspnoea.

- *Chronic dyspnoea:* COPD, bronchial asthma (Fig. 5.2), ILD, extensive fibrosis of the lung, chronic CCF.
- *Sudden and severe dyspnoea:* Spontaneous pneumothorax (Fig. 5.3), acute severe asthma (older term is status asthmaticus), accidental inhalation of foreign body, massive pulmonary thromboembolism (also known as acute cor pulmonale), acute LVF.

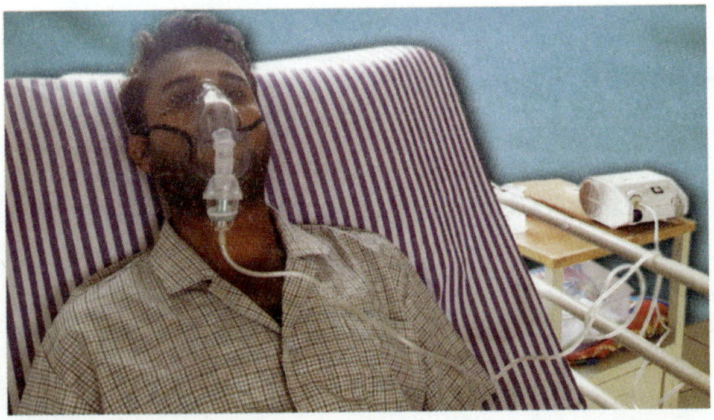

Fig. 5.2: Nebulisation in a patient of bronchial asthma with respiratory distress

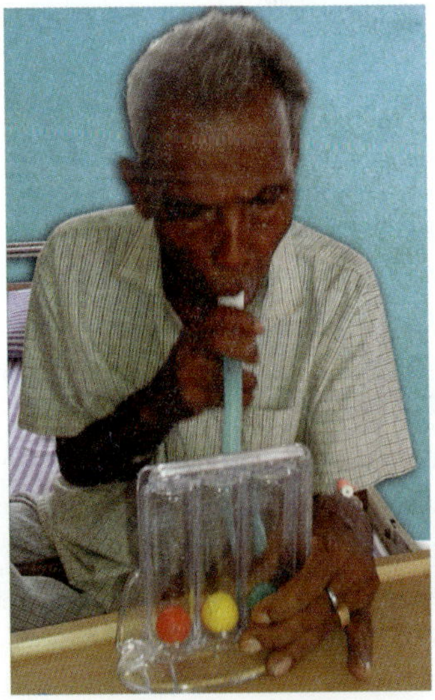

Fig. 5.3: Inflating incentive spirometer (breathing exercise) after recovering from pneumothorax

Q. What is 'Grading' of respiratory dyspnoea according to Medical Research Council (MRC) breathlessness scale?

Grades	*Features*
Grade 1	Becomes breathless when hurrying on the level or walking up a slight hill
Grade 2	Becomes breathless when walking with people of own age or walking on level ground
Grade 3	Walks slower than contemporaries on level ground due to breathlessness, or stops for breath when walking at own pace
Grade 4	Stops after walking 100 metres, or after a few minutes on level ground
Grade 5	Too breathless to leave the home, or too breathless when dressing or undressing

Q. Can you give a short account of cough?

Cough is the most important protective reflex (that clears the respiratory passages from mucus, fluid, irritants or foreign particles) of the respiratory system. It is divided into:

A. *Acute cough (<3 weeks):* Upper respiratory tract infection/URTI (e.g., viral), acute bronchitis/LRTI (e.g., bacterial), foreign body inhalation, lobar pneumonia or bronchopneumonia.

B. *Chronic cough (>8 weeks):* Cigarette smoking, bronchial asthma, COPD, pulmonary tuberculosis, ILD, bronchiectasis, lung abscess, bronchogenic carcinoma, ACE-inhibitor-induced.

Q. Different types of cough.

A cough is a sudden, usually involuntary, expulsion of air from the lungs with a characteristic sound with momentary loss of rhythm of respiration. It is the task of the clinician to analyse the types of cough to reach its aetiology.

- *Dry cough (non-productive):* Early URTI or LRTI, acute dry pleurisy, ILD, drug-induced.
- *Wet cough (productive):* Bronchiectasis, lung abscess, resolution stage of pneumonia, acute pulmonary oedema.
- *Bovine cough (laryngeal cough):* In recurrent laryngeal nerve palsy, the explosive nature of cough is lost.
- *Brassy cough:* Cough with a metallic sound is produced in carcinoma of larynx.
- *Hacking cough (pharyngeal cough):* In heavy smokers.
- *'Nocturnal' cough:* Chronic bronchitis, LVF, post-nasal drip, tropical eosinophilia, aspiration.
- *Barking cough:* A loud cough is common in laryngitis and hysteria.
- *Whooping cough (paroxysmal cough):* Rapid succession of dry cough is followed by a characteristic long inspiratory whoop (noise).
- *Nagging cough:* Post-nasal drip (rhinitis/sinusitis), ACE-inhibitor-induced, GERD, cough-variant asthma. These are the cases of chronic cough with normal chest X-ray or normal chest examination.

NB: 'Red flag signs' in cough are haemoptysis, dyspnoea, chest pain, loss of weight and pyrexia.

Q. How sputum or expectoration is analysed at the bedside?

Sputum should be analysed by these six points:

1. *Amount:* Normally ≤ 100 ml of tracheobronchial secretion is produced per day. A 'teaspoonful' or 'teacupful (> 100 ml)' of sputum production per day is respectively known as small sputum or profuse sputum. Profuse sputum is characteristic of bronchiectasis, lung abscess, alveolar cell carcinoma and acute pulmonary oedema.
2. *Character (or consistency):* Serous or watery in bronchoalveolar cell carcinoma, mucoid or grayish white in chronic bronchitis, mucopurulent or purulent in pneumonia or lung abscess. Frothy sputum is seen in pulmonary oedema and alveolar cell carcinoma while sticky, tenacious, jelly-like sputum is characteristic of bronchial asthma and COPD. If sputum of a bronchiectasis patient is kept for some time in a conical glass, it will separate into three arbitrary layers from top to bottom as mucoid (or serous), mucopurulent and purulent layer.
3. *Colour:* Yellow sputum in LRTI or bronchial asthma (due to large amount of eosinophils), green sputum in bronchial asthma or *Pseudomonas aeruginosa* infection of respiratory tract, black sputum in coal workers' pneumoconiosis, rusty sputum (i.e., tinge of blood in sputum) in pneumococcal pneumonia, pinkish in acute pulmonary oedema and anchovy-sauce like sputum is seen in ruptured amoebic liver abscess into lung.
4. *Odour or taste:* Foetid, offensive or foul-smelling expectoration is characteristic of bronchiectasis, lung abscess and infection with anaerobic organism.
5. Mixed with blood (haemoptysis) or not—see below.
6. Sputum production influenced by change of posture (e.g., bronchiectasis or lung abscess) or not.

Q. What is haemoptysis?

- Haemoptysis is the coughing out or expectoration of blood.
- Haemoptysis may be small or massive (>200 ml of blood in 24 hours). Massive haemoptysis is potentially very dangerous due to combined effect of blood loss along with asphyxia.
- Meaning of some specific phrases: 'Streaked' blood in sputum—from URT; blood 'mixed' with sputum—from LRT; 'frank' haemoptysis—no sputum, only blood; pseudohaemoptysis (or spurious haemoptysis)—blood coming from URT or oral cavity; recurrent haemoptysis—chronic bronchitis, bronchiectasis or bronchogenic carcinoma.

Q. Causes of haemoptysis.

1. *Pulmonary:* Bronchitis (acute or chronic), pulmonary tuberculosis, bronchiectasis, lung abscess, pneumonia, bronchogenic carcinoma, pulmonary infarction.
2. *CVS:* Mitral stenosis, acute LVF, primary pulmonary hypertension.
3. *Coagulation disorders:* Bleeding diathesis (e.g., haemophilia), anticoagulant therapy.
4. *Others:* Trauma, post-bronchoscopy or lung biopsy, vasculitis (e.g., Wegener's granulomatosis), idiopathic, hydatid disease of the lung, arteriovenous malformations.

NB: Five common causes of haemoptysis: Tuberculosis, chronic bronchitis, pneumonia, bronchiectasis and mitral stenosis.

Q. How to differentiate haemoptysis (i.e., coughing out of blood) from haematemesis (i.e., vomiting out of blood)?

Features	*Haemoptysis*	*Haematemesis*
• Content	Blood mixed with sputum; bright red and may be 'frothy'	Blood mixed with food-particles; may be coffee-ground in colour
• Premonitory symptoms	Cough or tickling in throat	Nausea, vomiting, retching or abdominal discomfort
• Amount	Relatively less than haematemesis; shock is less	Huge in amount; shock is not uncommon
• Melaena	Absent	Melaena may be present on next day
• Taste	Saline taste	Bitter taste
• Reaction	Alkaline; pH like blood	pH acidic
• Systems involved	Usually respiratory and CVS diseases	Gastrointestinal system

Q. What is anaphylaxis?

It is a systemic allergic reaction (IgE-mediated immediate hypersensitivity reaction) caused by liberation of histamine and many other vasoactive mediators released from mast cells. It is a life-threatening emergency and should be tackled immediately. Common features are bronchospasm, laryngeal oedema with severe dyspnoea, stridor and central cyanosis. An ideal example is penicillin injection producing anaphylaxis when given for the first time (if not given after proper skin test). This potentially fatal condition is being treated by parenteral adrenaline, corticosteroids and antihistaminics; in severe laryngeal oedema, assisted ventilation may be required.

Q. Common respiratory diseases with definition.

- *Pneumonia (i.e., consolidation):* Acute inflammation or exudative solidification of lung parenchyma.
- *Emphysema:* Permanent overinflation of air spaces in lung distal to terminal respiratory bronchioles as well as destruction of alveolar septae.
- *Chronic bronchitis:* Chronic cough with expectoration on most of the days for at least 3 consecutive months in a year, for more than 2 successive years.
- *Chronic obstructive pulmonary diseases (COPD):* Chronic obstruction to airflow (major site being the small airways) due to chronic bronchitis, emphysema and chronic bronchiolitis. The airflow limitation is usually progressive though it is treatable.
- *Chronic cor pulmonale:* RVH with or without RVF resulting from diseases affecting the structure (i.e., lung parenchyma and vasculature are being damaged by COPD) and function of lung (i.e., from severe kyphoscoliosis or ankylosing spondylitis). Acute cor pulmonale is synonymous with pulmonary thromboembolism.
- *Bronchiectasis:* Chronic necrotizing infection of bronchi and bronchioles proximal to terminal bronchioles, which leads to abnormal and permanent dilatation of the airways.
- *Lung abscess:* Localised parenchymal destruction due to suppuration within the lung.
- *Bronchial asthma:* Chronic inflammatory disorder of airways where the tracheobronchial tree shows increased responsiveness to multiplicity of intrinsic

and extrinsic stimuli, with reversible airflow obstruction, and are characterised by paroxysm of breathlessness, cough, wheezing and tightness of chest.

Acute severe asthma (older name is status asthmaticus): Severe airway obstruction where paroxysm of acute asthmatic attacks occur without any remission in between and is not manageable within 24 hours by conventional bronchodilators; often corticosteroids and respiratory assistance are required for remission.

- *Interstitial lung disease (ILD):* Disease of lung which affects the interstitium (i.e., the tissue and space around the alveoli). Prolonged ILD may give rise to pulmonary fibrosis.
- *Pleural effusion:* Accumulation of excess serous fluid within the pleural space.
- *Empyema thoracis:* Collection of pus within pleural cavity (Fig. 5.4).
- *Chylothorax:* Accumulation of a milky fluid within pleural cavity which is nothing but lymph (Fig. 5.5).
- *Pneumothorax:* Presence of air within pleural cavity.
- *Hydropneumothorax:* Collection of both serous fluid and air within pleural cavity. Similarly, pyopneumothorax is collection of pus and air, and haemopneumothorax is that of blood and air.
- *SVC syndrome:* Vide section on 'Neck vessels' in 'General examination'.

Q. Can you classify different respiratory disorders?

Obstructive pulmonary diseases	*Restrictive pulmonary diseases*
1. Examples: COPD, bronchial asthma, bronchiectasis, cystic fibrosis	Examples: Interstitial lung disease, pleural diseases, neuromuscular disorders (e.g., GB syndrome), thoracic cage abnormality (e.g., severe kyphoscoliosis)

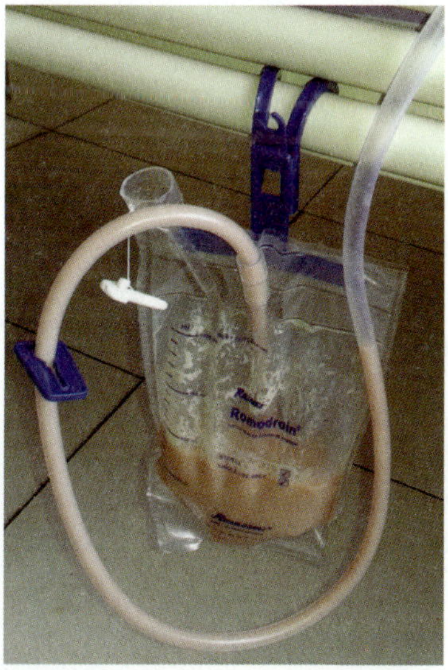

Fig. 5.4: 'Pus'—drained out from pleural cavity of a patient suffering from empyema thoracis

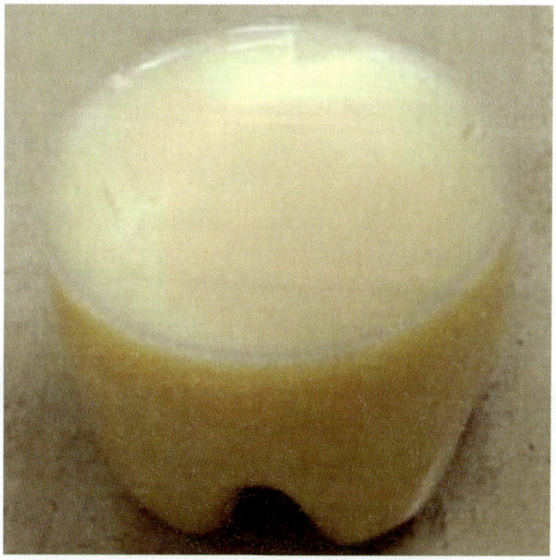

Fig. 5.5: 'Chyle' (the white lymph)—received after paracentesis thoracis from chylothorax

2. *Respiratory function tests:*	*Respiratory function tests:*
• FEV_1 ↓↓	• FEV_1 ↓
• VC normal or ↓	• VC ↓↓
• FEV_1/VC ↓	• FEV_1/VC normal or ↑

Q. How to palpate the trachea?

- The patient stands erect. Standing in front of the patient (may fix his head by your left hand), slide your right index finger from above downwards over trachea (slide from cricoid cartilage as trachea starts from lower border of cricoid cartilage). Henceforth again slide your right index finger in the space between sternomastoid muscle and trachea on both sides, and estimate on which side trachea has shifted (Fig. 5.6).
- In health, trachea remains central or slightly deviated to right side.

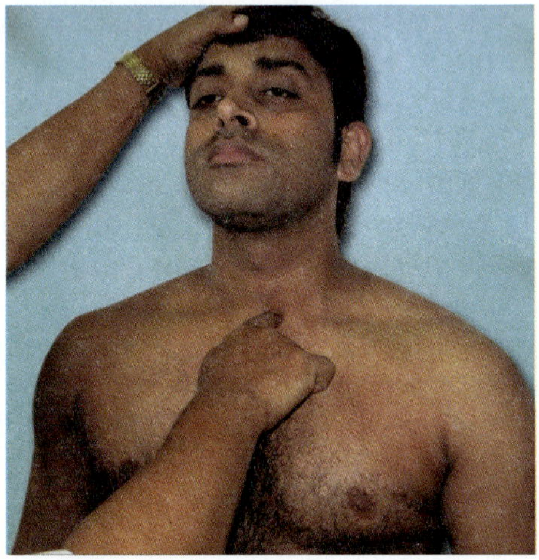

Fig. 5.6: Palpation of the trachea

NB: Upper mediastinum is symbolised by trachea, while the apex beat denotes lower mediastinum. In *dextrocardia* (right-sided heart from birth), the apex beat is on the right side but trachea remains central. However, in *dextroversion* (shifting of heart due to push-pull effects of lung i.e., left-sided pleural effusion, pneumothorax, or right-sided fibrosis or collapse of the lung), both apex beat and trachea shift to the right chest.

Q. What are the causes of shifting of trachea and apex beat?

To same side (pull effect)	*To opposite side (push effect)*
1. Fibrosis of the lung	1. Pleural effusion
2. Collapse of the lung	2. Pneumothorax
3. Thickened pleura (gross)	3. Hydropneumothorax
	4. Empyema thoracis, pyopneumothorax, haemo-pneumothorax

NB: There is no tracheal shifting in consolidation, bronchitis, emphysema, bronchial asthma, interstitial lung disease, bronchiectasis or lung abscess.

Normal intrapleural pressure is –2.5 to –6 mm of Hg. At the end of expiration, it is –2.5 mm of Hg which keeps the lungs apposed with the chest wall. At the height of inspiration the pressure becomes more negative i.e., –6 mm of Hg. It is the positivity or negativity of intrapleural pressure which shifts the trachea in different respiratory diseases i.e., negative intrapleural pressure draws trachea to same side while positive intrapleural pressure pushes trachea to opposite side.

Q. How the movement of the chest is recorded?

Both the palms are placed by the sides of lower rib cage in front in such a way that thumbs of both hands touch each other in the middle with a fold of skin in between the thumbs. Now, note the separation of thumbs at the height of inspiration. Normal expansion of chest in an adult is 5 cm (5–8 cm normally), and expansion of 2 cm or less is regarded as abnormal (Fig. 5.7). The movement can also be assessed at the back and apex of the lung.

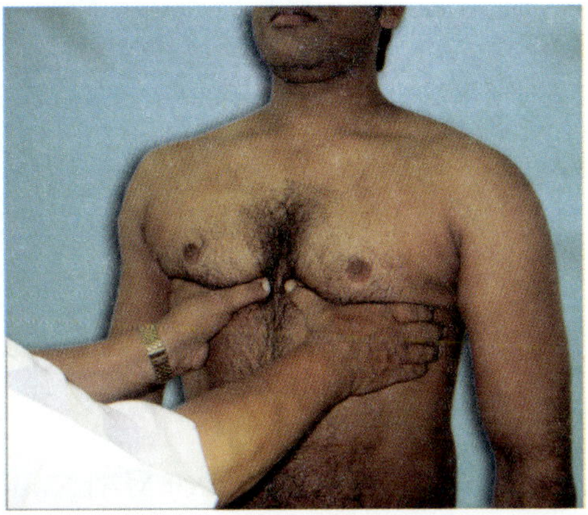

Fig. 5.7: Examining movement of the chest wall— anterior aspect

Q. Causes of restriction of movement of chest.

Unilateral	*Bilateral*
• Trauma in the chest • Pleural effusion, pneumothorax, hydropneumothorax • Consolidation, collapse or fibrosis of the lung	• Emphysema • Diffuse interstitial fibrosis • Hydrothorax (bilateral) • Ankylosing spondylitis, myasthenia gravis, obesity

Q. What are the different types of 'fremitus'?

Fremitus is a vibration felt by the hand when placed on a part of the body, especially over the chest. It determines the conductivity of the underlying tissue, which is picked up by hand. The different types of fremitus are:

- Vocal fremitus (it is the palpation of laryngeal vibrations when the patient speaks 'one, one' or 'ninety-nine, ninety-nine' in a constant tone and voice; always compare with the identical site on opposite side. Vocal fremitus is determined clinically by placing thenar-hypothenar eminences, or ulnar border of right hand over the intercostal spaces in front, sides and back of the chest.)*
- Ronchial fremitus (nothing but palpable rhonchi)
- Friction fremitus (synonymous with palpable pleural rub)
- *Tactile fremitus:*
  - Palpable coarse crepitations
  - Palpable subcutaneous emphysema (presence of air in the subcutaneous tissue due to rib fracture, pneumothorax, gas gangrene, etc.; also known as 'surgical emphysema')
  - Palpable pericardial rub.

*When this laryngeal vibration is auscultated, it is known as vocal resonance.

Q. What is percussion?

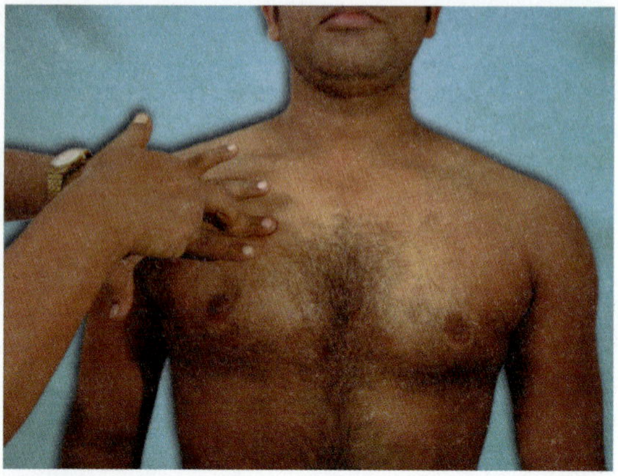
Fig. 5.8: Method of percussion over the anterior chest wall

While doing percussion, dorsal aspect of the middle phalanx of the middle finger of left hand (i.e., pleximeter finger) is kept firmly over a body surface (in the chest wall, it is kept over intercostal spaces i.e., ICS), and is struck suddenly with the tip of the middle finger of right hand (i.e., percussing or plexor finger) perpendicularly. Strike once or twice on the pleximeter finger and the whole movement should come from the wrist joint. Percussion in the chest wall is done in front (along midclavicular line or MCL), lateral wall (along midaxillary line or MAL), and at back along scapular line (a vertical line drawn from inferior angle of scapula). Always percuss from above downwards with comparing the note on the identical site on the opposite side while percussing the chest (Fig. 5.8). Students are advised to practice the method of percussion and to train their ears to recognise the different 'notes' of percussion sincerely from the initial days of their clinical rotation.

Q. What is midclavicular line (MCL)?

MCL is a vertical line drawn from the centre of clavicle i.e., above, the line passes midway between the middle of the suprasternal notch and the acromioclavicular joint; the lower point is the midinguinal point i.e., midpoint between anterior superior iliac spine and symphysis pubis.

Q. Different areas over chest to follow percussion.

A. Anterior chest wall (front bilaterally)—along MCL (Fig. 5.9)
- Clavicular (direct percussion)
- Infraclavicular (clavicle to 3rd rib)
- Mammary (3rd to 6th rib)
- Inframammary (6th rib to 7th ICS)

B. Lateral chest wall (right and left side)—along MAL (Fig. 5.10)
- Axillary (4th ICS to 6th rib; axilla starts from 4th ICS)
- Infra-axillary (6th rib to 8th ICS or lower costal margin)

C. Posterior chest wall (back bilaterally) (Fig. 5.11)
- Suprascapular (above the spine of scapula)
- Interscapular (between the medial border of scapula and spine—from T_2 to T_7)
- Infrascapular (from T_7 to T_{11}—along scapular line)

D. Apical or supraclavicular area: Always done by standing from the back of the patient (right and left side).

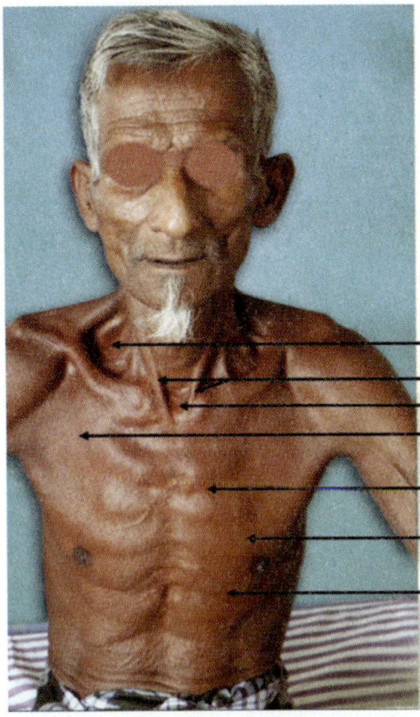

Fig. 5.9: Different areas of chest—the anterior aspect

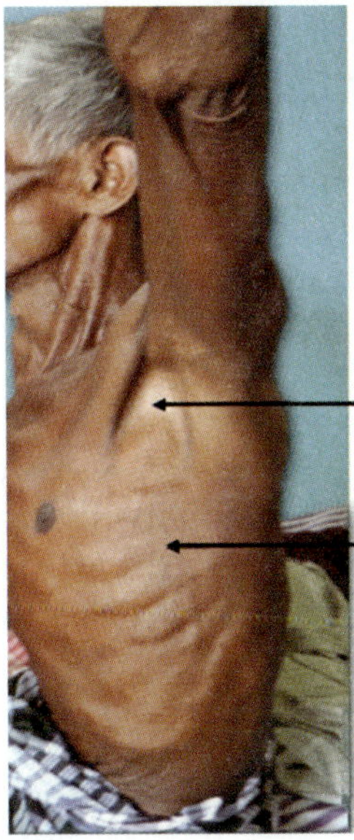

Fig. 5.10: Different areas of chest—the lateral aspect

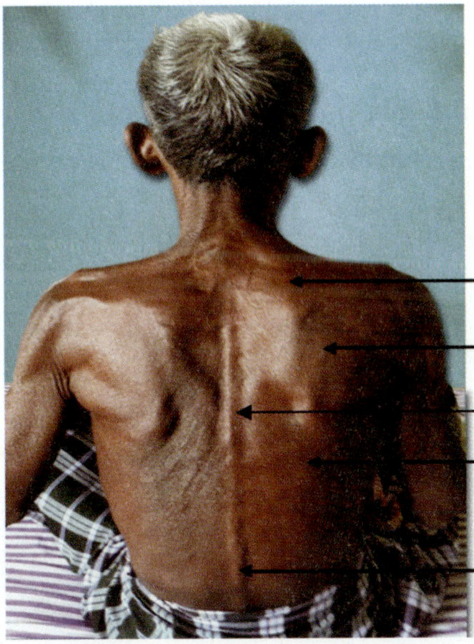

Fig. 5.11: Different areas of chest—the posterior aspect

Q. What is the purpose of percussion?

It is done to know the resonance (i.e., full of air or gas) or dullness (full of solid substance, fluid or blood) of the underlying organ being percussed, or in a broader sense:

A. *To know the:*
- Content (i.e., air or gas-filled)
- Contour (to delineate the border of the organ)
- Depth (to get an idea up to 2 inches depth).

B. *Purpose of percussion over chest:*
- *Conventional percussion (i.e., normal percussion over chest):* Done in front, sides, back and apex (see the format described in the question above).
- *Liver or cardiac dullness (i.e., in emphysema, their dullness is lost, and in liver abscess, upper border of liver dullness is elevated):* Upper border of liver dullness is delineated by percussing over right upper chest from above downwards; while cardiac dullness is losing its importance in modern medicine.
- *Shifting dullness (i.e., in hydropneumothorax):* The air-fluid interface changes its position when percussed in sitting position, after percussing in lying down position.
- *Coin percussion (i.e., in pneumothorax):* A typical metallic sound is audible when a coin is placed over the chest on the side of pneumothorax and being percussed by another coin.
- *Traube's space percussion (to know the tympanicity of fundus of stomach):* The Traube's space tympanicity is lost in splenomegaly, left-sided pleural effusion and carcinoma involving fundus of the stomach.
- *Tidal percussion (to know the movement of diaphragm):* Done at the back below inferior angle of scapula in inspiration and then in expiration to diagnose free diaphragmatic movements; it is also losing its value in clinical medicine.

*The upper border of liver dullness lies in the right 5th ICS in right MCL.

Q. What are the different percussion notes on different organs?

The table shows higher to lower notes from above downwards. The six common notes are:

Resonant note	*Dull note*
1. Tympanitic—abdomen, pneumothorax 2. Hyperresonant—emphysema 3. Resonant—normal lung 4. Impaired resonance—thickened pleura, fibrosis or collapse of the lung	5. Woody dullness—consolidation 6. Stony dullness—pleural effusion, empyema thoracis, 'hydro' part of hydropneumothorax

Q. Tenderness on chest percussion.

1. Empyema thoracis
2. Liver abscess (amoebic or pyogenic)
3. Recent injury to the chest
4. Malignant deposits in ribs.

Q. Outline of points of auscultation of chest.

Stand on the right side of the patient. Ask the patient to:
1. Turn the face to left side.

2. Breathe through open mouth.
3. Breathe regularly and deeply, without having any noise.

Now, put your diaphragm of the stethoscope over the patient's chest (anteriorly, over axilla and posteriorly but try to avoid over bony structures like clavicle, sternum or scapula). Try to compare auscultation with the identical site on the opposite side.

Q. What is the purpose of auscultation over chest?

Remember the 'rule of three' (to note the breath sounds, vocal resonance and adventitious sounds) while auscultating over chest:

Breath sounds	*Vocal resonance*	*Adventitious sounds*
• Vesicular • Bronchial – Tubular – Cavernous – Amphoric • Bronchovesicular (going to be obsolete)	• Bronchophony • Whispering pectoriloquy • Aegophony	• Crackles (older term is crepitations or rales) • Wheezes (older term is rhonchi) • Pleural rub

Q. Points to be noted in auscultation of respiratory system.

Breath sounds, vocal resonance and adventitious sounds are analysed in the following way:

- *Breath sounds* (Fig. 5.12)
  - Vesicular (rustling in character, intensity and duration of inspiration is greater than expiration, and no gap in between inspiration and expiration).
  - Bronchial (blowing, hollow or guttural in character, intensity of expiration is greater than inspiration, and a definite gap is present in between inspiration and expiration). It has three types:
    - Tubular (high-pitched, and found in consolidation, collapse with a patent bronchus, and sometimes above the level of pleural effusion)
    - Cavernous (low-pitched, and found over a superficial, big, empty cavity in lung connected with a patent bronchus)
    - Amphoric [low-pitched with tones and overtones or with a metallic tone, and is found in brochopleural fistula (i.e., open pneumothorax)].
  - Bronchovesicular (the term is rarely used nowadays. Here, inspiration is like vesicular, while expiration is like bronchial in character. In health, it is found over right infraclavicular area and interscapular area (it is the area of 'root or hilum of both the lungs' at the level of T_5, T_6, T_7 vertebrae on both sides). Pathologically, this type may be found in early consolidation or collapse of the lung).
- *Vocal resonance*
  - Quantitative change
    - Increased (bronchophony and whispering pectoriloquy are common in consolidation)
    - Decreased (pleural effusion, pneumothorax, thickened pleura)

  - Qualitative change (nasal intonation is added in vocal resonance and is known as aegophony; common in consolidation and while auscultating above the level of pleural effusion).
- *Adventitious sounds*
  - Crepitations/crackles
    - Fine (early pneumonia, LVF)
    - Coarse (resolving pneumonia, bronchiectasis)
  - Rhonchi/wheezes
    - Monophonic (foreign body or tumour in bronchus)
    - Polyphonic (dynamic compression of bronchus by bronchial asthma or COPD)
  - Pleural rub (found in pleurisy i.e., from tuberculosis, pneumonia, bronchogenic carcinoma).

NB: Go to the bedside: with the help of your teachers, try to be acquainted with the special 'characters' of the sounds like:

- Rustling character (sound like dry leaves blown by the wind) of vesicular breath sound—the normal breath sound in health.
- Blowing or hollow character of bronchial breath sound e.g., consolidation (just practice to auscultate over trachea of a person, and train your ear with the character of the sound, which is just bronchial).
- Nasal intonation of a sound mimicking bleating of a goat in aegophony e.g., in upper border of pleural effusion or consolidation
- Whispering words seem louder and heard distinctly by the clinician in whispering pectoriloquy, e.g., in consolidation. Bronchophony is simply louder vocal resonance.
- Uninterrupted, musical, whistling sound of rhonchi (wheezes) in smaller airway obstruction, e.g., bronchial asthma.
- Discontinuous bubbling or crackling sound of crepitations produced usually by passage of air through exudate-filled bronchi, bronchioles or alveoli, e.g., in acute bronchopneumonia, LVF.
- Leathery, scratchy or creaking sound of friction of visceral and parietal pleura in pleurisy gives rise to pleural rub. It is commonly found over antero-inferior part of lateral chest wall or lower part of back of the chest; better heard by pressing the chest piece of the stethoscope over the chest wall (remember, pericardial rub also increases by pressing the stethoscope).

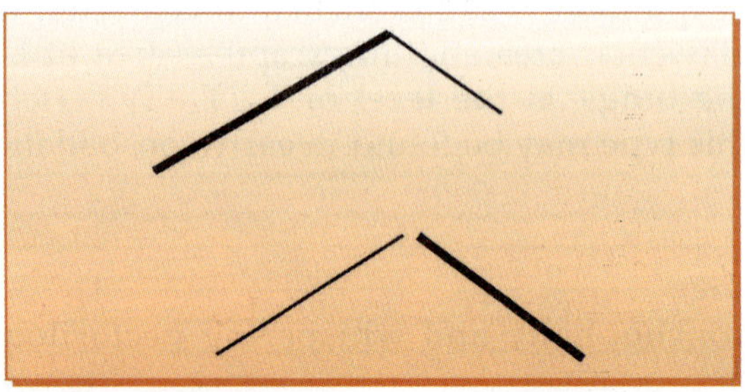

Fig. 5.12: Diagrammatic representation of vesicular (upper) and bronchial (lower) breath sounds

Q. A short note on tuberculosis.

- *Definition:* A chronic systemic infectious disease caused by *Mycobacterium tuberculosis* (MTb) complex. Robert Koch, a German physician and scientist, discovered the bacterium, *Mycobacterium tuberculosis.*
- Different organisms producing tuberculosis
  - *Mycobacterium tuberculosis* (MTb) complex:
    - *Mycobacterium tuberculosis* (commonest)
    - *Mycobacterium bovis*
    - *Mycobacterium africanum*
    - *Mycobacterium microti*
  - Atypical mycobacteria
    - *Mycobacterium avium intracellulare complex* (MAC)
    - *Mycobacterium kansasii*
    - *Mycobacterium fortuitum*
    - *Mycobacterium abscessus.*
- Two types: Pulmonary [primary and post-primary (reactivation or reinfection)] and extrapulmonary tuberculosis. Primary tuberculosis occurs in lungs, intestine and tonsils.
- Sources—Human strain and bovine strain.
- Routes of entry into body—nasal (respiratory droplet infection—commonest), oral, percutaneous, inoculation (direct) and transplacental.
- *Incubation period:* Usually 2–12 weeks.
- Sites of pulmonary and extrapulmonary tuberculosis
  - *Pulmonary:* Lungs.
  - *Extrapulmonary:* Lymph nodes, tonsils, intestine, pleura, peritoneum and meninges, genitourinary, bones and joints, eye, liver, adrenal gland.
- Clinical features of pulmonary tuberculosis
  - Symptoms
    - May be asymptomatic. Evening rise of temperature, anorexia, loss of weight, lassitude and may have palpitation.
    - Persistent cough with sputum production, may have haemoptysis, chest pain (due to pleurisy) and breathlessness.
  - Signs
    - Usually, there is no abnormal physical sign in chest; the earliest sign may be post-tussive crepitations (i.e., crepitations evoked after bouts of cough). Later on signs of tuberculous consolidation, cavitation, pleurisy, pleural effusion, spontaneous pneumothorax, collapse or fibrosis may be found.
- Allergic reactions to primary pulmonary tuberculosis
  - Erythema nodosum (Fig. 5.13).
  - Phlyctenular keratoconjunctivitis.
- Investigations done for diagnosis of pulmonary tuberculosis
  - Blood for Hb% (haemoglobin), TC (total count), DC (differential count), ESR (erythrocyte sedimentation rate).
  - Chest X-ray—PA and lateral view; CT scan of the chest, if required.

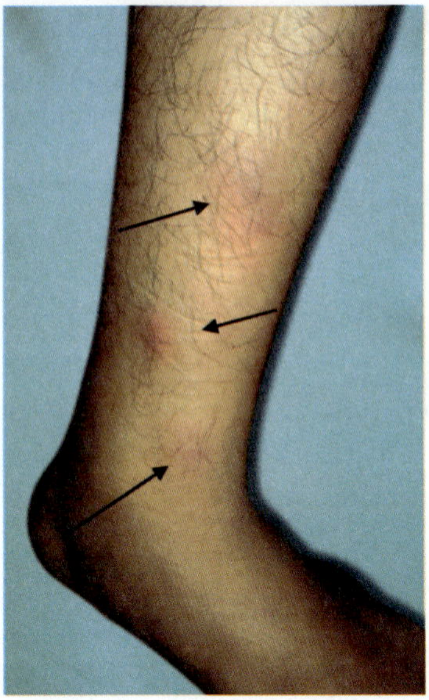

Fig. 5.13: Erythema nodosum (erythematous nodular lesion) in leg commonly seen in tuberculosis, sarcoidosis, leprosy and ulcerative colitis

- Mantoux test (tuberculin test).
- Sputum examination for AFB for consecutive 2 days (as per RNTCP) by Ziehl-Neelsen stain.
- Biopsy of cervical lymph nodes or examination of pleural fluid in selected cases.
- Culture of sputum for *Mycobacterium tuberculosis* in Lowenstein-Jensen media (result within 8–12 weeks).
- BACTEC test: Radioisometric blood culture test, which gives the result in 7 days.
- Polymerase chain reaction (PCR) for tuberculosis from sputum, blood or pleural fluid—to detect mycobacterial DNA.
- ELISA test for tuberculosis (IgG and IgM): Not helpful as the bacilii contains complex antigenic structure.
- Cartridge-based nucleic acid amplification test (CB-NAAT) is known in most countries as GeneXpert test. This is used for early diagnosis of tuberculosis, especially in tuberculosis and HIV co-infections. This test detects DNA sequences specific for *Mycobacterium tuberculosis* and rifampicin resistance by polymerase chain reaction, usually done from sputum samples.

- How to confirm pulmonary tuberculosis?
  - Demonstration of acid-fast bacillus (AFB) in sputum gives the surest diagnosis.
- Histological finding in tuberculosis anywhere in the body (i.e., 'tubercle')
  - Central area of caseation
  - Surrounded by epitheloid cells, Langhans' giant cells and lymphocytes, and
  - Varying degree of fibrosis.
- Common antituberculosis drugs (ATDs)
  - First-line drugs: Rifampicin, INH (isonicotinylhydrazide or isoniazid), pyrazinamide, ethambutol, streptomycin

- Second-line drugs: Ethionamide, prothionamide, amikacin, kanamycin, capreomycin, PAS (para-aminosalicylic acid), cycloserine, fluoroquinolones (ciprofloxacin, levofloxacin), linezolid, macrolides (clarithromycin, azithromycin), thiacitazone (not used nowadays)
- Newer ATDs: Rifabutin, rifapentine, bedaquiline.

❍ What are BCG, RNTCP, DOTS, MDR and XDR-TB in relation to tuberculosis?

- BCG: Bacillus Calmette-Guérin (BCG) vaccine is a life bacterial vaccine primarily used against tuberculosis, and is commonly used in those countries where tuberculosis is common. Tuberculosis is an endemic disease in developing countries like India, China and Africa (due to poor sanitation, overcrowding and poor public health measures). Usually BCG vaccine is given soon after birth or during the first 2 weeks of life. This vaccine protects against serious tuberculous disease (e.g., tuberculous meningitis or miliary tuberculosis) for up to 15 years after vaccination.
- RNTCP (Revised National Tuberculosis Control Programme): RNTCP is the state-run tuberculosis control initiative of the Government of India with a vision of achieving a 'Tuberculosis-free India'.
- DOTS (Directly Observed Treatment Short-course): DOTS chemotherapy is the backbone of RNTCP in India. The ATDs are given in an intermittent manner, under direct supervision of health personnel in a dosage of three times per week. For DOTS, patients are divided into three categories (Category I, II, III).
- MDR-TB: Multi-drug resistance tuberculosis is the resistance to INH plus rifampicin with or without other drug resistance.
- XDR-TB: Extensively drug-resistant tuberculosis (a rare type of high level MDR-TB) that is resistant to INH, rifampicin, fluoroquinolones, and at least one injectable second-line drugs (i.e., amikacin, kanamycin, or capreomycin).

*Tuberculosis is treated by 'multidrug treatment' to prevent drug resistance and achieve better patient's compliance. Conventionally, fixed dose combination (FDC) are used i.e., ATDs are present in fixed amount in a single tablet.

Q. Model description of clinical signs in common respiratory diseases.

1. *Pleural effusion (left-sided)*

❍ General survey: Patient prefers to lie in left lateral decubitus.

❍ *Inspection:*

- Diminished movement of chest in left side
- Intercostal spaces are full in left side of chest
- Apical impulse cannot be localised.

❍ *Palpation:*

- Less movement in left side of chest is corroborated
- Trachea and apex beat deviated to right side of chest
- Diminished vocal fremitus on left side of chest.

❍ *Percussion:* Stony dullness (i.e., dullness on percussion plus feeling of increased resistance by the percussing finger) on left side of chest which does not alter with change of posture i.e., shifting dullness is absent.

- *Auscultation:*
  - Diminished vesicular or absent breath sound on left side
  - Diminished or absent vocal resonance on left side
  - No adventitious sound heard i.e., rhonchi, crepitations or pleural rub is absent.

NB: The right side of chest is normal in all respect.

Rarely, bronchial breath sound may be heard at the upper border of moderate pleural effusion; in that situation, vocal resonance is increased in that part of the chest.

For earliest radiological detection of pleural effusion, 300 ml of fluid is required, while for earliest clinical detection the amount is 500 ml.

Q. Common causes of pleural effusion.

- Exudative: Pneumonia, tuberculosis, bronchogenic carcinoma, pulmonary infarction, lymphoma and leukaemias, SLE or other connective tissue diseases, Meig's syndrome.
- Transudative (called hydrothorax, which is often bilateral): CCF, nephrotic syndrome, cirrhosis of liver, hypoproteinaemia with severe anaemia (i.e., malnutrition), pericardial effusion, myxoedema.

NB: Haemothorax (from malignancy, trauma, tuberculosis, bleeding diathesis) have similar clinical finding like pleural effusion.

2. *Pneumothorax (right-sided)*

- *General survey:* Patient prefers to lie in right lateral decubitus. A water-seal drainage system is seen from upper part of right chest.
- *Inspection:*
  - Respiration: Rate is 28/minute
  - Diminished movement of chest in right side
  - Intercostal spaces are full in right side of chest
  - Apical impulse is seen much left to left nipple (i.e., deviated to left side).
- *Palpation:*
  - Less movement in right side of chest is corroborated
  - Trachea and apex beat deviated to left side of chest
  - Diminished vocal fremitus on right side of chest.
- *Percussion:* Tympanitic note on all over the right chest. Upper border of liver dullness is present in right 6th ICS in right MCL (normally, it is present in right 5th ICS in right MCL). Shifting dullness is absent.
- *Auscultation:*
  - Diminished vesicular or absent breath sound on right side
  - Diminished or absent vocal resonance on right side
  - No adventitious sound heard i.e., rhonchi, crepitations or pleural rub is absent
  - Coin sound: Present on right chest.

NB: The left side of chest is normal in all respect.

3. *Hydropneumothorax (right-sided)*

- *General survey:* A water-seal drainage system is seen from upper part of right chest.

- *Inspection:*
  - Respiration: Rate is 30/minute
  - Diminished movement of chest in right side
  - Intercostal spaces are full in right side of chest.
- *Palpation:*
  - Less movement in right side of chest is corroborated
  - Trachea and apex beat deviated to left side of chest
  - Diminished vocal fremitus on right side of chest.
- *Percussion:* In sitting position of the patient, the percussion note on air-containing upper part of right chest is tympanitic, while fluid-containing lower part is stony dull. Upper border of liver dullness is present in right 4th ICS in right MCL (the fluid in hydropneumothorax covers the actual upper border of liver).

  There is a horizontal fluid level detected all over the right chest on percussion.

  Shifting dullness is present in right chest i.e., change of fluid level is detected on change of posture.
- *Auscultation:*
  - Diminished vesicular or absent breath sound on right side. There may be bronchial (amphoric) breath sound in right chest in bronchopleural fistula.
  - Diminished or absent vocal resonance on right side. Vocal resonance is increased in the presence of bronchial breath sound.
  - No adventitious sound heard i.e., rhonchi, crepitations or pleural rub is absent. Occasional tinkling crepitations are found.
  - Succussion splash—audible when stethoscope is placed in air-fluid junction (detected by percussion) and the patient is shaken from side to side (sound mimicking splashing sound of intact coconut).
  - Coin sound: Present on right chest in the upper part.

NB: The left side of chest is normal in all respect.

4. *Pneumonic consolidation (left-sided)*

- General survey: Propped-up decubitus at 45° in bed. The patient is a bit breathless.
- *Inspection:*
  - Respiration: Rate is 36/minute
  - Diminished movement of chest in lower part of left side
  - Apical impulse is seen approximately 3 inches left to midline (i.e., no shifting).
- *Palpation:*
  - Less movement in left side of lower chest is corroborated
  - Trachea and apex beat are normal in position (i.e., no mediastinal shifting)
  - Increased vocal fremitus on left side of lower chest.
- *Percussion:* Dullness (woody) found on percussion over lower part of left chest.
- *Auscultation:*
  - Bronchial (tubular) breath sound on left lower chest.

- Increased vocal resonance (bronchophony and whispering pectoriloquy) on left side (lower part). Aegophony is audible in left chest.
- Adventitious sound heard i.e., pleural rub is present; a few crepitations are audible but rhonchi are absent.

NB: The right side of chest is normal in all respect.

Decoding Abbreviations

URTI	Upper respiratory tract infection
LRTI	Lower respiratory tract infection
COPD	Chronic obstructive pulmonary disease
ILD	Interstitial lung disease
FEV_1	Forced expiratory volume in first second
VC	Vital capacity
ELISA	Enzyme-linked immunosorbent assay
ICS	Intercostal space
AFB	Acid-fast bacillus.

Chapter

6

Gastrointestinal (GI) and Hepatobiliary System

SCHEME OF SYSTEMIC EXAMINATION: AN OVERVIEW

I. Examination of upper GI tract: Lips, teeth, gum, cheek (buccal mucous membrane), tongue, tonsils, palate, breath, and oropharynx; oesophagus cannot be examined.

II. Examination of the abdomen

A. *Inspection:*

- Shape of abdomen and appearance of skin [striae, ulcer, sinus, pigmentation, puncture marks, bluish discolouration around umbilicus (Cullen's sign) and bluish-red discoloration of flanks in acute pancreatitis (Grey Turner's sign)]
- Flanks—full (in ascites) or not
- Any localised lump seen or not
- Venous prominence (examine in standing position of the patient after coughing)
- Movement of the abdomen (respiratory movements, peristalsis and pulsation)
- Umbilicus (discolouration, nodules, venous prominence, sinus, hernia, and granuloma in and around umbilicus)
- Hernial sites, groin and hairs (e.g., pubic hair).

B. *Palpation:*

- Superficial palpation: Surface temperature, tenderness, consistency, localised lump, pulsation, divarication of recti while rising from bed, fluid thrill, direction of venous flow, cough impulse at hernia orifices
- Deep palpation: Palpation of liver, spleen, kidneys, gall bladder, colon, testes (though remain outside of the abdomen), urinary bladder, aorta, any lump or mass, hernia sites, deep tender spots e.g., McBurney's point or epigastric point.

C. *Percussion:*

- General note of abdomen (in health, there is tympanitic note)
- Upper border of liver dullness (in health, in the right 5th ICS in right MCL)
- Shifting dullness (i.e., to diagnose ascites)
- Percussion over urinary bladder (if distended).

D. *Auscultation:*

- Bowel sounds (i.e., peristaltic sounds)

- Hepatic or splenic rub
- Venous hum
- Bruit
- Foetal heart sound (in pregnancy).

III. Per rectal examination

Q. Mention the common presentations (chief complaints and H/o present illness) in GI and hepatobiliary system.

The patients having complaints of GI and hepatobiliary system commonly present with:

1. Anorexia (loss of appetite), dyspepsia (medical term which signifies indigestion; it may be reflux-like, ulcer-like or dysmotility-like).
2. Dysphagia (difficulty in swallowing) or odynophagia (painful deglutition).
3. Nausea (feeling or desire to vomit), vomiting, hiccough.
4. Heartburn (a sense of hot, burning, retrosternal discomfort)—in gastro-oesophageal reflux disease (GERD), where the oesophageal mucosa is exposed to acidic gastroduodenal contents for a prolonged period.
5. Jaundice (e.g., yellow eyes) or yellow urine.
6. Pain abdomen.
7. Haematemesis, melaena, haematochezia, bleeding per rectum.
8. Flatulence and/or flatus (too much gaseous distension is due to aerophagia or air ingestion, malabsorption or lactase deficiency; aerophagia is a repetitive pattern of swallowing or ingesting air, and belching).
9. Swelling in the abdomen (collection of fluid or presence of a tumour).
10. Constipation, diarrhoea, dysentery, alteration of bowel habit (sometimes, point towards carcinoma of the rectum), or mucus in the stool.
11. *Others:*
    a. Fever (intestinal tuberculosis, amoebic liver abscess, abdominal lymphoma, subphrenic abscess, spontaneous bacterial peritonitis, cholangitis).
    b. Loss of weight (intra-abdominal malignancy, tuberculosis, or lymphoma).
    c. Oral ulcers or halitosis (i.e., bad breath).
    d. Confusion, drowsiness, or inversion of sleep rhythm (hepatic encephalopathy i.e., neuropsychiatric manifestations from cirrhosis of liver).
    e. Low urine output or oliguria from hepato-renal syndrome (i.e., developing from cirrhosis of liver).
    f. Pedal oedema (with features of malnutrition and vitamin deficiency from severe anorexia or malabsorption).

Q. Queries in past, family, personal and treatment history in GI system.

Past history	*Family history*	*Personal history*	*Treatment history*
1. Jaundice 2. Blood transfusion (e.g., viral hepatitis B and C), recent tattooing	1. Any member of family suffering from similar type of illness (e.g., Wilson's disease)? 2. Family H/o tuber-	1. Dose of alcohol consumption (type, quantity with duration) 2. 'Substance abuse',	1. Drug history (rifampicin, INH, oral contraceptive pills, NSAID, or any herbal remedies)—NSAID

3. Alcohol consumption 4. Tuberculosis 5. Haematemesis or melaena 6. Fever (e.g., tuberculosis) 7. H/o exposure to STD	culosis, food poisoning, viral hepatitis 3. H/o consanguineous marriage in case of inherited metabolic liver disease (e.g., α_1-antitrypsin deficiency) 4. H/o familial polyposis coli, carcinoma of colon	especially IV drug abuse (e.g., hepatitis B and C infection) 3. Dietary habits	may induce haematemesis or melaena; rifampicin and INH are hepatotoxic 2. Acupuncture (for hepatitis B) 3. Vaccination against hepatitis B

Q. Possible causes of severe anorexia.

Any physical illness, infective illness, malignancy or psychological illness may give rise to anorexia. Marked anorexia is common in:

- Acute viral hepatitis
- Tuberculosis (especially gastrointestinal or pulmonary)
- Malignancy (especially stomach), lymphomas, leukaemias
- Any chronic illness like chronic renal failure (CRF), CCF, cirrhosis of liver
- Psychogenic e.g., severe depression, emotional upset, anorexia nervosa
- Drugs like chloroquine, digitalis, quinine, metronidazole.

Q. Common causes of halitosis (foul breath).

Bad breath is common in:

- Bad oral hygiene, food debris in between teeth, chain smoking
- Caries tooth, gingivitis
- Atrophic rhinitis
- Carcinoma of the tongue
- Bronchiectasis, lung abscess
- Diabetic ketoacidosis, renal failure, hepatic coma
- Intestinal obstruction.

Q. Causes of 'oral ulcers' in clinical medicine.

Oral ulcers, some are painless while some are painful, are prevalent in:

- Aphthous ulcers (idiopathic, superficial, painful ulcers)
- Candidiasis, herpes simplex infection
- Systemic lupus erythematosus (SLE) may have painless ulcers in palate, while painful oral ulcers are seen in Behçet's disease
- Carcinoma, leukaemia, Crohn's disease
- Use of cytotoxic drugs (i.e., for treatment of cancer) (Fig. 6.1)
- Kaposi's sarcoma, lichen planus, pemphigus, Stevens-Johnson syndrome.

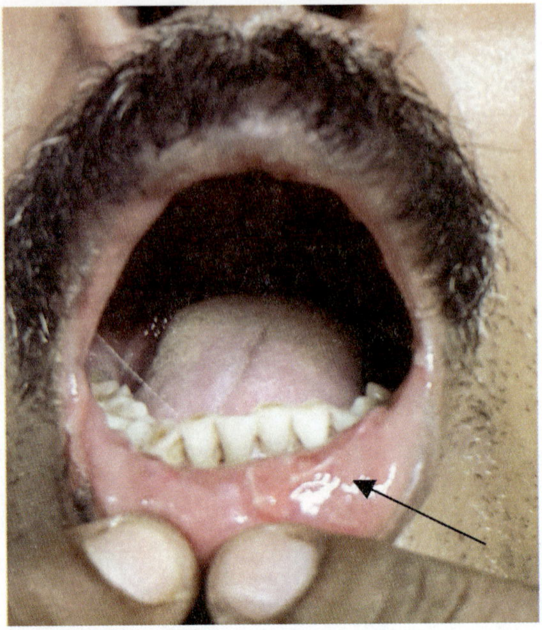

Fig. 6.1: Ulcers inside mouth and over lower lip as a result of cytotoxic drug therapy

Q. How tongue helps in diagnosing diseases in clinical medicine?

Previously, tongue was thought to be 'mirror of GI tract' only but it is now regarded as mirror of dysfunction of all systems in human body. Now examine tongue in the following ways:

1. Ask the patient to protrude the tongue: The patient cannot protrude it in 'tongue tie' (or ankyloglossia), malignancy of the tongue and bilateral XIIth cranial nerve paralysis.
2. Tremor (e.g., in anxiety neurosis, thyrotoxicosis) in tongue can be seen on protrusion, while fasciculation (e.g., in motor neuron disease or MND) is seen while tongue rests on floor of the mouth.
3. Large tongue is common in acromegaly, myxoedema, cretinism and Down's syndrome (macroglossia), while small tongue (microglossia) is seen in cerebral diplegia, MND, bulbar and pseudobulbar palsy.
4. Dry (dehydration, xerostomia) and moist (sialorrhoea, heavy metal poisoning) tongue.
5. Yellow (jaundice), pale (severe anaemia), blue (cyanosis), bluish-red (polycythemia), magenta-coloured (riboflavin deficiency, Fig. 6.2), black (ingestion of bismuth, charcoal, or Addison's disease), 'furred' (heavy smoking, sore throat), 'bald' (total loss of papillae is common in pernicious anaemia, tropical sprue) tongue, and candidiasis of tongue (common in immunodeficiency, Fig. 6.3).
6. Spastic (pseudobulbar palsy) and flaccid (bulbar palsy) tongue.
7. Raw-beefy (red, swollen and painful tongue in nicotinic acid and vitamin B_{12} deficiency), angry-looking (central coating with pointed tip in typhoid fever), geographical (denuded and migrating red patches due to loss of papillae, and of no

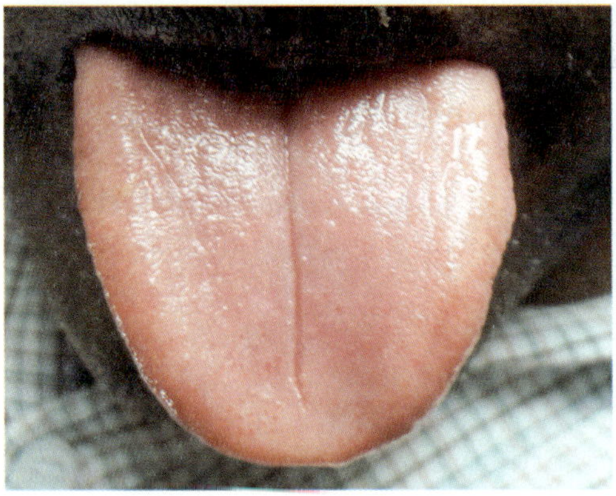

Fig. 6.2: Magenta-coloured tongue in riboflavin deficiency

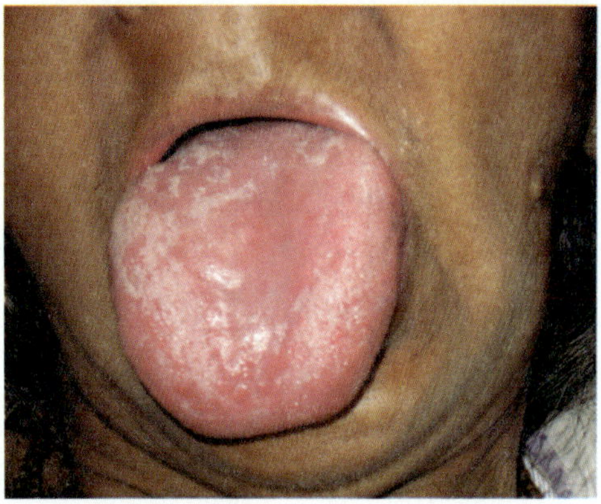

Fig. 6.3: Candidiasis of tongue in a patient of diabetes mellitus

clinical significance, Fig. 6.4), and strawberry and raspberry (scarlet fever) tongue; mushroom-like growth (malignancy of the tongue, Fig. 6.5), and ulcers (aphthous ulcer, Behçet's disease) in the tongue. Haematoma in the tongue may be seen in accidental tongue bite or coagulation disorders (Fig. 6.6).

8. Deviation of tongue while protruding and loss of power of tongue are seen in XIIth cranial nerve paralysis. Loss of taste sensation is found in VIIth (anterior two-thirds) and IXth (posterior one-third) cranial nerve paralysis.

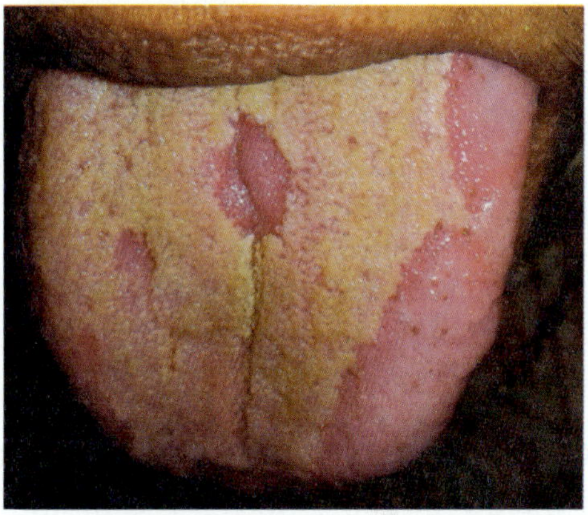

Fig. 6.4: Geographical tongue

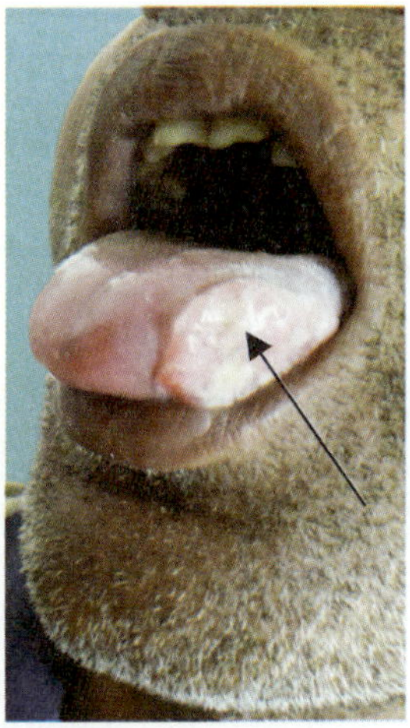

Fig. 6.5: Squamous cell carcinoma of the tongue

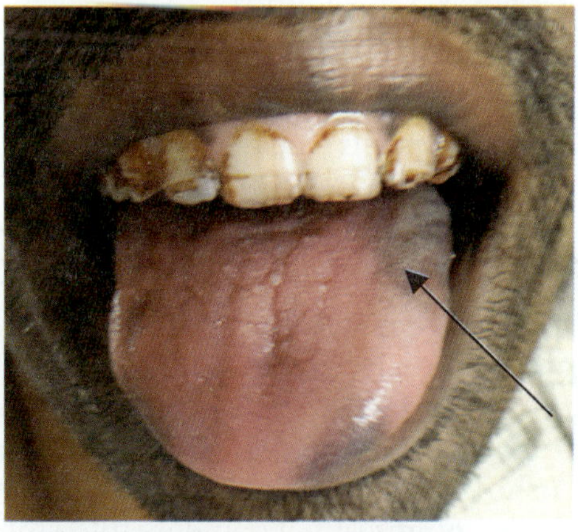

Fig. 6.6: Haematoma in the tongue in coagulation disorders; blood-stained teeth are evident

Q. Do you know the different types of dysphagia?

Difficulty in swallowing is of two types:
- Oropharyngeal (due to neuromuscular disorder): Bulbar and pseudobulbar palsy, myasthenia gravis.
- Oesophageal: Malignancy of oesophagus, peptic stricture, achalasia cardia, diffuse oesophageal spasm, mediastinal growth mechanically causing obstruction in oesophagus.

Q. Causes of persistent vomiting.

Nausea and vomiting (protracted) are commonly encountered in:
- Acute viral hepatitis, increased intracranial pressure (ICP), acute labyrinthitis, Ménière's disease, migraine, meningitis.
- CRF or uraemia, diabetic ketoacidosis, AMI, chronic alcoholism, hyperemesis gravidarum, drug-induced (e.g., digoxin), functional vomiting (psychogenic).
- Surgical: Acute pancreatitis, acute cholecystitis, intestinal obstruction, colics.

NB:
1. 'Pyloric stenosis' (or gastric outlet obstruction) is an intestinal obstruction at pylorus of stomach where the patients complain of projectile vomiting which is copious in amount, offensive and contains food taken 1–2 days back. It is diagnosed by a diffuse swelling in upper abdomen, visible peristalsis from left to right hypochondrium and succussion splash (splashing sound audible after shaking the patient's abdomen).
2. Vomiting of raised ICP occurs in the morning. It occurs suddenly without preceding nausea (i.e., projectile vomiting).

Q. 'Red flag' or 'alarming signs' in gastroenterology are:

Patients present with these symptoms/signs should immediately be investigated, especially if ≥ 55 years:
- Loss of weight (progressive)
- Anorexia (profound)
- Persistent dysphagia
- Protracted jaundice
- Haemaemesis/melaena
- Chronic diarrhoea.

Q. What is 'peptic ulcer disease (PUD)'?

PUD is a general term for ulcers that occur in the lower part of oesophagus, stomach (gastric ulcer) or duodenum (duodenal ulcer).

The aetiology of PUD is *Helicobacter pylori*, NSAID (non-steroidal anti-inflammatory drugs, e.g., aspirin), smoking, stress ulcer (e.g., Curling's ulcer from severe burn or Cushing's ulcer from raised ICP), gastrinomas (Zollinger-Ellison syndrome), or reflux of bile and intestinal contents into stomach.

Helicobacter pylori is a spiral, Gram-negative, flagellated, urease-producing bacillus which is transmitted through oral-oral or faecal-oral (enters through mouth by ingestion of contaminated food or drinks) route. It plays a vital role in the development of gastritis (chronic antral gastritis), peptic ulcer disease, gastric adenocarcinoma and MALToma (mucosa-associated lymphoid tissue—lymphoma) in human being.

The peptic ulcer is a break in superficial epithelial cells which is going deep into muscularis mucosae, while erosions are superficial breaks in the mucosa only.

Q. Enumerate the medical (non-surgical) causes of pain abdomen.

The medical causes of abdominal pain are:

- Peptic ulcer
- Acute pancreatitis
- Acute pyelonephritis
- Referred pain in abdomen: AMI (i.e., inferior wall myocardial infarction), basal pleurisy, caries spine (tuberculosis of the spine), herpes zoster infection (over skin)
- Miscellaneous: Diabetic ketoacidosis, adrenal crisis, hypercalcaemia, acute intermittent porphyria, Henoch-Schönlein purpura, sickle cell anaemia, hereditary angioedema.

NB: Pain arising out of acute appendicitis, acute cholecystitis, diverticulitis, ovarian cyst, ruptured ectopic pregnancy, pseudopancreatic cyst, biliary/renal/intestinal colic, perforation of an ulcer, or intestinal obstruction is of surgical/gynaecological interest.

Q. How pain abdomen is analysed?

Abdomen is regarded as a Pandora's box and it is often very difficult to diagnose pain abdomen in an agonising patient who does not allow examination of abdomen properly. However, an enquiry regarding pain abdomen should be made on:

- Site, e.g., epigastrium (slightly right for gastric ulcer, and slightly left for duodenal ulcer), right hypochondrium (e.g., acute cholecystitis), or right iliac fossa (acute appendicitis).
- Duration i.e., how long the patient is suffering from pain i.e., enquire for 'periodicity of attacks'.
- Time of onset and mode of onset—in gastric ulcer pain starts almost instantaneously after taking food, while in duodenal ulcer pain usually starts 2–2½ hours after taking food (i.e., when the stomach becomes empty of food, and is known as 'hunger pain'). The sudden onset of severe pain in abdomen which is rapidly progressive to be generalised indicate a hollow viscus perforation.
- Radiation: Epigastric pain radiating to back is common in pancreatitis. Colicky pain radiating from loin to groin and genitalia are diagnostic of renal colic.
- Relationship with food (e.g, in gastric ulcer, food initiates pain, while in duodenal ulcer food relieves pain).
- Character: Is the pain burning, dull-aching, agonizing (e.g., acute pancreatitis), or gripping (colicky pain) in nature; mild or severe?
- Aggravating factors: The pain of acute gastritis may aggravate after an alcoholic debauch. Abdominal pain which is accelerated by movement or coughing suggests inflammation (e.g., acute appendicitis, acute cholecystitis)

- Relieving factors: The pain may be relieved spontaneously, after meal, or after medication. Colicky pain is relieved by drawing the knees up to the abdomen and pressing the knees over the painful area during the painful spasms.
- Severity: It often depends on the pain threshold of the patient. However, severe excruciating pain, not relieved well even by opioids, points towards ischaemic vascular events like bowel infarction.
- Effect of pressure over pain: In colicky pain, pressure gives relief, while in inflammatory pain, application of pressure aggravates pain.
- Associated symptoms like nausea, vomiting, belching, gaseous distension of abdomen, loose motion, fever should be carefully accounted. Presence of breathlessness or palpitation points towards non-organic causes (i.e., functional pain).

Q. Characteristics of pain in peptic ulcer, acute pancreatitis and colic of any origin.

Character of each and every pain arising out of different organs are different. Let us have a look into it:

- *Peptic ulcer:* Episodic, localised to epigastrium, usually nocturnal, pointing sign positive (patent can pinpoint the site of pain), and having relationship with food. Upper gastrointestinal endoscopy can help visualising the ulcer (previously, barium meal examination of stomach and duodenum used to be done).
- *Acute pancreatitis:* Sudden onset, acute agonizing pain in epigastrium which pierces deep into the back; pain is often relieved by stooping forward position. Alcohol intake accelerates the pain. Profuse vomiting occurs, which may be associated with shock and collapse. Elevated serum amylase and lipase along with positive CT (computerised tomography) scan findings of pancreas clinch the diagnosis.
- *Colicky pain:* It is the sudden appearance of gripping pain, which comes and goes intermittently, and ultimately passes off as suddenly as it came. Common examples are biliary colic (a calculus or stone trying to cross common bile duct), renal colic (a calculus or stone trying to cross the ureter), or intestinal colic (e.g., infective enteritis with diarrhoea). Ultrasonography (USG) of abdomen can localise the calculus.

Q. Different causes of constipation.

It is the infrequent passage of hard stools which is very difficult to evacuate or a stool frequency <3 times/week. Constipation is commonly due to:

- Lack of physical activity, faulty toilet habit, less intake of dietary fibres.
- Chronic idiopathic constipation (most common cause and probably a colonic transit disorder).
- Surgical: Anal fissure, proctitis, carcinoma of the rectum, intestinal obstruction, acute abdomen.
- Metabolic: Hypokalaemia, hypercalcaemia, lead poisoning, autonomic neuropathy (e.g., diabetes mellitus).
- Disturbed motility: Irritable bowel syndrome (IBS), parkinsonism, pregnancy, spinal injury, cerebrovascular accidents (CVA).
- Drug-induced: Antidepressants (e.g., amitriptyline), anticholinergics, iron supplementation, codeine.

Q. What is diarrhoea and dysentery?

Diarrhoea and dysentery are very common gastrointestinal disorders. They are defined in the following ways:

- *Diarrhoea:* Frequent passage of liquid or unformed stool, or increase in the daily stool weight >200 g is diarrhoea. Diarrhoea is divided into acute (<2 weeks), persistent (2–4 weeks), and chronic (>4 weeks) according to duration.
  - Acute diarrhoea: Mainly comprises infective causes like bacterial (*Escherichia coli*, Salmonella, Shigella, staphylococcal enterocolitis, *Campylobacter jejuni*, *Vibrio cholerae*), viral (Rota), parasitic (*Entamoeba histolytica* or amoebiasis, *Giardia lamblia*), fungal (Histoplasma) and drug-induced (amoxicillin, erythromycin, colchicine, lactulose, etc). Acute diarrhoea, if not treated in time, may lead to hyponatraemia, hypokalaemia and metabolic acidosis.
  - Chronic diarrhoea: IBS (commonest cause), inflammatory bowel disease or IBD (ulcerative colitis and Crohn's disease), chronic pancreatitis, malabsorption syndrome, lactase deficiency (produces milk intolerance), celiac disease, intestinal tuberculosis, or persisting acute infections e.g., salmonellosis, giardiasis, amoebic colitis, hookworm infestations.
- *Dysentery:* It is characterised by diarrhoea with passage of blood and mucus with stool, and clinically manifested by colicky abdominal pain, fever and tenesmus (feeling of incomplete evacuation with a constant desire for defecation) as a result of acute inflammation of large gut. Basically it is of two types: Amoebic (by *Entamoeba histolytica*) and bacillary dysentery (shigellosis).

  Other than dysentery, **bloody diarrhoea** may also be due to IBD, campylobacter, *Escherichia coli* or *Clostridium difficile* infection.

NB: Irritable bowel syndrome (IBS), the commonest gastrointestinal disorder in clinical practice, is a non-organic, functional bowel disorder characterised by alteration of bowel habit (diarrhoea or constipation, or alternating diarrhoea and constipation), and pain in the abdomen (colicky or crampy pain, especially felt at lower abdomen, which is relieved after defecation).

Q. Define steatorrhoea and creatorrhoea.

These are defined as:

- *Steatorrhoea:* There is presence of fat in the stool, which is manifested by greasy, pale, frothy, bulky, offensive and oily stool. The stool is often difficult to flush from the toilet pan but once cleaned, it floats on the water of the pan. It is common in fat malabsorption in obstructive jaundice.
- *Creatorrhoea:* The passage of undigested muscle fibres (i.e., protein) in the stool, as seen in certain cases of pancreatic disease.

Q. What is haematemesis and what are the common causes?

Vomiting of blood is haematemesis; it is due to upper GI tract bleeding. The common causes are:

- Peptic ulcer (i.e., chronic duodenal ulcer): Most common cause
- Erosive gastritis (or gastric erosion i.e., NSAID-induced)

- Ruptured oesophageal varices (e.g., from cirrhosis of liver)
- Carcinoma of the stomach (coffee-ground vomitus) or oesophagus
- Mallory-Weiss syndrome (a vertical tear in cardia of stomach due to vomiting)
- Peptic oesophagitis
- Arteriovenous malformations in stomach
- Blood dyscrasias (e.g., leukaemia), anticoagulant therapy
- Miscellaneous: Uraemia, corrosive ingestion.

NB: So, in a patient of upper GI bleeding, look for shock (ashen-grey pallor, cold and clammy extremities, thready pulse with tachycardia, and hypotension), anaemia (anaemia takes some time to develop after acute blood loss), and stigmata of chronic liver disease, if there is any (jaundice, splenomegaly and ascites).

Q. What is melaena?

Melaena is the 'altered blood in stool' with characteristics of:
- Black, tarry, sticky stool (lysis of RBC → acid haematin → black stool)
- Offensive (foul smelling)
- Semisolid in consistency
- Red coloured fluid comes out from the stool after addition of water
- Usually associated with dizziness or syncopal attack during defecation.

NB: Haemaetemesis and melaena signifies bleeding from upper gut i.e., *proximal to ligament of Treitz*. The causes mentioned in haematemesis are also the causes of melaena too. Remember, black stool may also be due to iron ingestion (gives rise to hard stool), or after use of drugs like bismuth, licorice or charcoal.

Q. What is haematochezia (synonym with rectal bleeding)?

It is the passage of bright red blood per rectum mixed with or without stool. The bleeding in haematochezia occurs in the gut, *distal to ligament of Treitz*.

Q. Blood in stool—how a patient may present?

Blood in stool may remain in three forms like:
- Frank blood or haematochezia
- Altered blood or melaena
- Occult blood or invisible blood, which can be detected chemically.

Q. Causes of haematochezia or frank blood, or lower GI bleeding.

The common causes of lower GI tract bleeding are:
- Haemorrhoids, anal fissure and fistula, trauma, proctitis
- IBD (i.e., ulcerative colitis and Crohn's disease)
- Malignancy of the colon and rectum
- Diverticulitis, colo-rectal polyp, angiodysplasia of the colon
- 'Gay bowel syndrome' in male homosexuals.

Q. Some facts worth to remember in relation to GI bleeding.

1. To produce clinical signs, a patient of haematemesis should bleed minimally 500 ml of blood.
2. In GI bleeding, postural hypotension is produced after 1500 ml of blood loss.
3. In GI bleeding, shock is developed after 3000 ml of blood loss.
4. For an episode of 'single black stool' i.e., melaena, minimally 60 ml blood is to be lost and it should remain in intestine for at least 8 hours.

Q. How patients of IBD and intestinal tuberculosis presents?

At the onset, the clinician is confused between these diagnoses, especially in India but each of the disease has specific features to diagnose:

A. *Inflammatory bowel disease (IBD):* Diarrhoea with blood and mucus, sometimes associated with lower abdominal pain are the common presenting features. Constitutional features like malaise, lethargy, anorexia, nausea, vomiting, low-grade fever and loss of weight are more pronounced in Crohn's disease in comparison to ulcerative colitis.

B. *Intestinal tuberculosis:* Intestinal tuberculosis is very common in India. The pathological types of the disease are: Ulcerative (at ileo-caecal region), hyperplastic, and mixed. The patient may present with:
   - Signs of tuberculous toxaemia—anorexia, loss of weight, fever, night sweats
   - Pain in the abdomen
   - Alternating constipation with diarrhoea
   - Moving balls of air in the abdomen, gaseous distension
   - Ascites.

Q. What are the causes of viral hepatitis?

Necro-inflammation of the hepatic parenchyma is hepatitis, which is commonly due to viral hepatitis, drug (e.g., pyrazinamide)/poison (e.g., copper sulphate, mushroom)/alcohol-induced, or autoimmune in nature. Causes of viral hepatitis are:

- *Common viruses:*
  - Hepatitis A virus
  - Hepatitis B virus
  - Hepatitis C virus
  - Hepatitis D virus
  - Hepatitis E virus.
- *Less common viruses*
  - Herpes simplex virus
  - Cytomegalovirus
  - Epstein-Barr virus
  - Yellow fever virus
  - Coxsackie B virus.

NB: Other infective causes of hepatitis are Weil's disease (leptospira) and toxoplasma. Hepatitis A, C, D, E viruses are RNA virus, while hepatitis B is a DNA virus. Acute hepatitis is caused by hepatitis A, B ± D, and E virus, whereas hepatitis B, C and D are notorious for chronicity. Hepatitis C is the commonest cause of post-transfusion hepatitis. Hepatitis C virus very rarely produces acute hepatitis.

Route of entry: By faecal-oral route: Hepatitis A and E, parenteral route: Hepatitis B, C, and D.

Q. How a patient of acute viral hepatitis presents (enumerate symptoms and signs)?

The patient may present in any of the three stages like prodromal stage (fever, anorexia, nausea, vomiting, distaste for smoking, urticaria and arthralgia (especially, hepatitis B virus), myalgia, headache, malaise, discomfort in right hypochondrium, dark urine), icteric stage (jaundice*, mild/soft/tender hepatomegaly, splenomegaly in 10% patients, dark urine with pale stool—Fig. 6.7) or recovery stage (urine and eyes become less yellow, stool becomes yellow and there is return of appetite). The course of the disease is usually 2–4 weeks.

*Read 'Jaundice' from section of 'General examination'

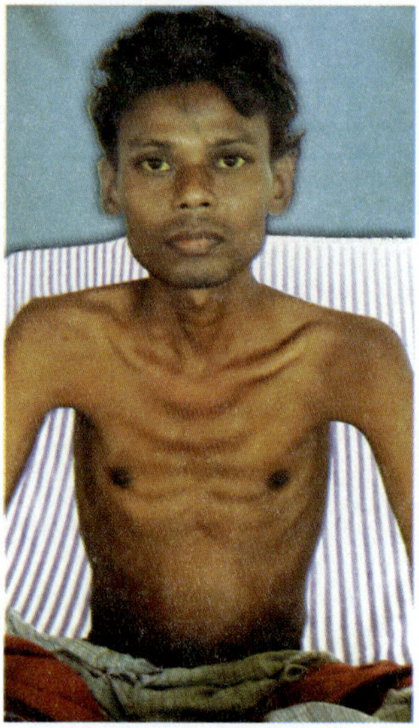

Fig. 6.7: Patient suffering from acute viral hepatitis with jaundice

Q. Common liver function tests done in clinical practice.

- Serum bilirubin (conjugated and unconjugated fractions)
- Aminotransferases (transaminases)—SGPT (serum glutamic pyruvic transaminase) is known as ALT (alanine aminotransferase), and SGOT (serum glutamic oxaloacetic transaminase) is known as AST (aspartate aminotransferase)
- Alkaline phosphatase
- Serum albumin and globulin
- Prothrombin time
- Gamma-glutamyl transpeptidase (GGT).

NB: Severity assessment of hepatic injury is best assessed by prothrombin time and partly by serum albumin.

Q. What is cirrhosis of liver?

Cirrhosis, by itself a pathological term, is the chronic and diffuse involvement of hepatic parenchyma of varied aetiology, and is clinically manifested by features of portal hypertension and hepatocellular failure in varying combination, and pathologically by irreversible necrosis, extensive fibrosis, and regenerative nodule formation in such a way that the normal hepatic architecture is totally lost. Cirrhosis is a classical example of chronic liver disease (CLD) and the other common CLD is chronic hepatitis (Fig. 6.8).

Aetiology of cirrhosis is alcoholic, biliary, cryptogenic (i.e., no cause found), cardiac, Wilson's disease, haemochromatosis, galactosaemia, Indian childhood cirrhosis, Budd-Chiari syndrome, drug-induced (e.g., methotrexate) and non-alcoholic steatohepatitis (NASH).

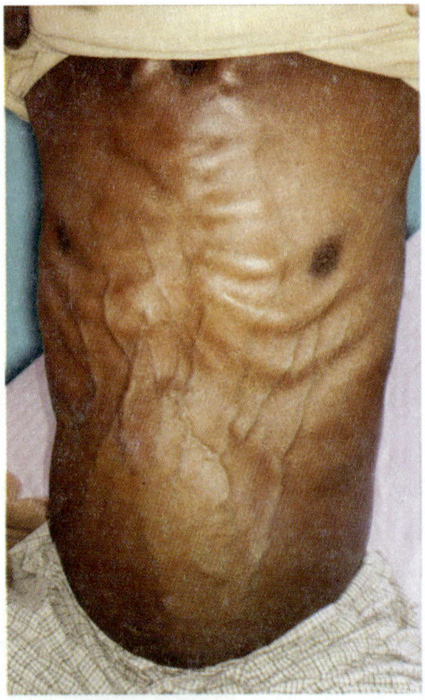

Fig. 6.8: Classical cirrhosis of liver—prominent and tortuous veins with ascites point towards chronic liver disease

Q. How to diagnose cirrhosis at the bedside?

A patient of cirrhosis will have features of both hepatocellular failure (i.e., liver failure) and portal hypertension. Both the subsets have some specific features which help in bedside diagnosis. The features of:

- Hepatocellular failure (i.e., hepatic failure)
  - Jaundice
  - Ascites and bipedal oedema
  - Fever, loss of muscle mass
  - Skin changes: Spider naevi* (Fig. 6.9), palmar erythema* (Fig. 6.10), white nails, diffuse pigmentation
  - Endocrine changes*: Gynaecomastia, testicular atrophy, loss of axillary and pubic hair, breast atrophy and menstrual irregularities, loss of libido (i.e., low sexual desire)
  - Fetor hepaticus: Sweetish-faecal smell in breath

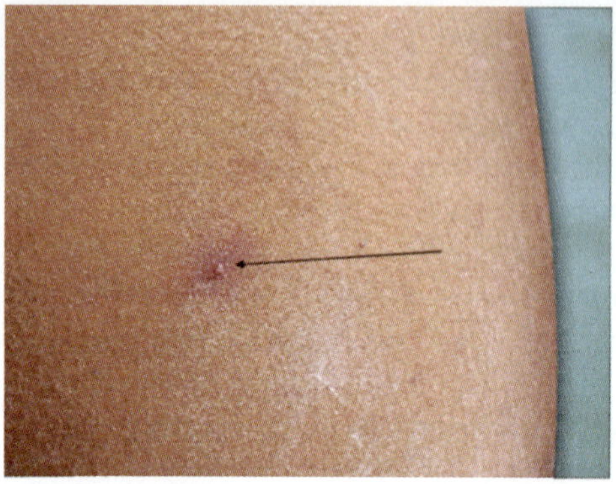

Fig. 6.9: Spider naevi over the upper part of back of chest—a hallmark sign of hepatocellular failure

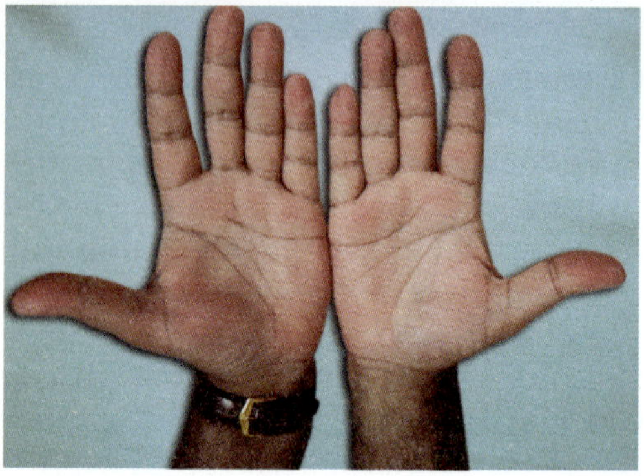

Fig. 6.10: Palmar erythema in a patient of cirrhosis of liver

- Hepatic encephalopathy (i.e., the neuropsychiatric syndrome): Inversion of sleep rhythm, confusion, flapping tremor (the toxins like NH_3, methionine, octopamine, etc. go directly to brain via collateral veins by-passing liver)
- Bleeding manifestations: Petechiae, purpura, ecchymoses (due to low prothrombin level)
- Circulatory changes: Capillary pulsation, clubbing, cyanosis.

*All endocrine changes along with spider naevi and palmar erythema are due to 'hyperoestrogenaemia'.

- Portal hypertension
  - Evidences of porto-systemic anastomosis (i.e., collateral circulation), that means engorged and tortuous veins seen at:
    - Lower end of oesophagus: Oesophageal varix (their rupture leads to haematemesis and melaena)
    - Around the umbilicus or over epigastrium (Fig. 6.11): Known as 'caput medusae' (looks like Greek Goddess Medusae's hair) when present around the umbilicus
    - Rectum and anal canal: Formation of haemorrhoids
  - Splenomegaly (cardinal feature at bedside)
  - Ascites.

NB: Feature common to hepatocellular failure and portal hypertension is ascites. Liver failure → hypoproteinaemia → low oncotic pressure → formation of ascites; portal hypertension only localises the fluid within the peritoneal cavity.

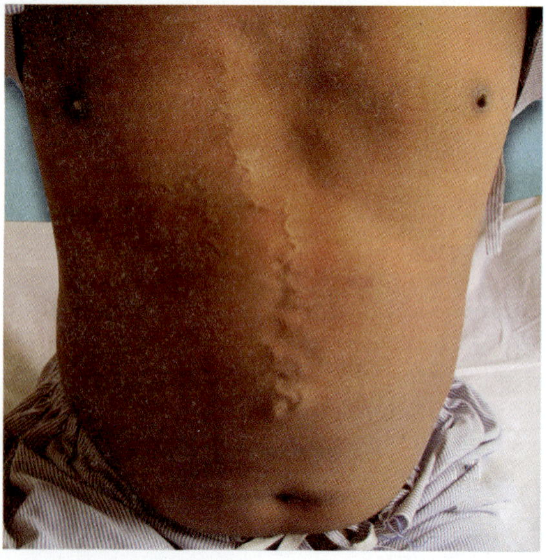

Fig. 6.11: Portal hypertension—venous collaterals are seen

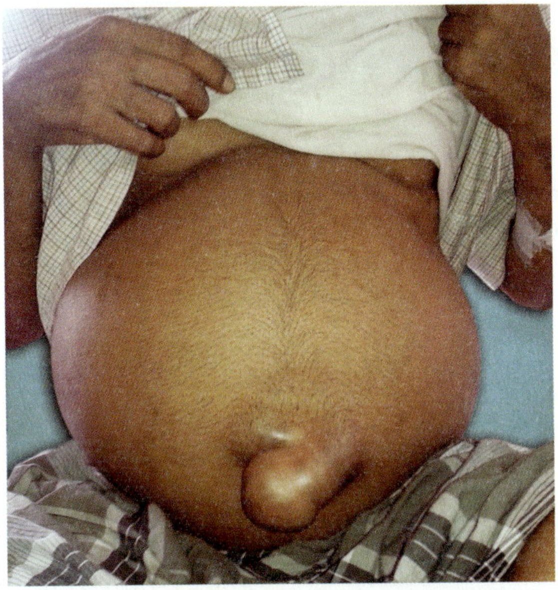

Fig. 6.12: Huge ascites with umbilical hernia

A huge ascites may have umbilical hernia associated with (Fig. 6.12).

Decompensated cirrhosis: Cirrhosis with one or more features of ascites, jaundice, GI bleeding and hepatic encephalopathy.

Compensated cirrhosis: Asymptomatic cirrhosis without those features.

Q. What is portal hypertension and its common causes?

As described in the previous question, portal hypertension is clinically diagnosed by venous collaterals in the abdomen, ascites and splenomegaly. To diagnose cirrhosis of liver in a patient, features of portal hypertension should be present along with features of hepatocellular failure. Portal hypertension is defined as:

- *Definition:* Normal pressure in the portal vein is 5–8 mm of Hg or 10–15 cm of saline. Portal pressure >30 cm of saline or >12 mm of Hg is known as portal hypertension.
- *Causes:* Cirrhosis of liver (commonest), Budd-Chiari syndrome (hepatic venous obstruction), portal vein thrombosis (e.g., umbilical sepsis in neonates, hyperviscosity syndrome), non-cirrhotic portal fibrosis (arsenic toxicity, schistosomiasis), veno-occlusive disease (by Jamaica bush tea).

Q. What are the causes of acute (fulminant) hepatic failure?

Acute hepatic failure is a fatal condition. It is caused by:

- Acute viral hepatitis (most common cause)
- Drug-induced (rifampicin, INH, paracetamol overdose, halothane), copper sulphate poisoning
- Shock and multi-organ failure
- Sepsis
- Acute fatty liver of pregnancy

- Budd-Chiari syndrome
- Weil's disease
- Eclampsia.

Q. What is the normal shape of the abdomen?

The normal shape of the abdomen is globular (neither scaphoid nor distended). In pathological conditions, the shape may be:

- *Scaphoid (sunken or boat-shaped):* Severe dehydration, emaciation, starvation, peritonitis (tuberculous or malignant).
- *Distended:*
  - Localised: Any intra-abdominal enlargement of viscus, neoplasm
  - Generalised—8 'F' i.e.,
    - Fat (obesity)
    - Faeces (intestinal obstruction)
    - Foetus (pregnancy)
    - Flatus (gaseous distension)
    - Fluid (ascites, any cyst, distended urinary bladder, Fig. 6.13)
    - Full (urinary) bladder
    - Fibroid or fatal tumour
    - Functional (IBS-like disorder associated with bloating).

Q. What is ascites and what are the common causes?

Ascites is defined as accumulation of 'free' fluid within the peritoneal cavity. The causes are:

- Exudative ascites: Peritonitis [tuberculous, malignant (Fig. 6.14), spontaneous bacterial], pancreatitis, lymphoma and leukaemias.
- Transudative ascites (may be associated with anasarca): Cirrhosis (Fig. 6.15), CCF, nephrotic syndrome, hypoproteinaemia with anaemia (nutritional), myxoedema.

NB: Common causes of ascites: Cirrhosis, malignant ascites, tuberculous peritonitis, CCF.

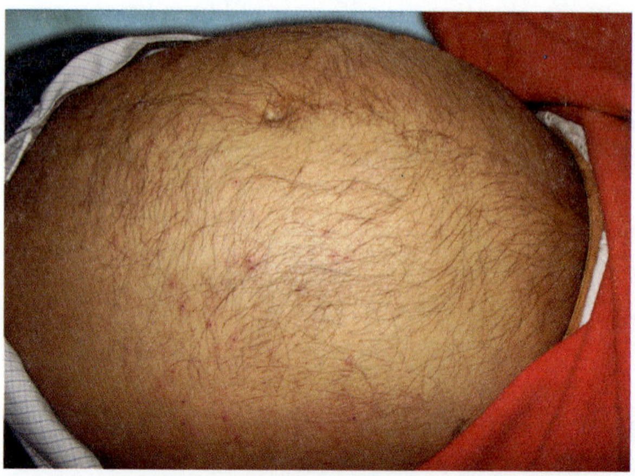

Fig. 6.13: Football-like distension of abdomen in ascites with scabies infection in the skin

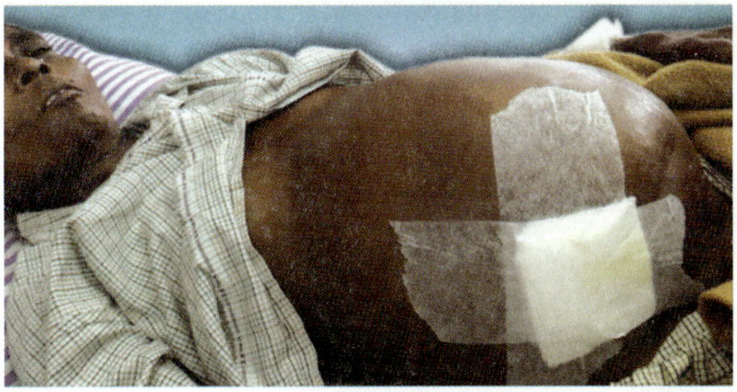

Fig. 6.14: Malignant ascites after paracentesis abdominis (i.e., tapping of abdominal fluid)

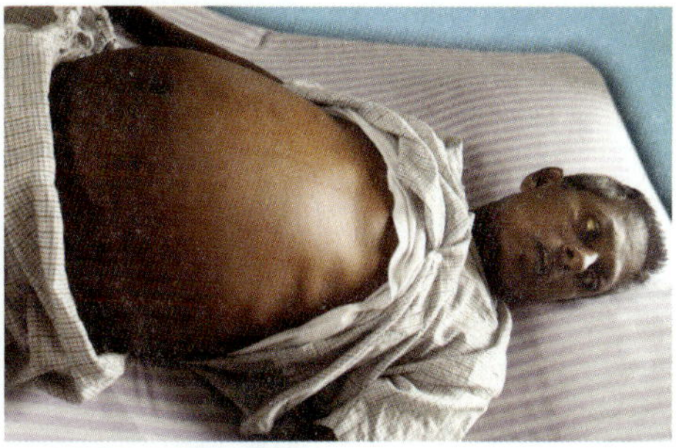

Fig. 6.15: A patient with ascites and jaundice—cirrhosis of liver

Q. Give an account of carcinoma of liver.

The liver is enlarged, hard, irregular and tender on palpation. Basically it is of two types:

- *Primary (known as hepato-cellular carcinoma or hepatoma):* From hepatitis B or C infection, or cirrhosis of liver. Age 40–50 years. Liver has single nodule without umbilication. Hepatic bruit ++, hepatic rub +.
- *Secondary:* Metastatic carcinoma is the most common carcinoma of the liver because of dual blood supply in liver (by hepatic artery and portal vein). The primary source may be in stomach, colon, bronchus, breast or thyroid. Liver has multiple nodules with umbilication. Hepatic bruit is usually absent but hepatic rub +++.

Q. How to divide the abdomen for the purpose of clinical examination?

The abdomen, the temple of surprise, is divided by two horizontal and two vertical lines into nine distinct areas. The upper horizontal line is in transpyloric plane (i.e., midway between suprasternal notch and symphysis pubis) and the lower horizontal line is known as inter-tubercular line (i.e., line joining tubercles on iliac crest). The two vertical lines pass from the femoral artery below to cross the lower costal margins close to the tip of the 9th costal cartilage (Figs 6.16 and 6.17).

The nomenclatures of different areas with content are:

1. Right hypochondrium: Liver, gall bladder
2. Epigastrium: Distal stomach, transverse colon
3. Left hypochondrium: Fundus of stomach, spleen, tail of pancreas
4. Right lumbar/flank: Kidney (right), adrenal gland, ascending colon
5. Umbilical: Small intestine, aorta, IVC, mesentery, head and body of pancreas
6. Left lumbar/flank: Kidney (left), adrenal gland, descending colon
7. Right iliac fossa: Caecum, appendix, terminal ileum, right ovary
8. Hypogastrium or suprapubic: Urinary bladder, uterus, rectum
9. Left iliac fossa: Sigmoid colon, part of descending colon, left ovary.

NB: 'Loin' means the part of the body on both sides of the spine between the lowest ribs and the hip bones, in the posterior abdominal wall.

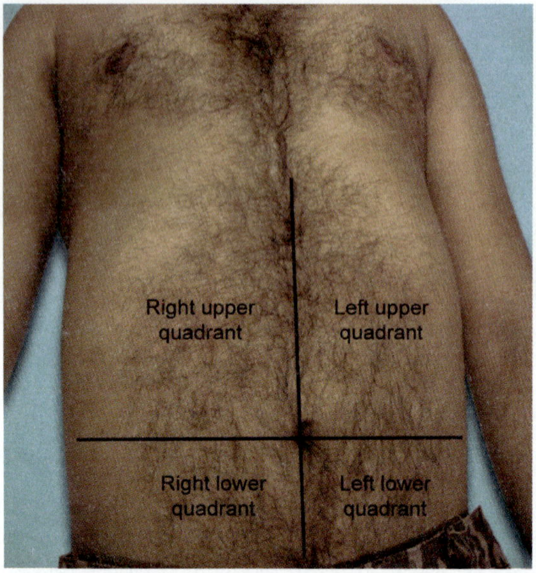

Fig. 6.16: Different quadrants of abdomen for the purpose of clinical examination

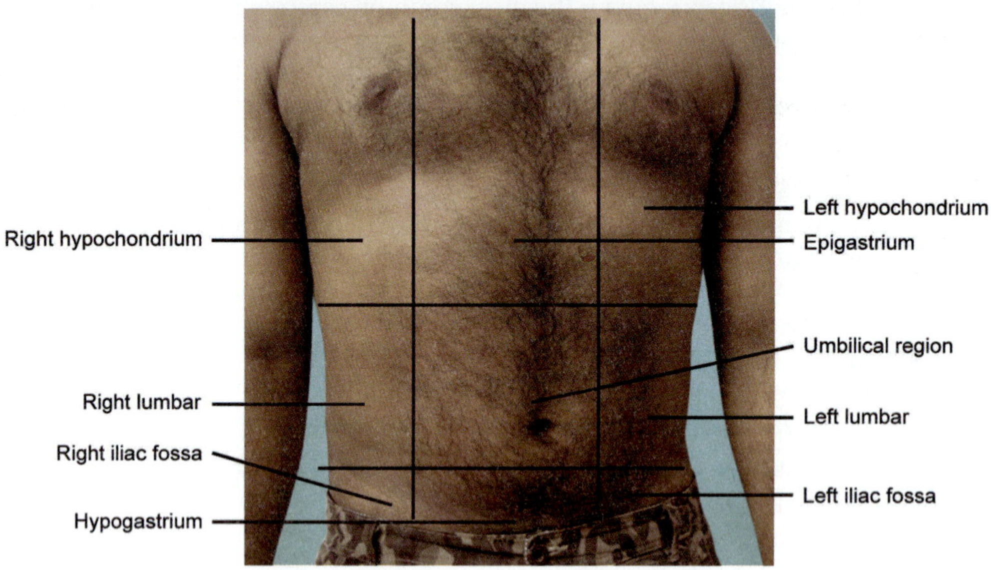

Fig. 6.17: Various (nine) regions of abdomen with anatomical correlations

Q. What are the significance/importance of dilated veins over abdomen/chest (Fig. 6.18)**?**

Dilated veins over abdomen is basically found in portal hypertension, SVC and IVC obstruction. Their presence in specific region of abdomen along with the direction of blood flow clinch the clinical diagnosis very promptly.

A. *Around umbilicus (caput medusae) or over epigastrium:* Portal hypertension where the direction of flow of blood is 'away from the umbilicus'; a venous hum (similar

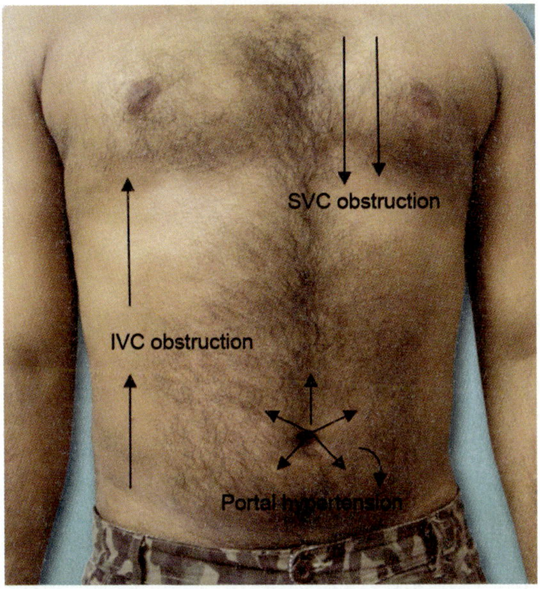

Fig. 6.18: Dilated abdominal wall veins with direction of blood flow (SVC—superior vena cava, IVC—inferior vena cava)

sound like bruit in arteries) may be audible over dilated abdominal wall veins around umbilicus.

B. *Over abdomen, lateral chest wall and back:* Inferior vena caval (IVC) obstruction where the direction of flow of blood is 'below upwards' i.e., from hypogastrium towards epigastrium.

C. *Over chest and upper arm:* Superior vena caval (SVC) obstruction where the direction of flow of blood is 'above downwards' i.e., from upper chest towards epigastrium.

NB: In health, the flow of blood is away from the umbilicus but one cannot see the venous prominences.

Q. How to palpate liver, spleen and gall bladder?

The patient should lie flat comfortably in bed. Proper light should be there for examination. Explain briefly to the patient what you are going to do. To gain confidence of the patient, a gentle palpation with proper care of the painful part is necessary. The prerequisites before palpation of abdominal viscera are (Fig. 6.19):

1. Stand on the right side of the patient as commonly we are right-handed (a left-handed clinician may stand on the left side of the patient for better palpation).
2. Hands of the patient should lie by his/her side (to prevent undue obliquity).
3. Flex the thighs (to relax the muscles of abdomen).
4. Turn the patient's face to opposite side and ask him/her to breathe deeply but regularly with open mouth.
5. Expose the abdomen from xiphisternum to just above the inguinal ligament.

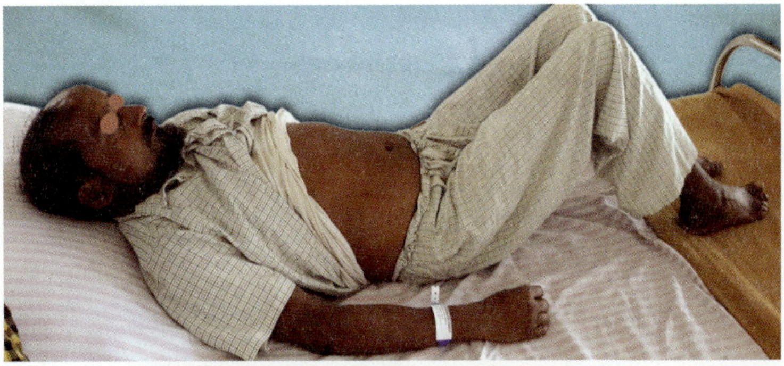

Fig. 6.19: Proper position of the patient before abdominal examination while the clinician will stand on the right side of the patient

Palpation of:

A. ***Liver:*** Stand on the right side of the supine patient. Place your right palm over the right iliac fossa (parallel to arbitrary lower border of liver, and lateral to right rectus abdominis muscle) and press the hand inwards and upwards. The liver can be felt at the height of inspiration, if enlarged, when the palpating hand gradually goes upwards towards right hypochondrium (conventional method). Now, try to palpate the left lobe of liver by moving the palpating hand from right hypochondrium to midline.

There are three methods of palpation of liver:

- *Conventional method* (described above; mostly practised in India) (Fig. 6.20).
- *Preferred method:* Place both hands side by side flat over right hypochondrium lateral to rectus abdominis muscle with fingers pointing upwards. If any resistance is felt (i.e., due to hepatomegaly), move the hands downwards till the resistance disappears. Now confirm the lower border of liver by asking the patient to inspire and moving the hands upwards and inwards. This method is preferred by rest of the world (Fig. 6.21).
- *Alternative method:* It is just like conventional method but the fingers of right hand are placed in the right iliac fossa directing upwards. This method is less sensitive than other two methods and thus not practised widely (Fig. 6.22).

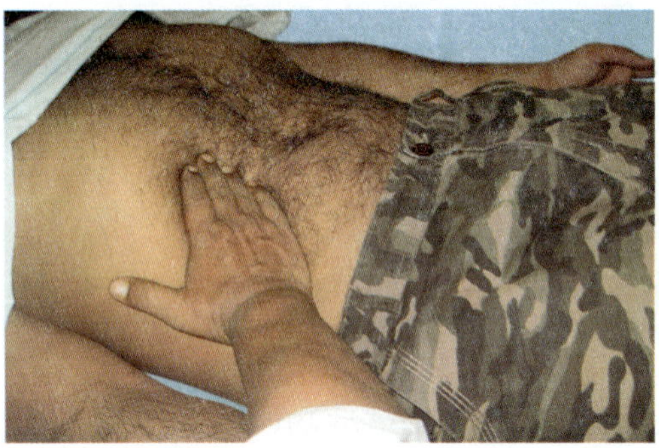

Fig. 6.20: Palpation of liver (conventional method)

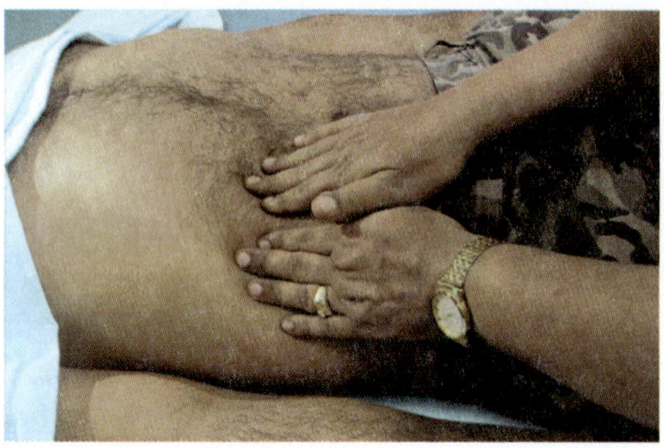

Fig. 6.21: Palpation of liver (preferred method)

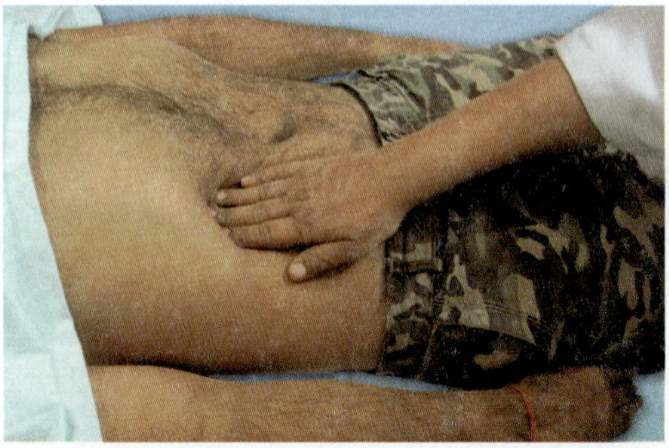

Fig. 6.22: Palpation of liver (alternative method)

In hepatomegaly, the points noted are:

- Degree of enlargement: The anterior liver span is 12–15 cm, measured from upper (determined by percussion) to lower border of liver at right MCL. It can also be expressed by distance (centimetres/inches) between right costal margin and lower border of liver at right MCL.
- Consistency: Soft (CCF) , firm (cirrhosis), hard (malignancy).
- Tenderness: Tender (viral hepatitis) or non-tender (fatty liver, cirrhosis).
- Surface: Smooth (CCF) or irregular (cirrhosis or malignancy).
- Margin or border: Sharp (cirrhosis) or rounded (fatty liver, CCF).
- Whether the left lobe is enlarged (e.g., amoebic liver abscess) or not.
- Any pulsation present (CCF) or not. Pulsatile liver (by placing right palm over enlarged liver and left palm over the back) may be felt in functional tricuspid incomptence (i.e., from CCF).
- Upper border of liver dullness: Percuss the right chest from above downwards. The upper border of liver dullness lies in the right 5th ICS in right MCL.
- Any hepatic bruit audible (hepatoma, haemangioma of liver), or hepatic rub palpable (after liver biopsy, metastatic carcinoma of liver)?

NB: It is very important to learn the art of palpation of liver and spleen (see below) from the initial days of clinical training.

B. ***Spleen:*** Stand on the right side of the supine patient and ask the patient to breathe deeply. Place your left palm firmly over left costal margin posterolaterally, and press it forward and medially. Start palpation with your right hand from right iliac fossa and proceed towards the left hypochondrium in search of palpable spleen (Fig. 6.23). Spleen becomes palpable when it is 2–3 times more than its normal size.

If spleen is not palpable in supine position, turn the patient in right lateral decubitus and palpate the spleen (Short's manoeuvre) (Fig. 6.24). If spleen is still not palpable, you can palpate it by standing on the left side of the patient with hooked fingers of left hand placed below left costal margin (Fig. 6.25).

In splenomegaly, the points noted are:

- Degree of enlargement: Spleen usually enlarges from left hypochondrium towards right iliac fossa (Fig. 6.26). The measurement is taken in centimetres/inches along

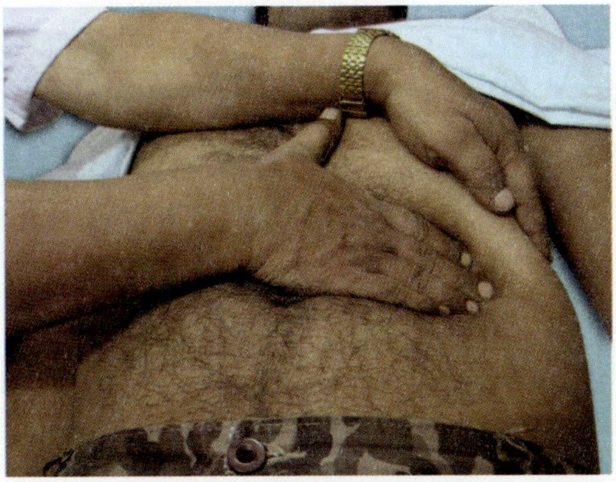

Fig. 6.23: Palpation of spleen

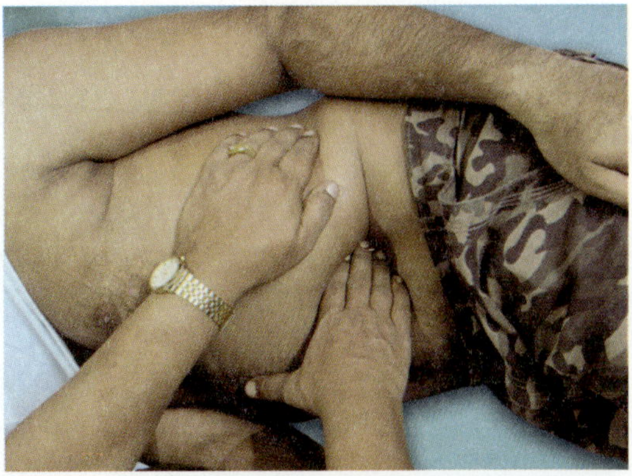

Fig. 6.24: Palpation of spleen in right lateral position

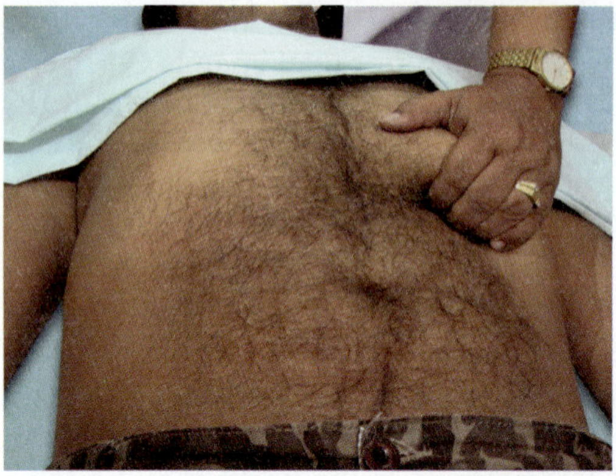

Fig. 6.25: Palpation of spleen by hooking method done from left side of the patient

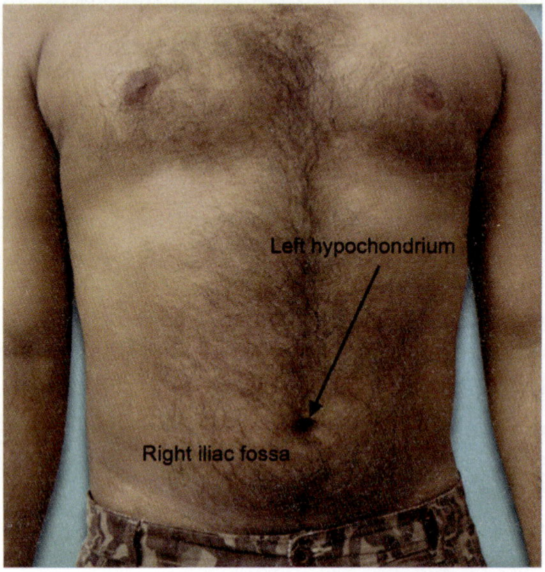

Fig. 6.26: Direction of splenic enlargement from left hypochondrium towards right iliac fossa

splenic axis by joining two points i.e., above where left costal margin is crossed by left MCL, and below up to the furthest apart point of spleen (Note: Left kidney enlarges towards left iliac fossa).

In health, spleen lies behind and below the left 9th, 10th and 11th rib, with its long axis along the line of 10th rib.

- Splenic notch: On its anterior border and very characteristic of splenic enlargement (helpful to differentiate kidney lump).
- Margin: Usually sharp.
- Consistency: Soft (acute malaria or acute kala-azar), firm (cirrhosis of liver), hard (chronic myeloid leukaemia/CML).
- Tenderness: Tender (SBE, infectious mononucleosis) or non-tender.
- Surface: Smooth (CML) or irregular (splenic cysts).

- Movement with respiration: Spleen freely moves with respiration (contrary to kidney lump).
- Fingers cannot be insinuated between left costal arch and the enlarged spleen (possible in case of kidney lump); spleen usually bulges forward.
- No band of colonic resonance on percussion over splenic swelling (present in case of left kidney lump).
- Any palpable or audible splenic rub present (present in chronic myeloid leukaemia/ CML, SBE or sickle cell anaemia)?

NB: Remember, a kidney (renal) lump is characteristically bimanually palpable and ballottable, which is not present in any other viscus.

C. ***Gall bladder:*** It is palpated in the same way as palpation of liver by conventional method i.e., start palpation from right iliac fossa and proceed towards right hypochondrium. In health, the gall bladder is not palpable. Gall bladder is palpable in mucocele/empyema/carcinoma of the gall bladder, or carcinoma of the head of pancreas (according to Courvoisier's law).

Q. Causes of hepatosplenomegaly.

Many systemic diseases, infective diseases or haematological malignancies are characterised by hepatosplenomegaly like:

- *Hepatomegaly:*
  - Mild (<2 fingers): Acute malaria, CCF, acute viral hepatitis.
  - Moderate (2–5 fingers): Chronic malaria/chronic kala-azar, lymphoma.
  - Massive (>5 fingers): Malignancy of liver, cystic disease of liver, amoebic liver abscess.
- *Splenomegaly*
  - Mild (<2 fingers): Acute malaria/acute kala-azar, SBE, haemolytic anaemia, miliary tuberculosis, acute leukaemias, immune thrombocytopenic purpura (ITP).
  - Moderate (2–5 fingers): Chronic malaria/chronic kala-azar, portal hypertension (e.g., cirrhosis), lymphoma, collagen vascular diseases (e.g., SLE).
  - Massive (>5 fingers): Chronic malaria/chronic kala-azar, thalassaemia major, CML, polycythemia vera, tropical splenomegaly syndrome, myelofibrosis, splenic tumour/cyst.
- *Hepatosplenomegaly*
  - Chronic malaria/chronic kala-azar
  - Haemolytic anaemia (congenital) e.g, thalassaemia major
  - Cirrhosis of liver
  - Chronic myeloid leukaemia (CML)
  - Lymphoma (Hodgkin's and non-Hodgkin's lymphoma)
  - Collagen vascular diseases e.g., SLE
  - Acute viral hepatitis
  - Enteric fever
  - Miliary tuberculosis
  - Polycythemia vera
  - Tropical splenomegaly syndrome (or, hyperreactive malarial splenomegaly).

Q. Different methods of palpation of abdomen.

Usually there are four methods of palpation of abdominal viscera. They are:

- *Conventional method (classical method):* Palpation of liver, gall bladder.
- *Hooking method (by hooked fingers):* Classically used in splenic palpation.
- *Bimanual method (using both hands):* Classically used for palpation of kidneys, or abdominal palpation in an obese or poorly relaxed patient*.
- *Dipping method (a sharp tap is given over abdomen by flexing the metacarpophalangeal joints of right hand suddenly):* Palpation of abdominal viscera in the presence of ascites.

*Palpation by using two hands, placing the left hand over the right hand, is necessary in patients who are obese, muscular or with poorly relaxed abdomen (Fig. 6.27).

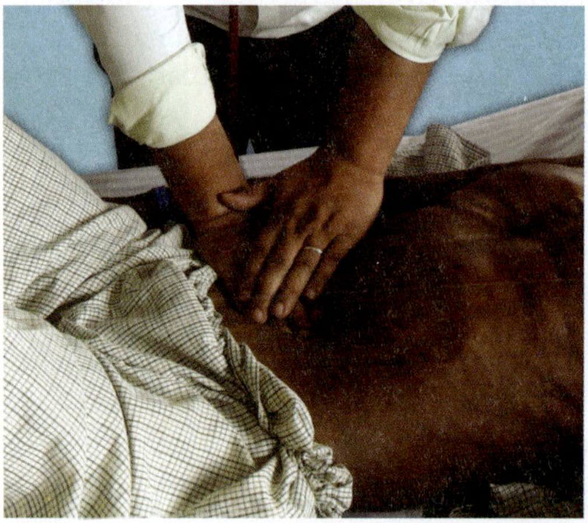

Fig. 6.27: Bimanual palpation of abdomen in an obese, muscular or poorly relaxed patient when the left hand is placed over the right hand

Q. Distension of the abdomen due to accumulation of fluid—causes behind?

Accumulation of fluid in abdomen may be due to collection of free fluid (ascites) or cystic fluid. Ascites is commonly due to cirrhosis of liver or tuberculous/malignant peritonitis. Cystic intra-abdominal swellings are due to distended urinary bladder, ovarian cyst, mesenteric cyst, pseudopancreatic cyst, hydatid cyst and polycystic kidney. Diagnosis of an abdominal lump (whether solid or cystic) is done by its site, size, margin, surface, consistency, movement with respiration, mobility, pulsation, or by the findings like whether it is bimanually palpable and ballottable.

Q. How to differentiate ascites from a cystic swelling?

There are two very sensitive methods for their diagnosis in clinical medicine. They are:

- *Fluid thrill: Fluid thrill is present both in ascites and encysted fluid.* For its presence, in case of ascites, fluid must remain under tension and should be large in volume (say, 2 litres). Tap or flick either flank of abdomen in a supine patient, while feel for a shock-like wave in other flank in case of presence of fluid thrill. Place ulnar border of one hand of the patient in the abdomen in the midline to prevent transmission of impulse through abdominal parietes (Fig. 6.28).

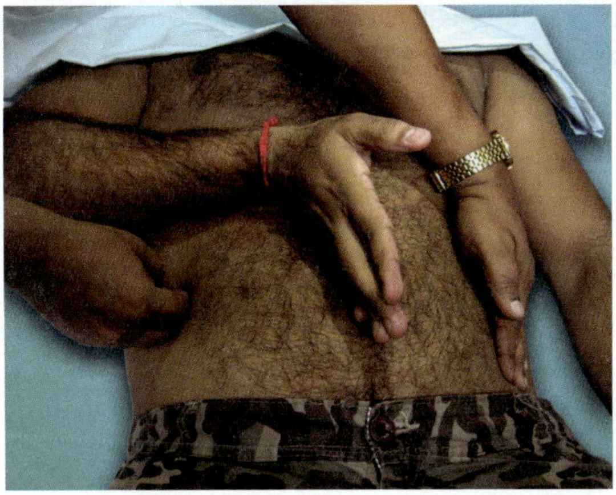

Fig. 6.28: Elicitation of fluid thrill

- *Shifting dullness:* It is the *surest bedside sign for ascites* (never found in encysted fluid). Collection of even ½–1 litre of free fluid can give rise to positive shifting dullness. Shifting dullness has good sensitivity as well as specificity both.
  Percuss the abdomen in the midline of a supine patient. In ascites, the midline will be tympanitic due to coils of intestine (air) floating over fluid, while flanks will be dull as a result of presence of fluid. Now, percuss from maximum point of tympanicity in midline towards the flank to determine the air-fluid interface; make a pencil mark there. The point of air-fluid interface (i.e., transition zone between tympany and dullness) will change its position when the patient changes his/her position to right or left lateral side (detected by percussion), and it is only possible when the fluid remains free in the abdomen i.e., in case of ascites.

NB: In a cystic swelling (e.g., ovarian cyst), the percussion note in the midline will always be dull and shifting dullness will never be present. Shifting dullness is a hallmark bedside sign for presence of free fluid in abdomen i.e., ascites. Remember, absence of fluid thrill and/or shifting dullness do not exclude the presence of ascites.

In a cystic swelling, fluid thrill may be present but shifting dullness is always absent.

Q. What is normal peristaltic sound?

'Bowel sounds' are produced by the movement of feces, fluid and flatus within bowel lumen as a result of peristaltic movements. Normal bowel sounds are intermittent low- or medium-pitched gurgles intermingled with occasional high-pitched tinkle. Place the stethoscope to one side of umbilicus minimally for one minute to listen these sounds. The sounds are:

- Increased (borborygmi)—mechanical intestinal obstruction and diarrhoeal diseases.
- Absent—paralytic ileus and peritonitis (i.e., abdomen is silent).

Q. Visible peristalsis—is it possible?

No peristaltic wave is seen in health. If peristalsis is visible, it signifies mechanical obstruction of intestine. Peristalsis can be evoked in a patient of suspected intestinal obstruction by:

- Flicking, stroking or gentle massage of anterior abdominal wall
- Drinking 1–2 glasses of water at a time
- Pouring a few drops of ether over the abdomen.

The site of obstruction in intestine can be obtained by analysing peristaltic waves like:

1. *Stomach:* Waves are golf-ball like, and moves from left to right hypochondrium; 2–3 waves are seen at a time. Commonly it is due to pyloric stenosis (or gastric outlet obstruction).
2. *Small intestine:* Seen as 'ladder pattern' (zigzag fashion) in periumbilical region; 10–12 waves formation/minute.
3. *Large intestine:* In obstruction of transverse colon, waves move from right to left hypochondrium. Waves are seen in right or left flank in obstruction of ascending and descending colon respectively. Waves are a bit larger i.e., cricket-ball like.

Decoding Abbreviations

IBD	Inflammatory bowel disease
IBS	Irritable bowel syndrome
SVC	Superior vena cava
IVC	Inferior vena cava.

Chapter 7

Genitourinary System

SCHEME OF SYSTEMIC EXAMINATION: AN OVERVIEW

It is desirable that a student will fill up the scheme of GI system examination with special reference to the following in a genitourinary case:

I. GI system: Tonsils are examined in a case of acute glomerulonephritis, and prostate should be examined per rectally in suspected obstructive uropathy.

II. Genitourinary system

A. *Inspection:* Genitalia (penis, vulva, testes, scrotal swelling, etc.), skin for nephrectomy or renal biopsy mark/scabies infection with pyoderma, abdominal swelling for ascites, scrotal oedema (e.g., nephrotic syndrome).

B. *Palpation:* Detailed examination of genitalia (with special reference to phimosis and testes), parietal oedema, fluid thrill, kidney mass and renal angle.

C. *Percussion*
- Shifting dullness in abdomen (for detection of ascites)
- Upper border of liver dullness (as hydrothorax may complicate nephrotic syndrome)
- Band of colonic resonance over left renal mass
- Percussion of urinary bladder (if distended).

D. *Auscultation*
- Bowel sounds (i.e., peristaltic sounds)
- Renal artery bruit (in mid-abdomen in renal artery stenosis)
- Venous hum

In a genitourinary case, other systems need special mention in relation to:

E. *CVS:* Neck veins may be engorged due to fluid overload, apex beat may be deviated due to left ventricular hypertrophy (LVH) as a result of hypertension, and pericardial rub or pericardial effusion may be evident.

F. *Respiratory system:* Respiratory rate may be high due to metabolic acidosis (e.g., uraemia), features of hydrothorax with evidence of respiratory tract infection may be present.

G. *Nervous system:* The patient may be drowsy (uraemia) or restless (hypertensive encephalopathy). Flapping tremor and signs of peripheral neuropathy (uraemia) may be present.

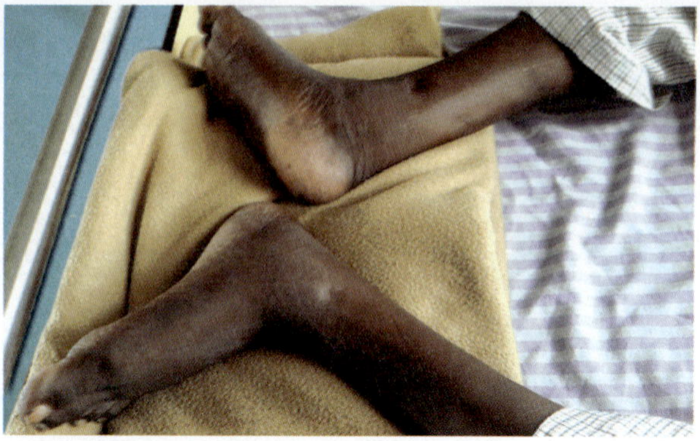

Fig. 7.1: Mild pitting pedal oedema in chronic renal failure (CRF)

NB: In general survey, pallor and oedema (Fig. 7.1) are two very important points to be examined; BP (i.e., in reference to hypertension) should also be given importance. Urine should be examined at the bedside for presence of albumin (heat coagulation test) and sugar (Benedict's test), if required.

Q. Mention the common presentations (chief complaints and H/o present illness) in genitourinary system.

The patients having complaints of genitourinary system commonly present with:

1. Oliguria (urine volume <400 ml/day).
2. Polyuria (urine volume >3 litres/day).
3. Anuria (passing urine <50 ml/day, or no urine formation for 12 hours).
4. Haematuria (passage of blood in urine).
5. Swelling of face, legs or whole body (i.e., anasarca).
6. Dysuria (feeling pain, discomfort or burning during micturition i.e., painful micturition); strangury is severe form of dysuria where there is painful urge for micturition but the patient is unable to pass urine.
7. Retention of urine.
8. Incontinence of urine.
9. Renal colic (acute colicky pain from loin to groin and often radiating towards testis or labium)/urinary pain (in loin, mid-abdomen or hypogastrium).
10. Swelling of abdomen (renal lump or formation of ascites from renal failure).
11. *Others:*
    a. Fever [urinary tract infection (UTI), pyelonephritis, renal tuberculosis, prostatitis].
    b. Sexual problems [sexual partners, loss of libido (i.e., low sexual desire), impotence, difficulty in ejaculation, dyspareunia (painful sexual intercourse), etc.].
    c. Any complaint regarding genitalia.
    d. *General:* Anorexia, nausea, vomiting, hiccough, fatigue, pruritus, breathlessness, tingling extremities.

NB: In health, the normal urine output in an adult is 1.5 litres (400 ml–3 litres).

Q. Common causes of oliguria, polyuria, anuria, nocturia, dysuria, haematuria, enuresis, retention and incontinence of urine.

- *Oliguria:* Acute gastroenteritis, acute glomerulonephritis (AGN), renal failure, CCF, hypovolaemia and shock.
- *Polyuria:* Chronic renal failure (CRF), diabetes mellitus, diabetes insipidus, hypercalcaemic and hypokalaemic nephropathy, psychogenic polydipsia (i.e., compulsive drinking of water), use of diuretics in oedematous states.
- *Anuria:* Rapidly pregressive glomerulonephritis (RPGN), bilateral ureteric obstruction, hypovolaemia, cardiogenic shock, end-stage renal disease (ESRD*).
- *Nocturia:* Passing more volume of urine during night-time is due to diabetes mellitus, BHP, polyuric states, salt-losing nephropathy, oedema-forming states, vesico-ureteric reflux.
- *Dysuria:* Infections in the urinary tract (UTI), stones in the urinary tract.
- *Haematuria:* AGN, UTI, malignant hypertension, infective endocarditis, renal infarction, renal tuberculosis, snakebite, blood dyscrasias.
  - Painless haematuria: AGN, infective endocarditis, hypernephroma, renal tuberculosis, malignant hypertension, coagulation disorders.
  - Painful haematuria: UTI, stones, trauma, renal infarction.
  - Medical causes of heaematuria: AGN, infective endocarditis (microscopic haematuria), malignant hypertension, snakebite, coagulation disorders or anticoagulant therapy, renal tuberculosis, renal infarction.
- *Enuresis:* Bed-wetting at night or during sleep, and is commonly due to a small bladder, stress, diabetes, UTI, sleep apnoea, spina bifida, etc.
- *Retention of urine:* Obstructive [benign hypertrophy of prostate (BHP), urethral stricture, kidney or bladder stone] or non-obstructive [spinal injury, paraplegia, stroke].
- *Incontinence of urine:* It is the leakage of urine, and is due to stress (urinary leak after stress e.g., coughing)/urge (uncontrolled passage of urine preceded by strong urge to void e.g., in severe UTI)/true or continual (e.g., continual urinary leakage due to vesico-vaginal fistula), or overflow incontinence (leakage of urine due to chronic retention of urine).

*ESRD is the last and final stage of chronic kidney disease (CKD) in which the kidneys no longer function enough to meet the needs of daily life, and dialysis or a kidney transplant is necessary for survival.

Q. Causes of red urine in clinical practice.

Red urine is commonly seen in:

- Haematuria (see the question above)
- Haemoglobinuria (i.e., in haemolytic disorders)
- Myoglobinuria (i.e., in rhabdomyolysis or breakdown of damaged skeletal muscles)
- Acute intermittent porphyria, alkaptonuria
- Drugs and others: Rifampicin, phenazopyridine, clofazimine; ingestion of beet root, senna and dyes used to colour sweets.

Q. Describe a classical attack of 'renal colic'.

Obstruction of ureter as a result of stone (calculi) is mostly responsible for renal colic; obstruction by blood clot, tumour or a sloughed renal papilla may also give rise to colicky pain.

Renal colic is an acute, severe pain which starts in the loin and then radiates round the flank to the groin, and often into the ipsilateral testis or vulva, and inner aspect of the thigh (i.e., along the distribution of genital branch of genitofemoral nerve). It is a gripping pain which steadily increases in intensity to reach its peak within a few minutes and passes off as suddenly as it came, only to appear again. The renal colicky pain is due to smooth muscle spasm or distension of ureter. The patient becomes restless and tries repeatedly to change position in bed in a false hope to get relief. Renal colic is often associated with nausea, vomiting, chill and rigor, and excessive perspiration.

Q. How to palpate the kidneys (Fig. 7.2)?

Prerequisites (i.e., preliminary preparation of the patient) are similar as done during palpation of liver and spleen (Fig. 6.19).

For palpation of right kidney, stand on the right side of the patient and place the right hand horizontally, lateral to rectus abdominis muscle, over right lumbar region anteriorly while the left hand is placed posteriorly in the right loin to trap the kidney bimanually (i.e., by both hands), at the height of inspiration (bimanual palpation).

Keep both of your hands over the patient as done in bimanual palpation; now a sharp tap is given by the left hand which is placed in the loin. The anteriorly placed right hand can feel the kidney (if enlarged), and the kidney then falls back by gravity on the posterior abdominal wall which is felt again by the left hand, which is known as ballottement (a confirmatory test for kidney lump).

The left kidney can be palpated from either side in the similar way.

A kidney lump is both bimanually palpable and ballottable.

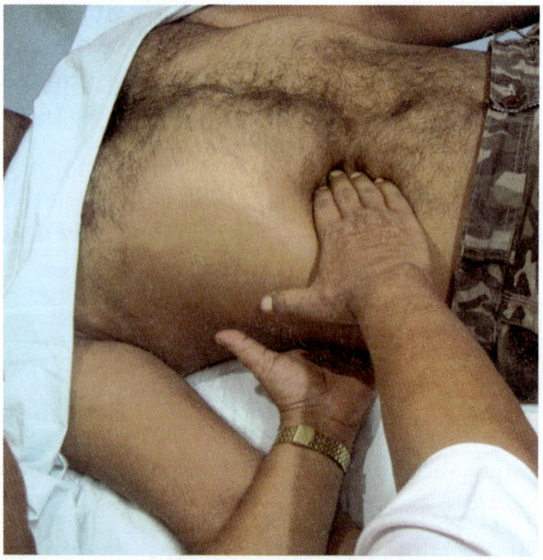

Fig. 7.2: Bimanual palpation of right kidney

Q. Causes of palpable kidney.

In health, the lower pole of right kidney may be palpable in thin patients for obvious reason (i.e., pushed by liver). The kidney is palpable in pathological conditions like:

- *Unilateral:* Dropped kidney, hydronephrosis, Wilms' tumour, hypernephroma, large cyst in kidney.
- *Bilateral:* Polycystic kidney, bilateral hydronephrosis (e.g., from BHP), bilateral dropped kidney, diabetic nephropathy in initial stage, acromegaly, amyloidosis.

Q. Importance of renal angle.

Renal angle is the angle formed by the lower border of 12th rib and lateral border of erector spinae muscles at back. Press it by ball of your thumb or thrust given by ulnar border of closed fist to note the tenderness (known as "Murphy's kidney punch"). Renal angle becomes tender in acute pyelonephritis, perinephric abscess, acute urinary obstruction, nephrolithiasis, etc. (Fig. 7.3).

Q. What is urinary tract infection (UTI)?

UTI is the multiplication of the organisms in the urinary tract. Predisposing factors are obstructive uropathy, renal stone, self-retaining catheter, diabetes, or any immunodeficiency; females are more susceptible because of shorter length of urethra, close proximity of urethra to perineum and urethral trauma during sexual intercourse.

Common organisms for UTI are *E. coli* (most common infection outside hospital), Streptococci, Staphylococci, Klebsiella, Proteus, Pseudomonas and *Chlamydia trachomatis*. The types of UTI are:

- Lower tract infection: Urethritis, cystitis, prostatitis.
- Upper tract infection: Acute pyelonephritis (infection of the pelvis of kidney and kidney; patients complain of loin pain).

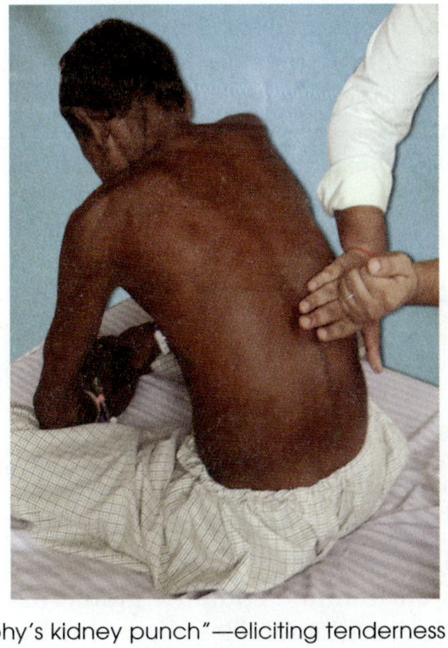

Fig. 7.3: "Murphy's kidney punch"—eliciting tenderness in renal angle

Common clinical features of UTI are:

- Increased frequency of micturition by day and night.
- Burning pain during micturition or painful voiding (i.e., dysuria).
- Urgency, strangury, suprapubic pain as well as tenderness, haematuria and foul-smelling urine
- Systemic: Fever with chill and rigor, nausea and vomiting

Diagnosis is done by routine examination (R/E), and culture and sensitivity (C/S) test of urine along with colony count. Demonstration of >10^5 organism/ml grown from a properly collected mid-stream 'clean catch' urine sample strongly suggests infection. Urine should be collected cautiously (i.e., aseptically), for examination in the laboratory.

Q. What is meant by proteinuria?

Presence of protein in urine is known as proteinuria. In health, an adult may excrete up to 150 mg of protein in urine/24 hours (physiological). Proteinuria (pathological) is classified into:

- *Mild:* 150–500 mg/day (+)
- *Moderate:* 500 mg–2 g/day (++)
- *Massive:* >2 g/day (+++); if crosses 3.5 g/day, it is known as 'nephrotic range' proteinuria. Urine may be frothy in massive proteinuria.

NB: Microalbuminuria—A normal person excretes <20 µg of albumin/minute i.e., <30 mg/24 hours. If daily excretion of albumin goes in the range of 20–200 µg/minute (i.e., 30–300 mg/day), it is designated as microalbuminuria. It is a sign of glomerular abnormality and is commonly found in diabetes mellitus with early renal involvement.

Q. What is GFR (glomerular filtration rate)?

The glomerular filtration rate is the amount of blood filtered by the glomerulus into the Bowman's capsule per unit of time (i.e., it is a calculation that determines how well the blood is filtered by the kidneys). In health, an adult have glomerular filtration rate (GFR) of 120 ml/min; with age, the GFR diminishes. CKD is divided into 5 stages according to GFR. ESRD is the last stage of CKD when the GFR becomes <15 ml/min.

Q. A synopsis of glomerulonephritis.

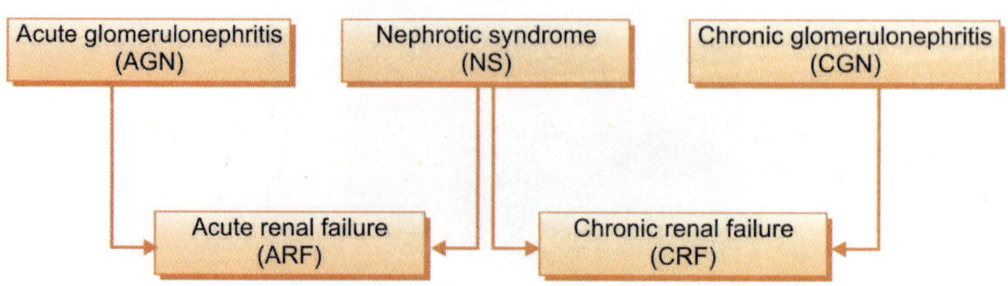

Acute glomerulonephritis (AGN), acute nephritis, type 1 nephritis, or acute nephritic syndrome (Fig. 7.4): It is an immune complex glomerulonephritis, where there is production of antibodies against glomerular antigen and thereby leading to deposition

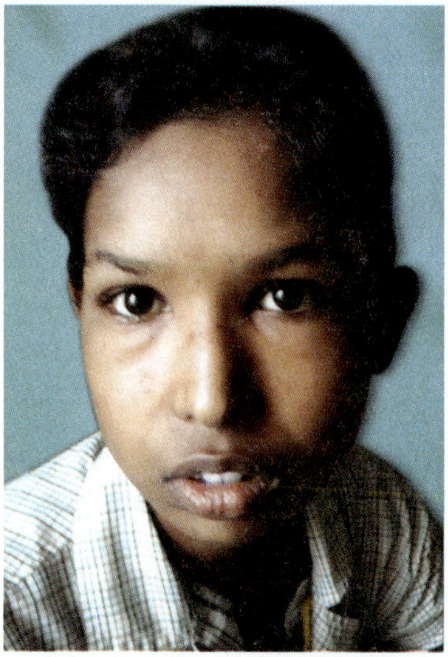

Fig. 7.4: Puffy face with mild swelling of lower eyelids from acute glomerulonephritis (AGN)

of immune complexes in the walls of glomerular capillaries, and developing into glomerular inflammation. The common causes are post-streptococcal (PSGN, most common), other bacterial (i.e., staphylococcal and pneumococcal) or viral (i.e., hepatitis B and C) infection, Henoch-Schönlein purpura, Goodpasture's syndrome (anti-glomerular basement membrane disease), IgA nephropathy, etc. The patient gives prior H/o pharyngeal infection (e.g., acute tonsillitis) or skin infection e.g., infected scabies, Fig. 7.5) in a case of PSGN. The 'latent period' in case of pharyngeal infection (H/o sore throat) is 1–3 weeks, whereas in cutaneous infection it averages 2–6 weeks. The patient of AGN, usually at the age of 5–15 years, presents with:

- Periorbital puffiness followed by generalised oedema (fluid retention)
- Oliguria (scanty urine)
- Haematuria (high-coloured/smoky/red/coca-cola like urine)
- Oedema and hypertension.

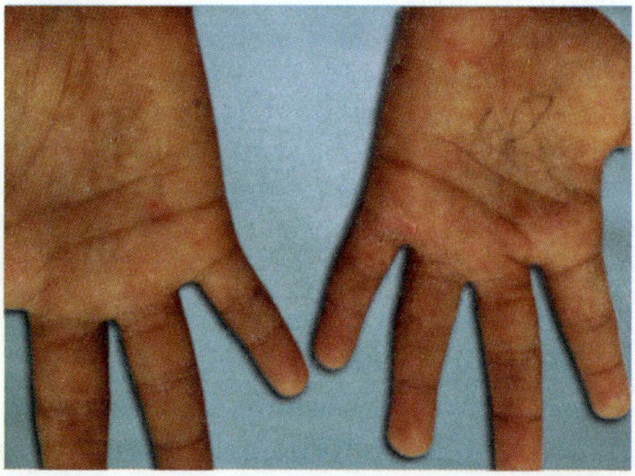

Fig. 7.5: Scabies—papules, pustules and impetigo are seen in hands. Infected scabies may give rise to acute glomerulonephritis

Complications of AGN are acute renal failure (ARF), acute LVF (patient may be breathless), hypertensive encephalopathy (patient may become unconscious) and electrolyte imbalance.

NB: Rapidly progressive glomerulonephritis (RPGN): A few patients of AGN show a little tendency to spontaneous recovery and develop renal failure within weeks or months are known as RPGN. The common causes are SLE, Goodpasture's syndrome and IgA nephropathy.

Nephrotic syndrome (NS, Fig. 7.6): It may be:

A. *Primary:*
- Minimal lesion or minimal change disease (most common cause in children)
- Membranous glomerulonephritis (most common cause in adults)
- Focal and segmental glomerulosclerosis
- Membranoproliferative glomerulonephritis
- Mesangial proliferative glomerulonephritis.

B. *Secondary:*
- Infections (post-streptococcal, malaria, infective endocarditis, HIV)
- Multisystem diseases—diabetes, SLE, vasculitis
- Drugs—penicillamine, gold, mercury, contrast media
- Heredofamilial—Alport's syndrome
- Neoplasms—lymphoma, leukaemia, carcinoma.

Definition of nephrotic syndrome: It is a clinical syndrome which is characterised by:
- Massive proteinuria (>3.5 g/day)
- Hypoalbuminaemia (i.e., serum albumin <3 g/dL)
- Generalised oedema or anasarca
- Hyperlipidaemia (i.e., serum cholesterol >300 mg/dL).

Complications of nephrotic syndrome are fluid retention, protein catabolism (i.e., wasting), susceptibility to infections, thromboembolic manifestations, accelerated atherosclerosis and chronic renal failure (CRF).

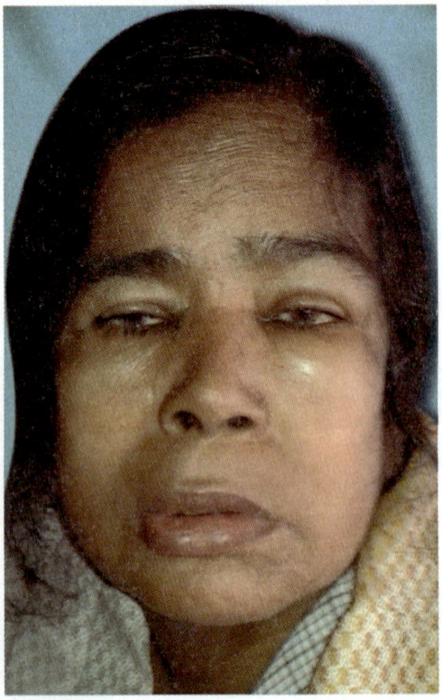

Fig. 7.6: Swelling of the face with periorbital oedema in nephrotic syndrome; the palpebral fissure of eyes are narrowed. The patient is suffering from dyspnoea as a result of bilateral hydrothorax

Chronic glomerulonephritis (CGN): The causes are idiopathic (most of the cases), SLE, vasculitis, hepatitis B or C infection, AIDS, or AGN after an interval of symptom-free period reappears as CGN. The patients present with facial puffiness in the morning, oedema, dyspnoea (as a result of anaemia), headache due to hypertension, or features of renal failure in severe cases e.g., nausea, vomiting, anorexia, hiccough, itching or easy bruising.

Q. Clinical differentiation between acute glomerulonephritis (AGN) and nephrotic syndrome (NS).

Features	*AGN*	*NS*
1. Age	5–15 years	1–5 years; also in adults
2. H/o pharyngitis or skin infection	Present	Absent
3. 'Acute onset' of oliguria	Present	Absent
4. Haematuria	Present	Absent
5. Hypertension	Present	Absent; may be present rarely
6. Generalised oedema (anasarca)	Absent	Present
7. Hydrothorax and scrotal oedema	Usually absent	May be present
8. Features of accelerated atherosclerosis (e.g., CVA)	Absent	May be present

Q. What is renal failure?

Renal failure is of two types: Acute and chronic.

- *Acute renal failure (ARF):* ARF is better known as acute kidney injury (AKI), which is manifested by sudden and usually reversible deterioration of renal function with rapid decline of GFR within hours to days with retention of nitrogenous waste products and disturbance of extracellular fluid balance, electrolytes, and acid-base homeostasis. The common causes are hypovolaemia (e.g., acute gastroenteritis, severe haemorrhage, acute pancreatitis), AGN, septicaemia, snakebite, hepatorenal syndrome, eclampsia.
- *Chronic renal failure (CRF):* Refers to long-standing, progressive, and irreversible deterioration of renal function classically developing over a period of years. The common causes are CGN, diabetes, malignant hypertension, collagen vascular diseases (e.g., SLE), interstitial nephropathy, obstructive uropathy (e.g., BHP), polycystic kidney disease, analgesic nephropathy (NSAID-induced).

NB: A patient of chronic kidney disease (CKD) may remain asymptomatic and suddenly detected to have high serum urea and creatinine on routine biochemical check-up. The CKD patient usually complains of anorexia, nausea, vomiting, hiccough and lethargy. Pallor (as a result of anaemia—which is multifactorial as a result of low erythropoietin, reduced red cell survival, reduced dietary intake, increased blood loss due to poor platelet function, diminished erythropoiesis, etc.), generalised pruritus, pigmentation, ecchymosis, drowsiness, convulsions, persistent hypertension, and coma may supervene when CRF appears (a few symptoms of CKD are due to CRF). Remember, the history is short in ARF in comparison to CRF, which is prolonged.

The terms CRF and uraemia are often used for the same purpose.

Q. What is renal replacement therapy?

'Renal replacement therapy' (RRT) is meant for replacing the function of the kidneys, when acute or chronic renal failure (ARF or CRF) sets in. Different types of RRT are:

- Haemofiltration (it removes waste products by convection when blood is passed through a set of tubing via a machine to a semipermeable membrane).

- Haemodialysis (it removes solutes by diffusion when the toxic elements in blood are filtered through a membrane while circulated outside of the body via a sophisticated machine).
- Peritoneal dialysis (here the peritoneum act as a filtering membrane; fluid is introduced within the peritoneal cavity and then drained afterwards).
- Renal transplantation (cadaveric or living donor transplantation).

NB: 'Dialysis': The most popular RRT is nothing but an artificial replacement (*see* above) for lost kidney function in renal failure.

Q. What are the normal serum sodium, potassium and calcium levels and their causes of aberrations?

Elements	*Normal level*	*Low level*	*High level*
Sodium	136–145 mmol/L	Hyponatraemia: Severe diarrhoea, vomiting, excess of diuretics, SIADH, renal failure	Hypernatraemia: Diabetes insipidus, infusion of hypertonic saline, Conn's syndrome
Potassium	3.5–5 mmol/L	Hypokalaemia: Severe vomiting, use of diuretics, metabolic alkalosis, DKA, Conn's syndrome	Hyperkalaemia: Renal failure, Addison's disease, metabolic acidosis, muscle crush
Calcium	9–11 mg/dL	Hypocalcaemia: Malabsorption, CRF, acute pancreatitis, hypopara-thyroidism, rickets or osteomalacia, use of bisphosphonates	Hypercalcaemia: Primary hyperparathyroidism, multiple myeloma, Paget's disease, malignant tumour with bony metastasis

Decoding Abbreviations

CKD	Chronic kidney disease
ARF	Acute renal failure
CRF	Chronic renal failure
BHP	Benign hypertrophy of prostate
SIADH	Syndrome of inappropriate antidiuretic hormone
RPGN	Rapidly progressive glomerulonephritis
PSGN	Post-streptococcal glomerulonephritis
GFR	Glomerular filtration rate
DKA	Diabetic ketoacidosis.

Chapter

8

Nervous System

SCHEME OF SYSTEMIC EXAMINATION: AN OVERVIEW

I. Whether the patient is conscious, alert and co-operative.

II. *Higher functions:* Level of consciousness, appearance and behaviour, orientation with time/place/person, personality and behavioural abnormality, illusion/delusion/hallucination, memory, intelligence, sleep, speech with handedness.

III. Cranium and spine.

IV. Neck rigidity, Kernig's sign, Brudzinski's sign, straight leg raising (SLR) test, and examination of carotid arteries.

V. *Cranial nerves:* From I to XII cranial nerves (motor and sensory functions, and reflexes).

VI. *Motor functions:* Nutrition, tone, power, co-ordination and involuntary movements.

VII. *Sensory functions*

- Superficial: Pain, touch, temperature
- Deep: Vibration (Fig. 8.1), muscle, pressure, joint and position sense
- Cortical: One point localisation, two point discrimination, stereognosis, graphaesthesia, perceptual rivalry.

VIII. *Reflexes*

- Superficial: Abdominal, cremasteric, plantar response
- Deep: Biceps, triceps, supinator, knee and ankle jerk; clonus (patellar and ankle) present or not?

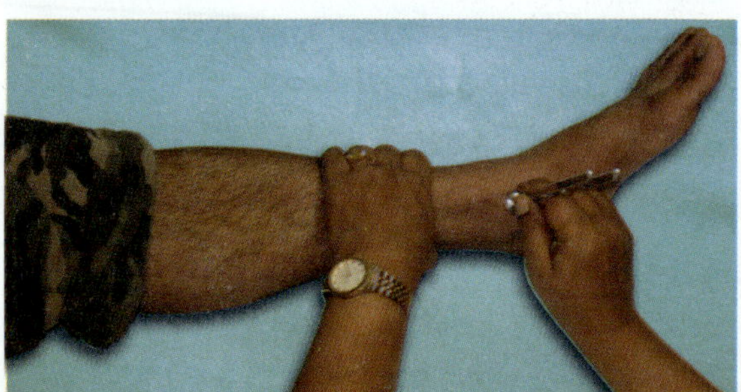

Fig. 8.1: Testing vibration sense at the ankle

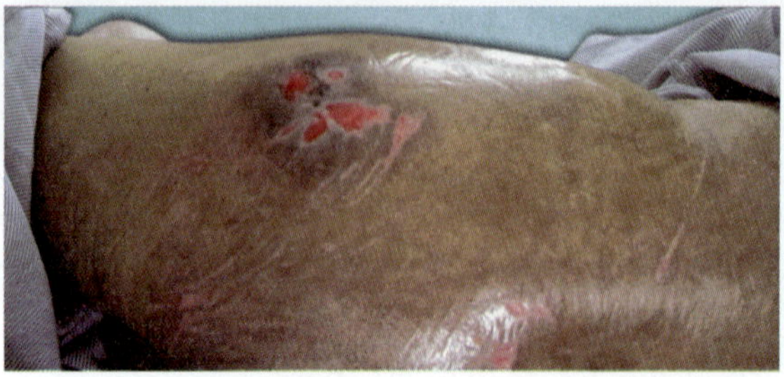

Fig. 8.2: Bedsore (denuded skin over bony prominences) in a chronic debilitated patient

- Visceral: Swallowing, bladder, bowel.
- Others: Glabellar tap, grasp reflex, palmo-mental reflex, sucking reflex.

NB: Motor, sensory functions and reflexes are tested for upper and lower limbs for both the sides. Cranial nerves are tested for both the sides.

IX. *Trophic changes:* Bedsore (in pressure points like over sacrum, Fig. 8.2) trophic ulcer (Fig. 8.3), Charcot joint, changes in skin and hair.

X. *Cerebellar functions:* Scanning speech, intention tremor, dysdiadochokinesia, nystagmus, dysmetria, rebound phenomenon, pendular knee jerk, etc.

XI. *Autonomic functions:* Postural hypotension, impotence, nocturnal diarrhoea, abnormal sweating, Horner's syndrome, etc.

XII. *Stance* and gait (including Romberg's sign):* For example, wide base stance; festinant, waddling, hemiplegic, reeling or stamping gait, etc.

NB: After the examination of central nervous system (CNS), peripheral nervous system (PNS) should be examined in the following way.

Peripheral nervous system: Peripheral nerves e.g., great auricular nerve at neck, ulnar nerve at elbow and common peroneal nerve at the neck of fibula are examined for thickening, nodularity and tenderness (reference: Leprosy).

*Stance (attitude of the patient on standing) and gait (posture of the patient during walking) should be tested in all patients, if possible. Tandem gait (i.e., heel to toe gait gives early diganosis of gait instability, Fig. 8.4).

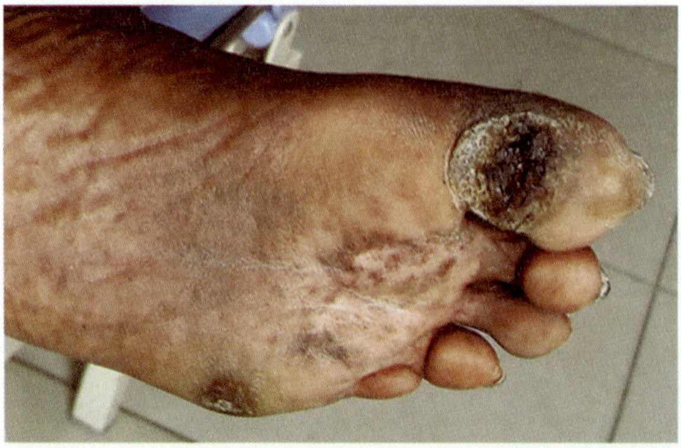

Fig. 8.3: Trophic ulcer in a case of peripheral neuropathy

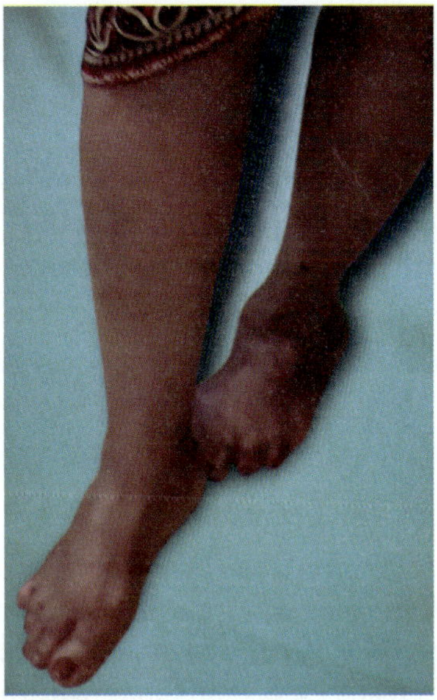

Fig. 8.4: Heel to toe walking (tandem gait) testing

Q. Mention the common presentations (chief complaints and H/o present illness) in nervous system.

The major symptoms regarding all sectors in neurology are:

A. *Higher function:* Unconsciousness, behavioural abnormality, sudden difficulty in speech, loss of memory, delirium or emotional disturbances.

B. *Cranial nerves:* Disturbance in smell, visual abnormality, diplopia, sudden drooping of eyelid, difficulty in mastication, facial asymmetry, loss of taste sensation, vertigo, hearing loss, nasal intonation or regurgitation, dysarthria, wasting of the tongue.

C. *Motor system:* Loss of power, wasting, muscle pain, abnormal movements (e.g., fasciculation or flexor spasms), unsteady gait.

D. *Sensory system:* Anaesthesia, paraesthesia, tingling, numbness, analgesia, root pain*, girdle-like sensation, or like walking on cotton wool.

E. *Increased intracranial tension (IIT):* Headache, vomiting, convulsions, coma.

F. *Cerebellar system:* Swaying while walking, weakness (i.e., for hypotonia), shaking of hands when reaching for an object, difficulty in shaving, etc.

G. *Autonomic nervous system:* Retention of urine, urinary incontinence, precipitancy or hesitancy during micturition, impotence, diarrhoea or constipation.

H. *Others:* Fever (meningitis, brain abscess), seizure [epilepsy or cerebrovascular accidents (CVA)], psychological aberration (e.g., sudden euphoria or agitation), nuchal pain (neck pain is due to meningitis or subarachnoid haemorrhage), stiffness of the body (parkinsonism), abnormal movements (chorea), discharging ear (meningitis).

NB: *Other symptoms in neurology:*

- Symptoms *in the limb* complaint by the patient—pain, weakness, paraestheia and root pain*.
- Difficulty in *loss of power in the motor system of limbs:*

- Upper limb: Proximal weakness (lifting of arm above head), distal weakness (writing, sewing).
- Lower limb: Proximal (squatting and getting up from squatting position), distal (slipper falling from the feet).

- Symptoms *in the head* complaint by the patient—abnormality in smell and taste, visual loss, hearing loss, headache (headache of IIT, migraine, or headache with neck pain in meningitis or subarachnoid haemorrhage), syncope or black-out, dizziness and vertigo.

*Root pain is the sharp, stabbing, electric shock-like pain aggravated by coughing, jolting, sneezing or movement of spine. It is due to irritation or compression of posterior nerve roots (also known as radicular pain).

Q. 'Evolution' of symptoms in clinical neurology.

1. *Sudden onset and rapidly evolving neurodeficit:* Vascular or traumatic.
2. *Gradually progressive course:* Over months (intracranial space occupying lesion or ICSOL) or over years (e.g., Parkinson's disease, Alzheimer's disease).
3. *With waxing and waning i.e., relapse and remissions:* Multiple sclerosis (a demyelinating disease).
4. *Episodic weakness with full recovery:* Epilepsy, periodic paralysis.
5. *Temporary focal weakness:* Transient ischaemic attack (TIA), Todd's palsy (i.e., paralysis following epilepsy recovers within 24 hours).

Q. What is meant by the following terminologies?

Remember: **'Plegia'** means complete paralysis, while **'paresis'** means partial paralysis or weakness.

1. *Hemiplegia:* Paralysis of one-half of the body (especially of face, arm and leg), and usually the cause remains within the brain. If face is involved, it is complete hemiplegia and if not, it is incomplete hemiplegia. Hemiparesis is weakness of one-half of the body.
2. *Paraplegia:* Paralysis of both the lower limbs (commonly due to lesion in the spinal cord). Paraparesis is weakness of both the lower limbs.
3. *Monoplegia:* Paralysis of one limb. Paralysis of one upper limb is called **brachial monoplegia**, while that of one lower limb is known as **crural monoplegia**.
4. *Quadriplegia:* Paralysis of all the four limbs (commonly a feature of cervical cord lesion).
5. *Crossed hemiplegia:* Paralysis of ipsilateral cranial nerve (lower motor neurone or LMN type) with contralateral hemiplegia (due to a brainstem lesion).

Q. What are upper motor neuron (UMN) and lower motor neuron (LMN)?

In neurological disorders, one has to determine whether it is UMN lesion or LMN lesion. Each type of lesion has specific clinical features (*see* Table below).

- *UMN:* The pyramidal cells in the motor area of cerebral cortex and their axons up to the cranial nerve nuclei (i.e., corticonuclear or corticobulbar tract), or anterior horn cells in the spinal cord (i.e., corticospinal tract) are known as UMN.

- *LMN:* The anterior horn cells of the spinal cord and its dendrite up to the motor end plate, and cranial nerve nuclei in the brainstem with the cranial nerves constitute LMN. LMN is the final common pathway of all types of motor impulses.

Q. How to differentiate between UMN and LMN paralysis?

Signs	*UMN palsy*	*LMN palsy*
1. Muscle involvement and power	Muscle groups are involved Muscles are weak	Individual muscles are involved Muscles are more weak than UMN palsy
2. Wasting and fasciculation	Absent (only disuse atrophy may be present)	Present. Atrophy and wasting are prominent features
3. Tone	Hypertonia (clasp-knife spasticity)	Hypotonia (flaccidity)
4. Reflexes	Superficial reflexes lost. Deep reflexes (i.e., jerks) are brisk	Superficial reflexes lost. Deep reflexes (i.e., jerks) are lost or diminished
5. Plantar response	Extensor (i.e., Babinski's sign present)	Flexor

Q. What is a 'stroke'?

The term stroke usually identifies all forms of 'cerebrovascular accidents (CVA)'. A stroke or CVA is defined as 'focal neurological deficit of abrupt onset due to a vascular lesion, lasting >24 hours, and is manifested, either as cerebral infarction or haemorrhage'.

So, stroke may be haemorrhagic (20%) or ischaemic (80%). Cerebral thrombosis and cerebral embolism result in cerebral ischaemia, which ultimately lead to **cerebral infarction**. Most common cause of hemiplegia in the elderly is cerebral infarction.

In a stroke, commonly the patient presents with impaired consciousness, aphasia (loss of speech), hemiplegia or hemiparesis, hemisensory loss, or even coma. Visual field defects or signs of involvement of brainstem are obtained. Features of increased intracranial tension (IIT) are always associated with cerebrovascular accidents (see below).

As majority of pyramidal fibres cross in the medulla, right-sided cerebral haemorrhage/infarction in the brain will give rise to left-sided hemiplegia, and vice versa for left-sided cerebral haemorrhage/infarction.

Q. Diseases under cerebrovascular accidents (CVA, producing hemiplegia).

- ***Pathological classification***
  - *Cerebral thrombosis:* Thrombus obstruct intracerebral vessels (anterior, middle and posterior cerebral arteries and their branches); usually hypertensive and atherosclerotic.
  - *Cerebral embolism:* Embolism from cardiac source (e.g., MS with atrial fibrillation, mitral valve prolapse) obstruct intracerebral vessels.
  - *Cerebral haemorrhage:* Almost all patients are hypertensive. Headache and vomiting occur at the onset of paralysis; prognosis is bad.
  - *Subarachnoid haemorrhage:* Commonly in young adults with a bursting occipital headache, and is due to rupture of berry aneurysm or arteriovenous malformations in the brain; neck rigidity and Kernig's sign are present.

- *Hypertensive encephalopathy:* An acute syndrome with severe hypertension along with nausea, vomiting, excruciating headache, convulsions, confusion, speech or vision difficulty and coma. The neurodeficit is totally correctable.
- *Others (subtle stroke):* Multiple sclerosis, Todd's palsy, cerebral metastasis, subdural or epidural haematoma.

NB: These are the CVAs or diseases under CVA.

- ***Clinical classification*** (on the basis of evolution and duration)
  - *Transient ischaemic attack (TIA):* Abrupt onset of focal neurological deficit due to cerebral ischaemia occurring in atherosclerotic vascular disease complicated by hypertension, where symptoms last for <24 hours and the patient recovers completely. It is postulated that the definition of TIA is unsatisfactory as ischaemic changes occur after 1 hour.
  - *Stroke in evolution:* The symptoms worsen gradually or in a step-wise pattern over hours or days.
  - *Completed stroke:* The neurological deficit is completed from the beginning and persists for weeks or months, and often permanently.
  - *Minor stroke:* Usually the patient recovers within a week.

NB: Hemiplegia occurs due to lesion in cerebral cortex (commonly monoplegia), subcortex (i.e., corona radiata), internal capsule (most common site for CVA), brainstem (crossed hemiplegia) and upper spinal region (incomplete hemiplegia i.e., face is not involved)). *In CVA, the hemiplegic side of the body is the opposite side of cerebral involvement;* in spinal hemiplegia, ipsilateral side of the body is involved.

Q. Common risk factors for CVA.

- *Major risk factors:*
  - Systemic hypertension
  - Smoking
  - Diabetes mellitus
  - Hyperlipidaemia
  - Cardiac diseases (valvular and ischaemic heart diseases)
  - Obesity.
- *Minor risk factors:*
  - Strong family H/o CVA
  - Oral contraceptive pills
  - Trauma
  - High alcohol consumption
  - Sleep apnoea.

Q. What is meant by 'strokes in young'?

CVA or strokes are common above 40 years of age where atherosclerosis is the main cause. On the other hand, strokes in young occurs <40 years of age where the causes are a bit different from aged population, and they are:

- Cerebral embolism
- Subarachnoid haemorrhage

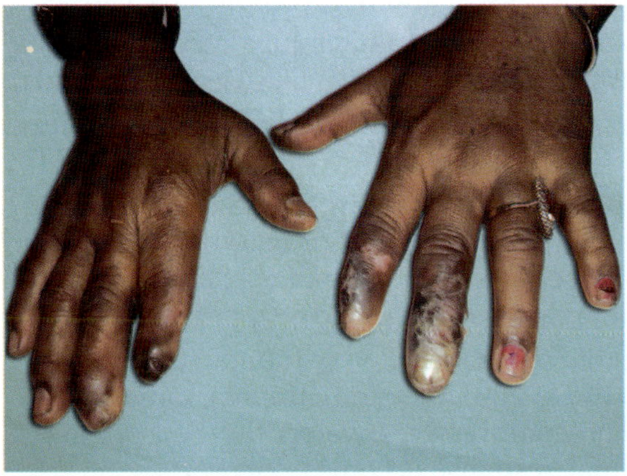

Fig. 8.5: Periungual erythema, nail dystrophy and small ulcerations are seen in distal end of fingers in anticardiolipin antibody syndrome

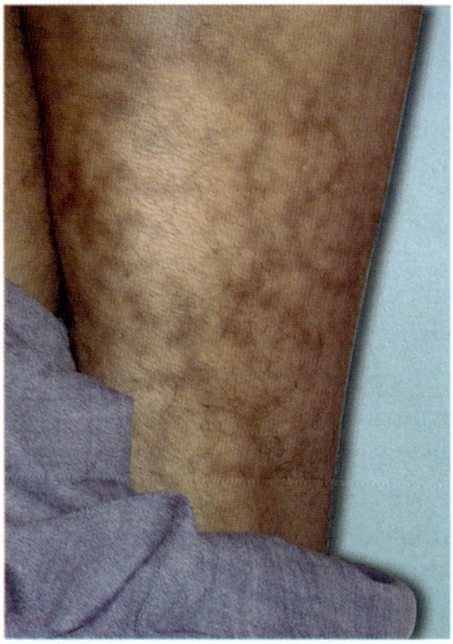

Fig. 8.6: Livedo reticularis in leg seen in anticardiolipin antibody syndrome

- Vasculitis or arteritis (e.g., Takayasu's disease)
- Demyelinating disease (e.g., multiple sclerosis)
- Intracranial space occupying lesion (ICSOL or brain tumour)
- Procoagulant states like antithrombin III deficiency, antiphospholipid antibody syndrome (or anticardiolipin antibody syndrome, Figs 8.5 and 8.6)
- Head injury
- *Miscellaneous:* Encephalitis, cerebral malaria, cerebral abscess, drug abuse (e.g., cocaine), anticoagulant therapy, hyperviscosity syndrome (e.g., polycythemia, thrombocythemia), hemiplegic migraine.

Q. What are the different causes of paraplegia?

- *Paraplegia commonly develops from lesions in spinal cord (cerebral causes are rare).* Spinal causes may develop into *spastic (UMN type lesion)* or *flaccid (LMN type lesion)* paraplegia. Again each of spastic and flaccid paraplegia may be of *compressive* or *non-compressive* in origin. Proper history and evolution of paralysis very often clinch the aetiological diagnosis.

Aetiology of paraplegia:

- *Cerebral causes:* Cerebral diplegia, superior sagittal sinus thrombosis, parasagittal meningioma, hydrocephalus.
- *Spinal causes:*
  - Spastic paraplegia
    - Compressive (transverse lesion in spinal cord): 'Cord compression' due to glioma, meningioma, neurofibroma, syringomyelia, caries spine (i.e., Pott's paraplegia due to spinal tuberculosis: Probably the most common cause in India), patchy meningitis, multiple myeloma, leukaemic/lymphomatous/ metastatic deposits in spine, trauma, prolapsed intervertebral disc (PID).

    - Non-compressive (longitudinal lesion in spinal cord): Acute transverse myelitis, multiple sclerosis, motor neuron disease (MND), lathyrism, Friedreich's ataxia, subacute combined degeneration (SCD), hereditary spastic paraplegia.
  - Flaccid paraplegia (including both compressive and non-compressive causes):
    - Spastic paraplegia in 'neural shock stage' (e.g., spinal injury, acute transverse myelitis; in neural shock stage, spastic paraplegia behaves like flaccid paraplegia).
    - Guillain-Barré (GB) syndrome, poliomyelitis, trauma, lumbar plexus injury, periodic paralysis due to hypo- or hyperkalaemia.

NB: ***GB syndrome:*** An immune-mediated, acute post-infective demyelinating polyradiculoneuropathy which gives rise to *flaccid paraplegia* or quadriplegia. It is an example of flaccid paraplegia. There will be no sensory loss and plantar response becomes flexor. Complete or near complete recovery occurs in 80% patients.

Acute transverse myelitis: Acute onset of total transection of the spinal cord due to infection (most common and commonly due to viral infection), trauma, radiation, etc. resulting in *spastic paraplegia*; it is also a non-compressive myelopathy. Sensory loss is present below the level of lesion and plantar response becomes extensor.

Acute transverse myelitis and GB syndrome are two common causes of paraplegia in clinical practice.

Q. What are conus medullaris and cauda equina?

There are 31 pairs of spinal nerve i.e., cervical 8, thoracic 12, lumbar 5, sacral 5, and coccygeal 1. At the level of L_1 vertebra, spinal cord ends and tapers to form 'conus medullaris'. The spinal roots below L_1 vertebra emerge at their respective foramina, and form 'cauda equina'.

Q. What do you mean by seizure, epilepsy and convulsions?

- *Seizure:* A seizure is a sudden surge of electrical activity in the brain due to paroxysmal, excessive and synchronous discharge from CNS neurones. Seizures are divided into two broad categories: Generalised e.g., grand mal epilepsy, and partial or focal e.g., in brain tumour.
- *Epilepsy*:* It is a chronic disorder which is characterised by recurrent, unprovoked seizures.
- *Convulsions (fits):* It is an abnormal violent and involuntary contraction, or series of contractions of the muscles of extremities, trunk and head. On the other way, convulsions are the motor component of a seizure.

*Status epilepticus: When convulsions and unconsciousness recur without any intervening normal period in between.

Q. What are delirium and dementia?

- *Delirium:* It is an acute confusional state due to acute or subacute brain failure with global impairment of cognitive functions, where impairment of attention is accompanied by abnormality of perception and mood. The patient may be violent and talkative.

The common causes of acute confusion are CVA, septicaemia, head injury, encephalitis, alcohol intoxication/withdrawal, illicit drug intake, organ failure (hepatic, renal or respiratory), hyponatraemia, and hypoglycaemia/hyperglycaemia.

- *Dementia:* It means loss of reasoning or more particularly, a deterioration of all intellectual and cognitive functions without alteration of consciousness, and is usually due to chronic progressive degenerative disease of brain where memory is affected in the early stage.

The common causes of dementia (or loss of memory) are cerebral atherosclerosis (e.g., multi-infarct dementia), chronic subdural haematoma, Alzheimer's disease, alcoholism, Wernicke-Korsakoff syndrome, pellagra, Wilson's disease, 'normal pressure' hydrocephalus, vitamin B_{12} deficiency, Huntington's disease, and AIDS.

Q. What is Mini-Mental State Examination (MMSE)?

It is a simple bedside test to assess difficulty in cognitive functions (i.e., mental or intellectual functions), and is performed by 10 simple questions, while the results are scored numerically.

Q. What are the clinical features and causes of increased intracranial tension (IIT)?

Anywhere in clinical medicine, a clinical feature means combination of symptoms and signs. Features of IIT are:

Symptoms

- Headache (pain in and around the vertex is headache; there is early morning dull aching pain in head which is increased by coughing/sneezing/exertion/bending forward).
- Vomiting (sometimes there is 'projectile vomiting' i.e., without warning symptoms of nausea).
- Convulsions (usually generalised convulsions).
- Altered consciousness to coma.

Signs

- Pulse: Bradycardia; may be irregular pulse.
- BP: There may be hypertension.
- Respiration: To start with it is slow and deep respiration which ultimately becomes rapid and shallow breathing to end with Cheyne-Stokes respiration.
- Pupil: Unequal or abnormally reacting; papilloedema on fundus examination by an ophthalmoscope.
- False localising signs like bilateral Babinski's sign, or VIth cranial nerve palsy (unilateral or bilateral).
- Anterior fontanelle is bulged in infants.

Causes

- Cerebrovascular accidents (CVAs).
- Meningitis, encephalitis, meningism.
- Intracranial space occupying lesions (SOL) like cerebral tumour, cerebral abscess, cerebral haematoma.
- *Others:* Head injury, cerebral oedema, hydrocephalus, cerebral venous sinus thrombosis, and benign intracranial hypertension.

Q. What are meningitis and meningism?

- ***Meningitis:*** It is the inflammation of meninges. Common causes of meningitis in the community are viral meningitis, tuberculous meningitis and bacterial (e.g., meningococcal) meningitis, which results from acute infection of meninges by different virus and bacteria. The common symptoms are high fever, headache (commonly nuchal i.e., at nape of the neck), photophobia, nausea and vomiting, with signs of meningeal irritation like neck rigidity, Kernig's sign and Brudzinski's sign. Signs of meningeal irritation are demonstrated by:
  - *Neck rigidity* (Fig. 8.7)*:* Stand on the right side of supine patient. Try to lift the patient's head from the bed by placing your left hand behind the patient's head. In health, the neck is supple and can be easily flexed but in meningitis, the neck cannot be flexed easily due to spasm of extensor muscles of neck.

    Neck rigidity and Kernig's sign are present in meningitis, meningism, subarachnoid haemorrhage, meningoencephalitis, and tetanus.
  - *Kernig's sign* (Fig. 8.8)*:* In meningitis, extension of the knee with the hip joints flexed at 90° gives rise to painful spasm of hamstring muscles, and it is impossible to straighten the leg.
  - *Brudzinski's sign (in children):* In meningitis, passive flexion of the neck causes reflex flexion of the hip, or knee of one or both the limbs.
- ***Meningism:*** It is synonymous with meningeal irritation as a result of local or systemic infection without any direct infection of CNS. The symptoms of meningism and meningitis are very often similar though in meningism, neck rigidity is present but Kernig's sign is less pronounced. The common causes of meningism are enteric fever (typhoid fever), pneumonia, tonsillitis, or any viral illness.

In meningism, the macroscopical, chemical, microscopical and bacteriological examination of cerebrospinal fluid (CSF) examined after lumbar puncture is absolutely within normal limits, while in meningitis all the findings of CSF remain abnormal; only the CSF pressure remains high in meningism.

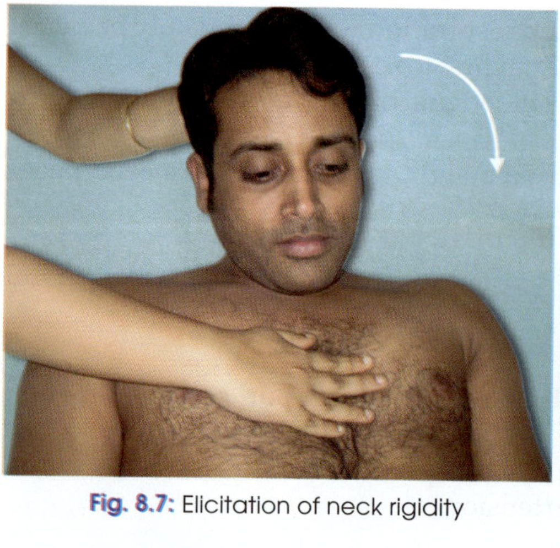

Fig. 8.7: Elicitation of neck rigidity

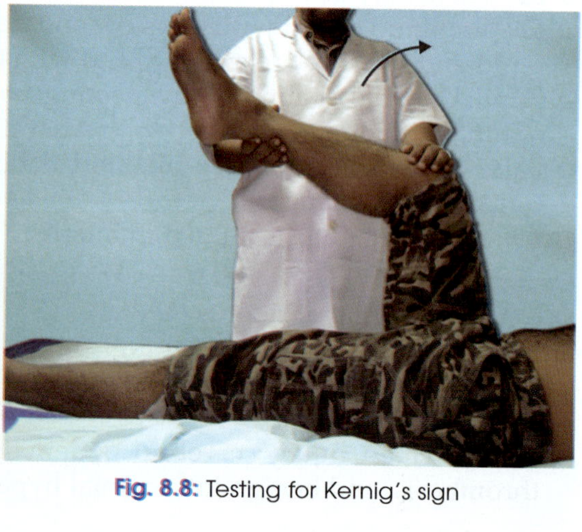

Fig. 8.8: Testing for Kernig's sign

Q. What are different causes of coma?

Coma is the persistent loss of consciousness where the patient cannot be aroused by external or internal stimuli. Structural lesions in the brain, toxic or metabolic derangements, and cardiac problems are the main causes of coma such as:

- CVA (e.g., cerebral haemorrhage, massive cerebral infarction with oedema, subarachnoid haemorrhage, hypertensive encephalopathy), encephalitis, subdural or extradural haematoma, cerebral malaria, head injury, post-epileptic fits.
- Diabetic ketoacidosis, hypoglycaemia, hyponatraemia, renal failure, hepatic failure, respiratory failure, adrenal crisis, pituitary apoplexy, eclampsia.
- Stokes-Adams syndrome (develops from complete heart block), arrhythmia, tight aortic stenosis, cardiogenic shock (i.e., from AMI), severe hypotension.
- Poisoning (e.g., barbiturate), drug or alcohol overdose, hypothermia, heat stroke, snakebite, severe sepsis, psychogenic (e.g., hysteria).

Q. Can you explain illusion, delusion and hallucination?

They are:

- *Illusion:* Abnormal perceptions or false interpretations of real stimuli which is corrected by proper explanation i.e., a rope can mimic a snake but the false impression immediately goes after proper clarification.
- *Delusion:* False beliefs which can never be corrected with facts i.e., here the rope will always be taken as a snake and never corrected by proper explanation.
- *Hallucination:* False perceptions through a special sense i.e., auditory, visual, olfactory or gustatory, in the absence of any external stimulus i.e., a person hears voices when none is present around him/her.

*Also read the 'Level of consciousness' in the section of 'General examination'.

Q. What are the enquiries and tests for cranial nerves done at bedside?

1. *Olfactory (I):* Enquire about changes in smell (or taste). Testing is done ideally with oil of peppermint or oil of cloves but in clinical practice it is done with common familiar objects like soap, toothpaste, scent, etc. Most common cause of bilateral anosmia (i.e., loss of smell sensation) is due to coryza (i.e., inflammation of nose, commonly due to cold), and not as a result of neurological insult; unilateral anosmia may result from head injury. Test separately on each nostril.
2. *Optic (II):* Ask for any visual difficulty. Inspect the eyes closely and test for acuity of vision (near vision is tested by Jaeger's chart and distant vision by Snellen's chart), field of vision (assessed clinically by 'confrontation perimetry', and ideally by Bjerrum's screen perimeter), colour vision (clinically tested by any colouring agent, and ideally tested by Ishihara's chart) and fundoscopy (the fundi of both eyes are examined by an ophthalmoscope). The common visual field defects are homonymous hemianopia (mostly due to CVA) and bitemporal hemianopia (typically by a pituitary tumour).
3. *Oculomotor (III), trochlear (IV), abducens (VI):* Enquire for diplopia, observe for ptosis (drooping of the upper eyelid) and squint, and test for voluntary ocular movements, nystagmus and pupillary reflexes (direct light reflex, consensual light reflex,

accommodation reflex). Unilateral ptosis is commonly due to oculomotor palsy (e.g., from diabetes mellitus) or Horner's syndrome (cervical sympathetic palsy), and bilateral ptosis is due to myasthenia gravis, myotonia dystrophica, snakebite (Elapidae group) and congenital. Partial ptosis results from Horner's syndrome and recovering oculomotor palsy. In IVth cranial nerve palsy, the patient cannot look down from neutral position of eyes, and in VIth nerve palsy, the patient has limitation of lateral movement of the eyeball.

4. *Trigeminal (V):* Test for sensory functions (pain, touch and temperature) over face (ophthalmic, maxillary and mandibular division of trigeminal nerve), and power of 'muscles of mastication' (i.e., temporalis, masseter and pterygoids; these muscles are tested by clenching the teeth, and opening the mouth against resistance). Elicit the corneal reflex of both the sides (afferent pathway is ophthalmic division of trigeminal and efferent pathway is facial nerve, Fig. 8.9) and jaw jerk—both afferent and efferent pathways pass though trigeminal nerve; jaw jerk is increased in bilateral UMN lesion above Vth nerve nucleus at pons, Fig. 8.10). Muscles of mastication are wasted in MND. Herpes zoster ophthalmicus affects the ophthalmic division of trigeminal nerve of one side, which may end fataly with loss of vision (Fig. 8.11).
5. *Facial (VII):* Look for palpebral fissure, frowning, symmetry of blinking, eye closure, nasolabial folds, angle of the mouth, blowing of the cheek, showing the teeth, and dribbling of saliva. Try to assess the function of muscles of facial expression like frontalis (wrinkling the forehead), corrugator superciliaris (frowning), orbicularis oculi (closing the eyes forcibly), buccinators (blowing or whistling), orbicularis oris (purse the lips shut). Ask the patient to show his/her upper teeth, and note the deviation of the angle of mouth towards the healthy side. One can assess the taste sensation of anterior two-thirds of the tongue. Facial nerve palsy is the most common cranial nerve palsy encountered in clinical practice. It is desirable to differentiate between LMN (e.g., Bell's palsy) (Fig. 8.12) and UMN type e.g., CVA or stroke, of VIIth nerve palsy; in UMN type of VIIth nerve palsy, the forehead is spared while in LMN type palsy, forehead is affected on the paralysed side.

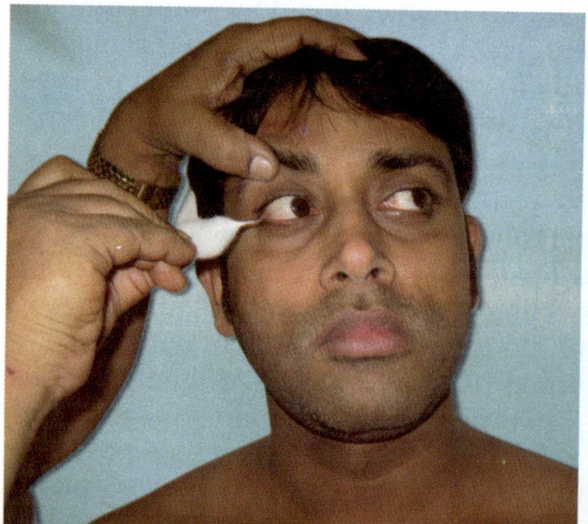

Fig. 8.9: Demonstration of corneal reflex

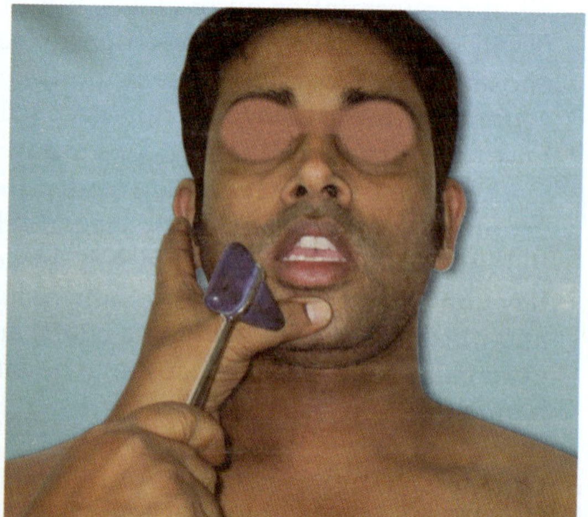

Fig. 8.10: Elicitation of jaw jerk

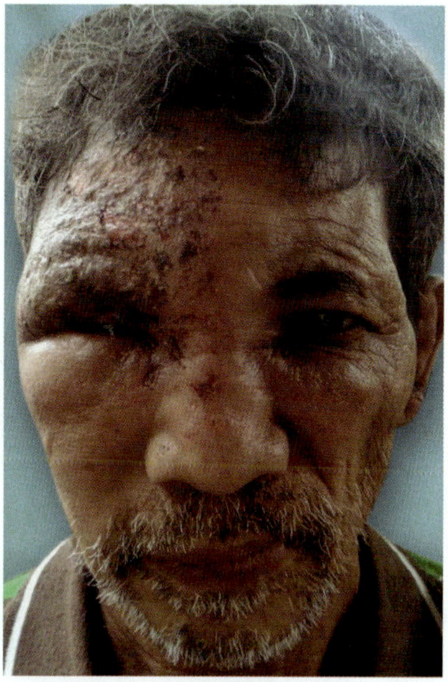

Fig. 8.11: Herpes zoster ophthalmicus affecting the right side

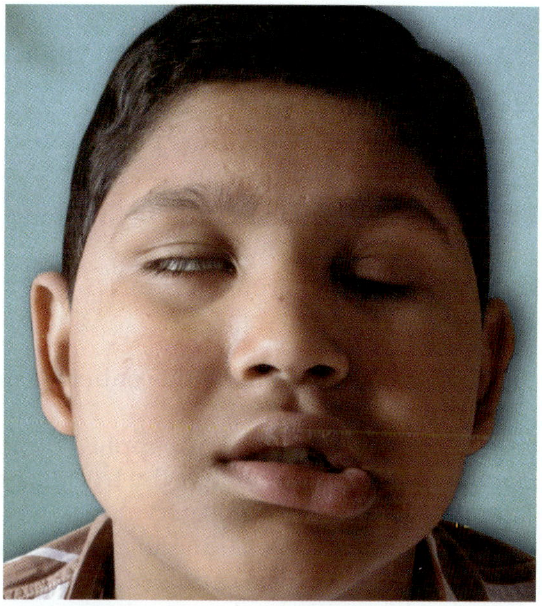

Fig. 8.12: Right-sided Bell's palsy (lower motor neuron VIIth cranial nerve palsy) with deviation of face to left side on showing the teeth; there is incomplete eye closure on right side

6. *Vestibulocochlear (VIII):* Ask for deafness, tinnitus i.e., ringing in the ears, and vertigo. Test for hearing by whisper test, Rinne's and Weber's test, if necessary. Vestibular function is tested by positional nystagmus and caloric test. Deafness is of two types: conductive deafness is commonly due to diseases of outer and middle ear, while sensorineural deafness is usually attributable to presbycusis, Ménière's disease, etc.
7. *Glossopharyngeal (IX) and vagus (X):* Examine patient's voice, movement of soft palate (tested by asking the patient to say 'Aaah'), and 'gag reflex'; one can test the taste sensation of posterior one-third of the tongue (supplied by IXth cranial nerve). Lesions of IX, X, XII, XII cranial nerves usually occur in combination (read bulbar and pseudobulbar palsy).
8. *Accessory, spinal part (XI):* Assess the power of trapezius (tested by opposing the shrugging of the shoulders of the patient, standing behind the patient) and sternomastoid muscles (tested by turning the face to opposite side against resistance applied over chin) on both the sides.
9. *Hypoglossal (XII):* Inspect the tongue for wasting, fasciculation and position within the oral cavity. Ask the patient to protrude the tongue out of the oral cavity to see the tremor, if there is any. Examine the power of the tongue.

Q. How to differentiate 'ptosis' due to third nerve palsy and Horner's syndrome?

Ptosis is the drooping of one or both upper eyelids.

Oculomotor palsy

- Usually complete ptosis (commonly unilateral; due to paralysis of levator palpebrae superioris)

- Lateral or divergent squint (due to unopposed action of lateral rectus)
- Fixed (loss of light and accommodation reflex) and dilated pupil.

Horner's syndrome

- Pseudoptosis (it is a partial ptosis; due to paralysis of Muller's muscle)
- Miosis (constricted pupil)
- Anhidrosis (ipsilateral loss of sweating over face, neck, upper chest and arm)
- Enophthalmos (shrunken eye)
- Loss of ciliospinal reflex.

NB: In oculomotor palsy, the patient complains of diplopia.

All extraocular muscles are supplied by occulomotor nerve except superior oblique (by trochlear nerve) and lateral rectus (by abducens nerve).

Horner's syndrome is due to paralysis of cervical sympathetic nerve. The causes of Horner's syndrome are central (hypothalamic cause, brainstem infarction, syringomyelia), peripheral (carcinoma of apex of the lung, mediastinal mass, carotid artery thrombosis), and others (congenital, idiopathic).

Ptosis is commonly due to oculomotor palsy, Horner's syndrome, myasthenia gravis, Elapidae snakebite, myotonic dystrophy or congenital (Fig. 8.13).

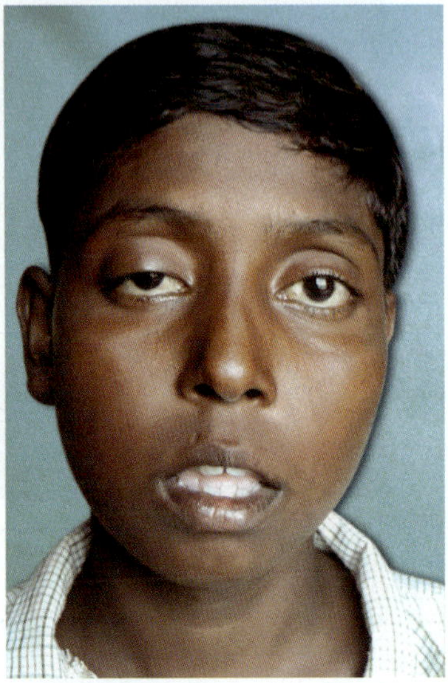

Fig. 8.13: Unilateral partial ptosis (congenital)

Q. Pupil in health and diseases.

The normal size of pupil is 3–5 mm. If it is <3 mm, it is called **miosis**, and if >5 mm, it is **mydriasis**. Pin-point pupil is very small (1 mm or less).

Mydriasis

- Occulomotor palsy
- Optic atrophy
- Glaucoma
- Dhatura poisoning
- Deep coma
- Application of mydriatic.

Miosis

- Pontine haemorrhage
- Horner's syndrome (unilateral)
- Organophosphorus poisoning
- Old age.

Remember, sphincter pupillae and ciliaris muscle are supplied by occulomotor nerve, while dilator pupillae is innervated by sympathetic trunk.

Q. What is Bell's palsy (Fig. 8.12)**?**

It is the acute onset of idiopathic, unilateral LMN type of facial nerve palsy due to non-suppurative inflammation (may be viral e.g., herpes simplex virus) of the nerve within the facial canal above the stylomastoid foramen. There is sudden onset of facial weakness on the affected side without any sensory loss (as sensory supply of face is done by trigeminal nerve). There will be facial asymmetry, more prominent on speaking and expressing emotional movements, which is diagnosed on clinical ground.

Bell's phenomenon occurs on the paralysed side i.e., eyeball rolls upwards and inwards on attempted forced eye closure.

Q. Can you give an outline of bulbar and pseudobulbar palsy?

Old name of medulla oblongata is 'bulb' and it contains the IX, X, XI and XII cranial nerve nuclei. *Bulbar palsy* is LMN type of lesion of IX, X, XI and XII cranial nerves (affection of cranial nerve nuclei or those nerves), while *pseudobulbar palsy* is UMN type of lesion of IX, X, XI and XII cranial nerves (i.e., bilateral affection of corticobulbar fibres). The muscles supplied by those cranial nerves are affected i.e., it is a palato-labio-glosso-pharyngo-laryngeal paralysis. In bulbar palsy, the affected muscles are virtually paralysed though in pseudobulbar palsy, the voluntary control over those muscles is impaired.

In pseudobulbar palsy, the tongue becomes spastic, jaw jerk is brisk and plantar response is extensor while in bulbar palsy they are respectively flaccid tongue, absent jaw jerk and flexor plantar response. Emotional instability is common in pseudobulbar palsy.

The common causes of bulbar palsy are:
- Motor neuron disease (MND)
- Poliomyelitis
- Syringobulbia
- Guillain-Barré (GB) syndrome
- Encephalitis
- Brainstem tumours
- Diphtheria
- Others: Snakebite (Elapidae group), myasthenia gravis and botulism.

Pseudobulbar palsy is commonly due to:
- Diffuse cerebral ischaemia (multiple lacunar infarction): Bilateral stroke
- Diffuse atherosclerosis (cerebral atrophy)
- Chronic motor neuron disease (MND)
- Multiple sclerosis.

Q. What is the importance of cranium and spine examination in neurology?

They are examined for:

1. *Cranium*
   a. Microcephaly (i.e., cerebral palsy), macrocephaly (e.g., hydrocephalus) or turricephaly (i.e., premature synostosis of sutures).
   b. Elevation, depression, haematoma, secondary metastases or mass in multiple myeloma.

c. Bruit: Bruit in cerebral arteriovenous malformation may be auscultated over cranium or closed eye.
d. Fontanelle (in children, tense fontanelle is common in IIT and hydrocephalus).

2. *Spine*
   a. Tenderness (e.g., trauma, acute transverse myelitis)
   b. Kyphoscoliosis (e.g., poliomyelitis, syringomyelia, neurofibromatosis)
   c. Gibbus (e.g., carries spine)
   d. Spina bifida (known by presence of tuft of hair or dimpling of skin), bruit and movement (forward, backward or sideways) of spine.

Q. What are the different types of 'tone' in muscles in different neurological disorders?

Tone is the partially contracted condition of a muscle.

Tone is *examined clinically* by handling the limbs and moving them passively at their various joints while feeling the resistance during passive movement (e.g., flexibility of joints is found in hypotonia, while stiffness of joint is common in hypertonia). It is basically of two types:

Hypotonia (flaccidity)

- LMN lesion, UMN lesion in shock stage, cerebellar lesion
- Chorea (only extrapyramidal lesion with hypotonia)
- Myopathy, myasthenic crisis, polyneuropathy
- Hypnotics, muscle relaxants, deep sleep
- Down's syndrome, rickets, emaciation due to any cause.

Hypertonia (spasticity and rigidity)

- UMN lesion (*clasp-knife spasticity*)
- Extrapyramidal lesion except chorea (*lead pipe or cogwheel rigidity*)
- Tetanus, strychnine poisoning, tetany, non-cooperative patient, myotonia
- Decerebrate rigidity, hysterical hypertonia.

Q. What are different reflexes in neurology?

Reflex is the involuntary and nearly instantaneous motor response in response to a sensory stimulus. The different reflexes tested in clinical neurology are:

Reflexes	*Types*	*Root value*
Superficial	• Abdominal	• T_8–T_{12}
	• Cremasteric	• $L_{1,2}$
	• Plantar response	• S_1
Deep/tendon reflex, or jerks	• Upper limb	
	– Biceps jerk (Fig. 8.14)	• $C_{5,6}$
	– Supinator jerk (Fig. 8.15)	• $C_{5,6}$
	– Triceps jerk (Fig. 8.16)	• $C_{6,7}$
	• Lower limb	
	– Knee jerk (Fig. 8.17)	• $L_{2,3,4}$
	– Ankle jerk (Fig. 8.18)	• $S_{1,2}$

Visceral	• Swallowing • Bladder • Bowel
Others	• Glabellar tap • Grasp reflex • Palmo-mental reflex

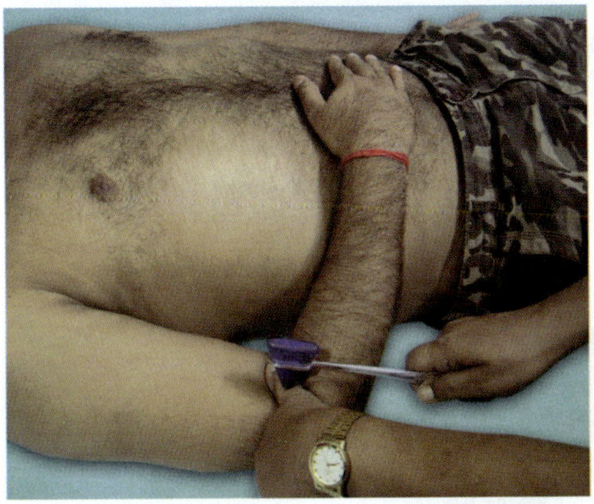

Fig. 8.14: Testing for biceps jerk

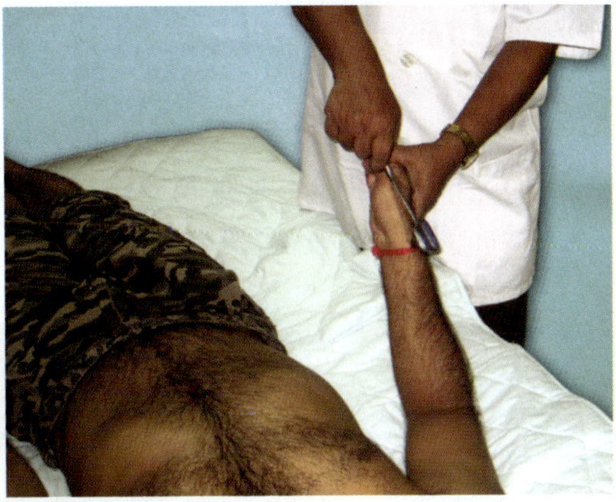

Fig. 8.15: Testing for supinator jerk

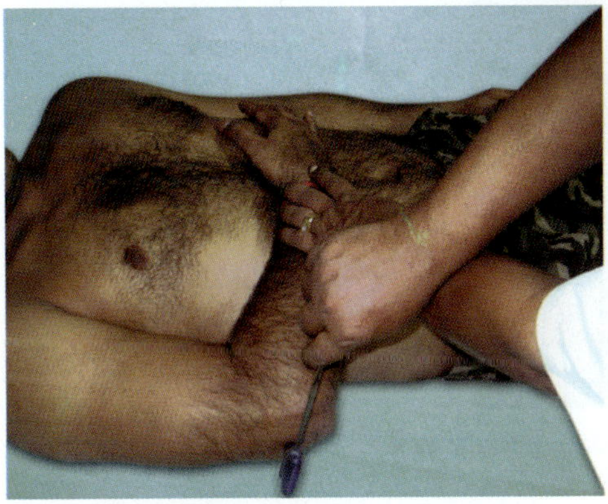

Fig. 8.16: Testing for triceps jerk

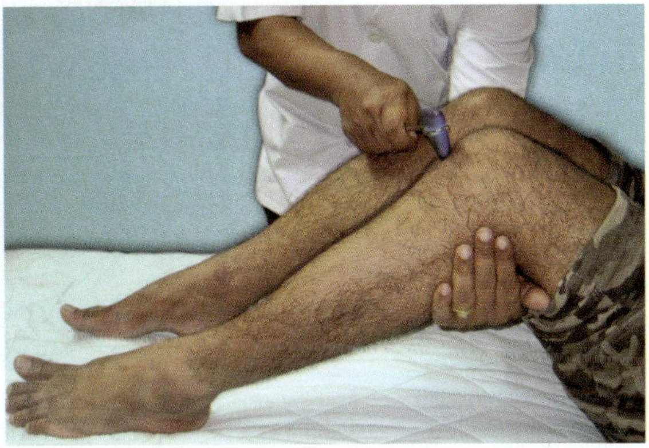

Fig. 8.17: Elicitation of knee jerk

NB: 'Reinforcement' or **"Jendrassik's manoeuvre"** are adopted by the clinician when deep reflexes or jerks are not elicited by routine methods. Ask the patient to clench his/her teeth (Fig. 8.19), or interlock the fingers of two hands together and then pull them as hard as possible while eliciting the jerks (Fig. 8.20). This 'reinforcement' increases the excitability of anterior horn cells and increases gamma fusimotor drive.

Q, What is clonus?

It is the rhythmical contraction of a group of muscle in response to sudden and sustained stretching. Clonus is a sign of corticospinal tract lesion (i.e., UMN palsy), which is associated with brisk jerks, spasticity and Babinski's sign. It is the duty of a clinician to

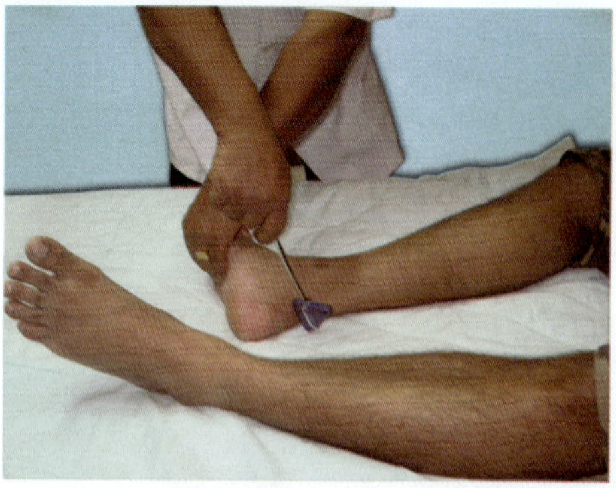

Fig. 8.18: Elicitation of ankle jerk

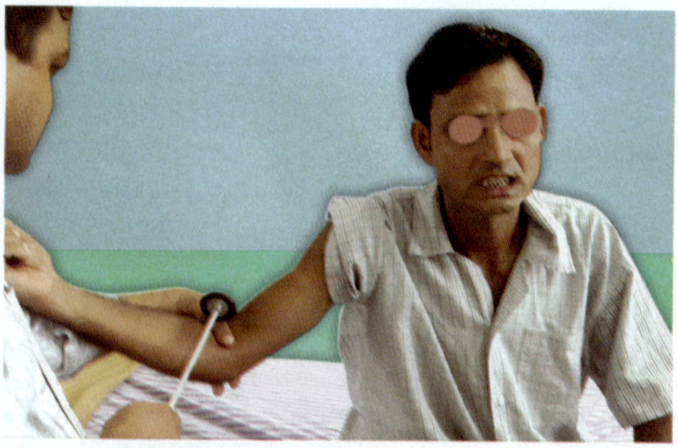

Fig. 8.19: Reinforcement test by asking the patient to clench the teeth while eliciting jerks of upper extremity

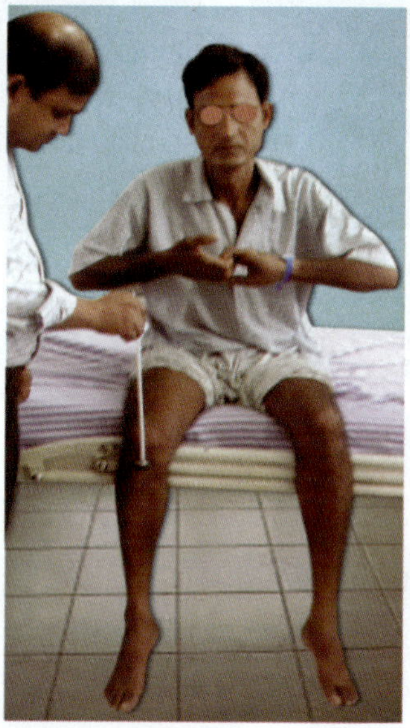

Fig. 8.20: Reinforcement test by asking the patient to interlock the fingers of two hands and pull them as hard as possible while eliciting jerks of lower extremity

test for clonus if jerks are brisk. Commonly ankle clonus, patellar clonus and jaw clonus are tested in neurology.

Q. What is plantar response (Fig. 8.21)?

In health, when the lateral part of the sole of a foot is scratched gently but firmly by the tip of a key, stick of a percussion hammer or a needle, there is flexion of all five toes with dorsiflexion and inversion of foot along with contraction of adductors of thigh (known as 'flexor' response). It is the most important reflex in neurology. The 'extensor' response is:

- *Dorsiflexion or extension of the great toe*
- Fanning (i.e., spreading out), and extension of outer four toes

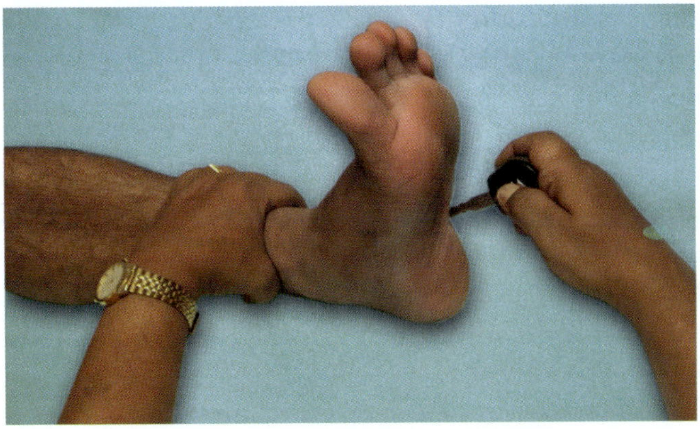

Fig. 8.21: Testing for plantar response

- Dorsiflexion of the ankle, and flexion of the knee and the hip
- Contraction of tensor fascia lata.

Plantar response extensor is also known as **"Babinski's sign"**, which is present in:

1. Pyramidal tract lesion or UMN paralysis
2. Children below 1 year of age, deep sleep
3. Deep coma due to any cause, anaesthesia, metabolic encephalopathy
4. Hypoglycaemia
5. Immediately after generalised convulsions (post-ictal period).

NB: In UMN palsy, the jerks are brisk and plantar response is extensor.

Q. What is peripheral neuropathy (or polyneuropathy) and how the patients present?

It is a diffuse symmetrical disease process of peripheral nerves (peripheral means outside central nervous system) involving the peripheral parts of body and gradually progressing proximally.

The patients present with sensation of pins and needles (i.e., tingling and numbness, or paraesthesia) and pain in 'gloves and stockings' distribution along with weakness of distal parts of limbs. Common causes of peripheral neuropathy are:

- Vitamin B_1, B_6 and B_{12} deficiency
- Leprosy
- Diabetes mellitus
- Chronic renal failure (or uraemia)
- Alcohol
- Drugs and toxins: INH, vincristine, nitrofurantoin, arsenic, lead
- Others: Disseminated malignancy, HIV infection, SLE, GB syndrome.

Q. Can you enumerate the different signs of cerebellar disorder?

Cerebellum regulates the rate, rhythm, range and force of muscular contractions, and moreover it maintains posture, equilibrium and co-ordination. Cerebellum has ipsilateral (i.e., same-sided) control over the body. The cerebellar signs are:

1. Titubation (i.e., head-nodding)
2. Nystagmus (horizontal, jerky type)
3. Scanning speech
4. Intention tremor
5. Hypotonia
6. Dysmetria (i.e., inability to judge distance, speed and power of movement, and is assessed clinically by 'finger-nose test')
7. Dyssynergia (i.e., decomposition of movements)
8. Dysdiadochokinesia (inability to perform rapid, repeated and alternating movements smoothly)
9. Rebound phenomenon
10. Pendular knee jerk
11. Ataxia i.e., clumsiness of movements without any motor or sensory deficit, and is manifested by unsteady gait (or reeling gait).

Common cerebellar disorders are multiple sclerosis, neoplasms, cerebellar haemorrhage, spinocerebellar degeneration, Friedreich's ataxia, etc.

NB: Romberg's sign is positive in sensory ataxia (i.e., a test of posterior column function). The basic feature of this sign is that the patient becomes more unsteady standing with his eyes closed than the eyes are kept open. Romberg's sign is not a test for cerebellar ataxia.

Q. Do you know different involuntary movements?

The common involuntary movements in clinical neurology are:

1. *Tremor:* It is the involuntary, repetitive, rhythmic, oscillatory movement of a part of the body around a fixed point. Tremor is probably the most common involuntary movement. It is classified clinically by:
   - Static tremor: Seen in a resting patient e.g., parkinsonism
   - Action tremor: Tremor seen in outstretched hands e.g., anxiety, thyrotoxicosis, chronic alcoholism, sympathomimetics-induced or familial tremor (Fig. 8.22)
   - Intention tremor: Tremor at the goal point of any action e.g., cerebellar disorder
   - Flapping tremor (asterixis or bat's wing tremor) e.g., in failure of vital organs like hepatic pre-coma, renal failure, respiratory failure or cardiac failure.

   NB: Tremor may be classified as fine (7–10/second) and coarse (4–6/second).

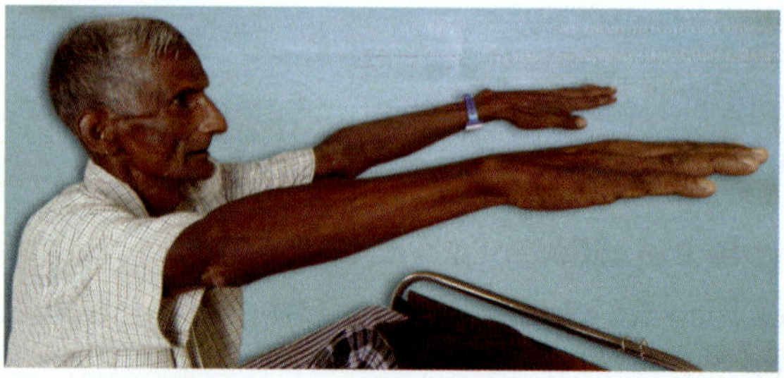

Fig. 8.22: Demonstration of action tremor

2. *Chorea:* It is the brief, rapid, jerky, quasi-purposive involuntary movements mainly affecting face, limbs and tongue. Examples of chorea are rheumatic fever (Sydenham's chorea), Huntington's chorea (incurable, autosomal-dominant fatal brain disorder), Wilson's disease, kericterus, etc.
3. Athetosis: Slow, sinuous, writhing involuntary movements affecting distal part of limbs e.g., kernicterus, post-hemiplegic state (infantile), Wilson's disease, cerebral palsy.
4. Myoclonus (sudden, rapid, electric shock-like jerky movements of muscles).
5. Dyskinesia (extrapyramidal syndromes i.e., axial tortional movements involving neck muscles or perioral muscles by use of drugs like metoclopramide, phenothiazines, etc).
6. Dystonia (abnormally maintained posture).
7. Hemiballismus (violent ballistic and flinging movement of one side of body).
8. Myokymia (or benign fasciculation): Commonly seen as twitching of muscles around the eye.
9. Torticollis (persistent abducted and rotated posture of neck).
10. Asterixis (flapping tremor: See tremor above in point No.1).
11. Tetany (increase in neuromuscular irritability due to low serum ionic calcium level; there may be carpo-pedal spasm, Chvostek's sign or Erb's sign. It is commonly due to hypocalcaemia resulting from malabsorption syndrome, hypoparathyroidism or alkalosis due to hyperventilation).
12. Fasciculation (fine, rapid, twitching of large group of muscle fibres i.e., involving the whole motor-unit, and is seen in degeneration of anterior horn cells in motor neuron disease (MND), cervical spondylosis or syringomyelia). However, *fibrillation* is the contraction of single muscle fibre, and is rarely seen in tongue (as tongue lacks submucous coat) in LMN type of XIIth cranial nerve palsy.
13. Tics or habit spasm (unintentional, fast and repetitive muscle movements, which is often embarrassing for the person).
14. Others: Titubation, akathisia (motor restlessness with inability to sit still), opisthotonus (e.g., in tetanus).

Q. What is parkinsonism?

It is a clinical syndrome with bradykinesia (slow movements), tremor (oscillatory movements of fingers), rigidity (increased tone) and postural instability (resulting in falls). The patient adopts a posture of 'universal flexion'. The patients have characteristic 'festinant gait' which starts with a rapid, short, shuffling steps as if the patient is trying to catch-up his centre of gravity. Glabellar tap is positive (i.e., if a series of finger tap is applied over glabella, continuous blinking of both eyeballs occurs; normally, the response is inhibited after 3–4 blinks). It is predominantly a disease of old age and is more common in males. The basal ganglia is the site of lesion (i.e., extrapyramidal system) and dopamine loss is the main pathology. It is said that in parkinsonism, there is delay in initiation, slowness in expression and paucity in execution (i.e., the affected person becomes slow in performing every action). There are different kind of drugs to treat this condition.

Q. What are the muscle disorders?

Muscle disorders are classified under:

- *Dystrophic:* Muscular dystrophy (Duchenne type) or myopathy
- *Myotonic* (i.e., sustained contraction with slow relaxation): Myotonic dystrophy
- *Inflammatory:* Polymyositis, dermatomyositis, sarcoidosis
- *Endocrine causes:* Cushing's syndrome, hypo- and hyperthyroidism, corticosteroid or statin therapy
- *Myasthenic:* Myasthenia gravis (a neuromuscular junction disease which produces fatigable weakness which is worse on exercise)
- *Others:* Periodic paralysis, alcohol abuse.

Q. What are the causes of sudden onset of muscle weakness without loss of consciousness?

They are:

- Transient ischaemic attack (TIA)
- Hypoglycaemia
- GB syndrome
- Poliomyelitis
- Electrolyte imbalance (e.g., hypokalaemia, hypercalcaemia)
- Snakebite (Elapidae group)
- Periodic paralysis (hypokalaemic or hyperkalaemic)
- Hysterical.

Q. What are the common causes of muscle wasting?

Generalised

- LMN lesion due to any cause (neurogenic atrophy)
- UMN lesion: May develop into disuse atrophy
- Muscular dystrophy (i.e., myopathy)
- *Causes of emaciation:* Disseminated tuberculosis, diabetes mellitus (especially, type 1), thyrotoxicosis, advanced malignancy, AIDS (acquired immune deficiency syndrome), malabsorption syndrome, severe malnutrition or anorexia nervosa.

Wasting of the small muscles of hands

- Leprosy (Hansen's disease)
- Motor neuron disease (MND)
- Poliomyelitis
- Syringomyelia
- Cervical spondylosis or cervical rib
- Tumours of the spinal cord (e.g., glioma)
- Nerve injuries involving median or ulnar nerve (e.g., trauma, carpal tunnel syndrome).

NB: Examine a patient of neurology step by step by strictly following the scheme of examination. Do not skip a single point whether it is related to symptoms or signs. It is difficult for a beginner to grasp a huge subject like neurology but with time all the clinical methods will be in your fingertips if you are methodical.

Decoding Abbreviations

CNS	Central nervous system
PNS	Peripheral nervous system
IIT	Increased intracranial tension
HIV	Human immunodeficiency virus.

Chapter

9

Endocrine System

Q. Describe the major glands in the endocrine system.

It comprises:

- Hypothalamus and pituitary gland
- Thyroid gland
- Parathyroid glands
- Islet cells of pancreas (i.e., endocrine part of pancreas)
- Adrenal glands
- Gonads (testes and ovaries)

[*Adipose tissue* or mass may represent the largest endocrine organ (adipocytes are endocrine cells, which secrete bioactive peptides, termed 'adipokines')].

Q. What are the effects of hypo- and hyperfunction of these endocrine glands?

Endocrine gland	*Hyperfunction*	*Hypofunction*
1. Pituitary (the 'Master Gland')	• Growth hormone: Gigantism (Fig. 9.1) (before puberty)/ acromegaly (after puberty) • Vasopressin (ADH): SIADH	• Growth hormone: Dwarfism (pituitary dwarf) • Vasopressin (ADH): Diabetes insipidus • All hormones: Panhypopituitarism (e.g., Sheehan's syndrome)
2. Thyroid	Thyrotoxicosis	Hypothyroidism (cretinism/ myxoedema)
3. Parathyroid	Hyperparathyroidism	Hypoparathyroidism
4. Islet cells of pancreas	Insulinoma (β-cells)/glucagonoma (α-cells)	Diabetes mellitus (β-cells)
5. Adrenal gland	Cushing's syndrome (adrenal cortex) Pheochromocytoma (adrenal medulla)	Addison's disease (adrenal cortex)

*ADH is antidiuretic hormone, SIADH is syndrome of inappropriate antidiuretic hormone

**Hypothalamus (part of brain, which is the control and relay centre of whole endocrine system), pineal gland (secretes melatonin, which regulates sleep cycle and wakefulness) and thymus (activates the immune system by activating T-cells) are glands within endocrine system.

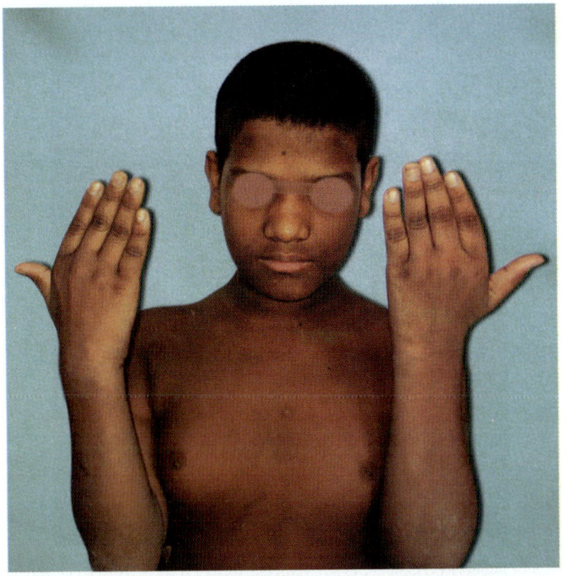

Fig. 9.1: A rare case of gigantism in a boy of 7 years of age

Q. Can you directly examine these endocrine glands?

The endocrine glands (i.e., ductless glands) secrete their products (hormones) directly into the blood rather than through a duct, in contradiction to exocrine glands which secrete substances by way of a duct. The pituitary, parathyroid, pancreas, adrenal glands and ovaries cannot be examined directly. Thyroid gland and testes can be examined physically in details. In the endocrine system, it is the hypo- and hyperfunction of the glands reflected by the deficiency or excess secretion of hormone respectively by the specific gland is translated into different clinical manifestations, and easily picked up by the clinicians at the bedside.

The testes can be thoroughly examined by palpation. Moreover, by Prader orchidometer, testicular size <3 cm indicates atrophy (normal adult testis size is 4–7 cm). Normal pre-pubertal males have small and rubbery testes; bilateral small and soft testes (atrophied testes) are characteristic of leprosy and cirrhosis of liver; a patient of Klinefelter's syndrome has small and firm testes; testis feels lobulated in testicular tumour. An adult penis is 8–12 cm long and in hypogonadism the penis size is 2.5 cm (Fig. 9.2).

Q. Discuss the common symptoms (chief complaints and H/o present illness) of endocrine disorders.

Symptomatology	*Possible endocrine disorder/s*
• Loss of weight	Diabetes, thyrotoxicosis, adrenal insufficiency, hypogonadism
• Gain in weight	Cushing's syndrome, hypothyroidism
• Coarsening of (body) features	Acromegaly, hypothyroidism
• Protrusion of the eyeball	Graves' disease

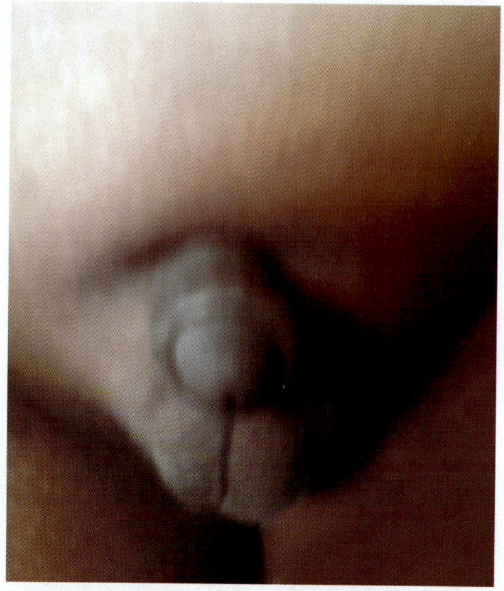

Fig. 9.2: Cryptorchidism (absence of testes from the scrotum) with a small penis

• Tiredness or lassitude	Diabetes, hypothyroidism, Cushing's syndrome, hypogonadism, hyperparathyroidism, adrenal insufficiency
• Palpitations	Thyrotoxicosis, pheochromocytoma, menopausal syndrome
• Heat intolerance	Thyrotoxicosis, menopausal syndrome
• Headache	Acromegaly, pheochromocytoma (from hypertension), any other pituitary tumour, osteomalacia (vitamin D deficiency)
• Large tongue	Acromegaly, cretinism, myxoedema
• Muscle weakness (proximal)	Thyrotoxicosis, Cushing's syndrome, hyperparathyroidism, primary hyperaldosteronism (i.e., Conn's syndrome leading to hypokalaemia)
• Visual problem	Diabetes (i.e., retinopathy), pituitary tumour (i.e., pressure effects)
• Hirsutism	Cushing's syndrome, acromegaly, polycystic ovarian disease (PCOD)
• Polyuria	Diabetes (mellitus and insipidus both), hyperparathyroidism
• Paraesthesia (i.e., tingling extremities)	Hypoparathyroidism, diabetic neuropathy, acromegaly (carpal tunnel syndrome)
• Loss of libido	Male hypogonadism, hypothyroidism, acromegaly
• Amenorrhoea or menstrual irregularities	Thyrotoxicosis, hyperprolactinaemia, Cushing's syndrome; (remember, menorrhagia in hypothyroidism), PCOD
• Recurrent renal calculi	Hyperparathyroidism
• Striae (purple) over body	Cushing's syndrome, corticosteroid therapy

Q. Hypothyroidism and hyperthyroidism—describe in a nutshell.

Hypothyroid (Fig. 2.26)	*Hyperthyroid* (Fig. 9.3)
Failure of the thyroid gland (reduced circulatory level of thyroid hormones) after puberty is known as *myxoedema*.	'Hyperthyroidism' indicates glandular hypertrophy of thyroid with excess function of thyroid, while *thyrotoxicosis* indicates increased circulating free

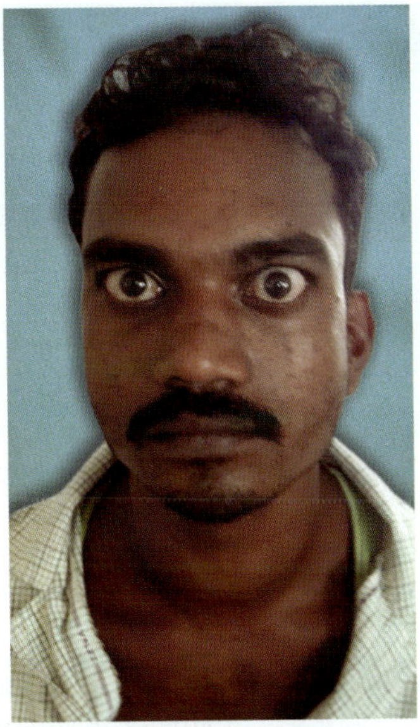

Fig. 9.3: Thyrotoxicosis revealed by exophthalmos; enlargement of thyroid gland is seen at neck

Usually it develops due to autoimmune Hashimoto's thyroiditis. There is reduced level of thyroid hormones (T_3 and T_4), and females are more commonly affected than males (M:F = 6:1).

Common features are—dull and expressionless face, baggy lower eyelids, dry/scaly and coarse skin, increased sensitivity to cold, hoarseness of voice, pallor (e.g., due to carotenaemia), lethargy and tiredness, weight gain, non-pitting oedema (due to deposition of mucinous materials like mucopolysaccharides, hyaluronic acid and chondroitin sulphate), constipation, menorrhagia, effort angina, sinus bradycardia, loss of libido, carpal tunnel syndrome*, depression, delayed relaxation of ankle jerk, and may have a goitre. The symptoms and signs develop over many years and thus diagnosis is delayed.

The patient may suffer from myxoedema coma or myoedema madness (psychotic manifestations). Goitre is more common in thyroid hormones (T_3 and T_4) along with toxic features. Graves' disease, an autoimmune disease, is the commonest cause of hyperthyroidism. It is much more common in females.

Common features are—anxiety, irritability, heat intolerance (i.e., preference for cold), perspiration, loss of weight in spite of increased appetite, tremor (fine), palpitations, angina, atrial fibrillation, hyperdefecation (diarrhoea), goitre, proximal myopathy, and oligomenorrhoea. *Graves' disease* may have pretibial myxoedema (non-pitting oedema over shin bones with raised, thickened, hyperpigmented and indurated plaques), exophthalmos (increased protrusion of the eyeball from the orbit exposing sclera above and below the cornea; synonym with proptosis—Fig. 9.4), and thyroid acropachy (clubbing with bony changes of distal phalanges resembling hypertrophic osteoarthropathy).

Loss of weight in thyrotoxicosis is due to increased metabolic rate.

On examination, there is fine tremor, tachycardia

*It is entrapment of median nerve when it passes through carpal tunnel at wrist. The patient C/o nocturnal hand pain, paraesthesia and numbness of radial three-and-a-half fingers of hand.

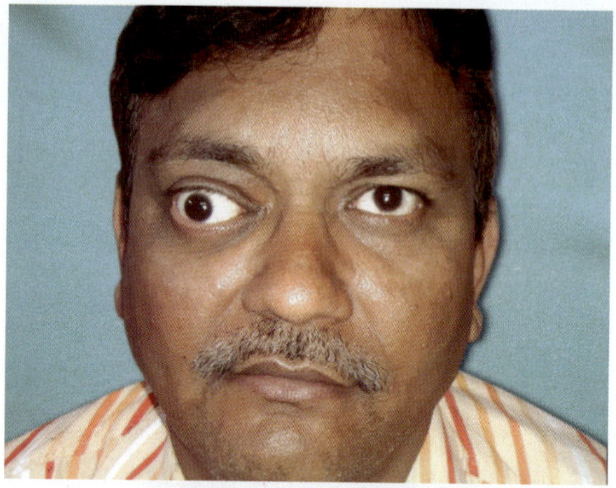

Fig. 9.4: Unilateral proptosis (exophthalmos) of right eye probably due to thyrotoxicosis

hyperthyroidism (Graves' disease) than in myxoedema.
Hypothyroidism since birth due to complete or partial failure of thyroid gland is *cretinism*.

with increased pulse pressure (gives rise to water-hammer pulse), proximal muscle weakness with exaggerated deep reflexes (e.g., knee jerk), systolic murmur at the apex; one may get a systolic bruit over enlarged thyroid gland.

Q. Primary and secondary hypothyroidism: What do they mean?

They are described as below:

- *Primary hypothyroidism:* Disease in the thyroid gland (e.g., iodine deficiency in sub-Himalayan regions). The patient will have weight gain and other myxoedematous features. Here, serum T_4 will be low and TSH will be high.
- *Secondary hypothyroidism:* Disease in the pituitary gland or hypothalamus. The patient will be lean and thin. Here, both T_4 and TSH will be low.

Q. What are the hormones secreted from different parts of adrenal gland?

Adrenal gland is divided into outer cortex and inner medulla. The cortex is a part of hypothalamo-pituitary-adrenal axis, which secretes cortisol and androgen after getting proper signal from above. The division of adrenal gland goes like this:

- *Cortex:*
  - Zona glomerulosa: Principally secretes aldosterone (mineralocorticoids)
  - Zona fasciculata: Mainly secretes glucocorticoids
  - Zona reticularis: Predominantly secretes sex steroids (testosterone, oestrogen and progesterone).
- *Medulla:* Produces catecholamines (adrenaline, nor-adrenaline and dopamine).

Q. Short notes on acromegaly, Cushing's syndrome and Addison's disease.

Acromegaly

- *Ask the patient:* Whether his facial character has changed/what people say about it? Or, inquire whether he/she had to change to larger wedding rings, or larger size of shoes over the years? Or, check the serial passport-size photographs for last few years. The patient has large head with change of facial features over years, and large hands and feet.

- *The facies* (Fig. 9.5): Coarse facies (enlarged face with prognathism i.e., prominent lower jaw, wide-spaced teeth, frontal bossing, prominent supraorbital ridges and malar bones, stubby nose and large ears, thick lips, bushy eyebrows with hyperhidrosis, and enlarged tongue; acne, hirsutism; deep and husky voice).
- *Characteristic features:* Hands and feet are large and spade-like (Fig. 9.6), thick skin with excessive sweating, visual field defect (e.g., bitemporal hemianopia), headache, joint pain, hypertension, diabetes, organomegaly (e.g., hepatomegaly, cardiomegaly), carpal tunnel syndrome, or obstructive sleep apnoea syndrome. Other features are increased heel-pad thickness, galactorrhoea (in females), acanthosis nigricans, loss of libido and osteoarthritis. Polyps in colon and colonic carcinoma are common in acromegaly.

Cushing's syndrome

- *Cushing's syndrome* is excess glucocorticoid production from zona fasciculata of adrenal cortex due to any cause. *Cushing's disease* is excess ACTH secretion from pituitary gland, which is resulting in excess glucocorticoid production from adrenal gland (i.e., Cushing's syndrome due to pituitary adenoma).
- *The facies:* The face looks bloated and rounded, like the full moon, and is known as 'moon face'. The face is dusky and plethoric, and may have hirsutism (Fig. 9.7) and acne. There is short and thick neck with supraclavicular pad of fat.
- *Characteristic features:* Moon face, buffalo hump in the region of nape of the neck, truncal obesity, plethoric appearance, thin limbs, hyperpigmentation, thin and atrophic skin with easy bruisability, striae (purple or red) (Fig. 9.8), poor wound

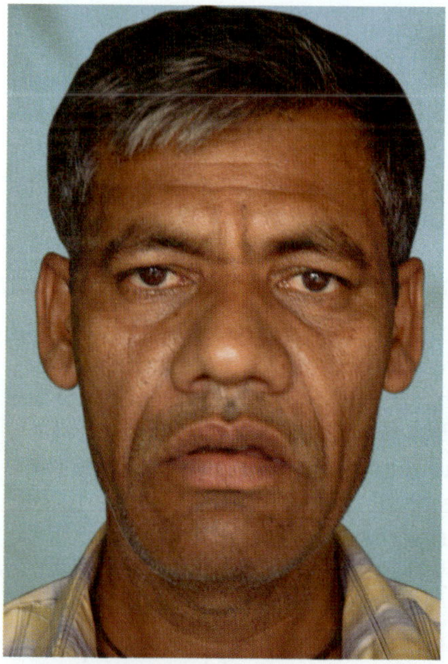

Fig. 9.5: Face in acromegaly

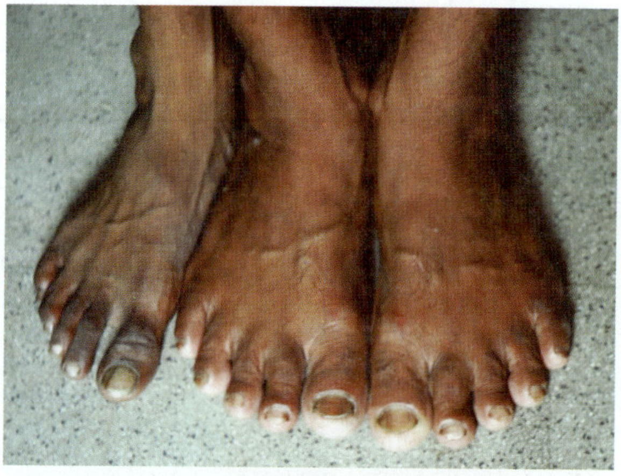

Fig. 9.6: Wide and large feet in acromegaly compared with a normal foot on its right side

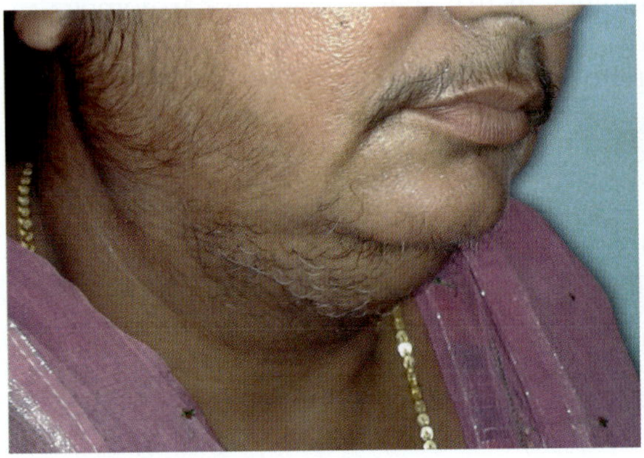

Fig. 9.7: Hirsutism

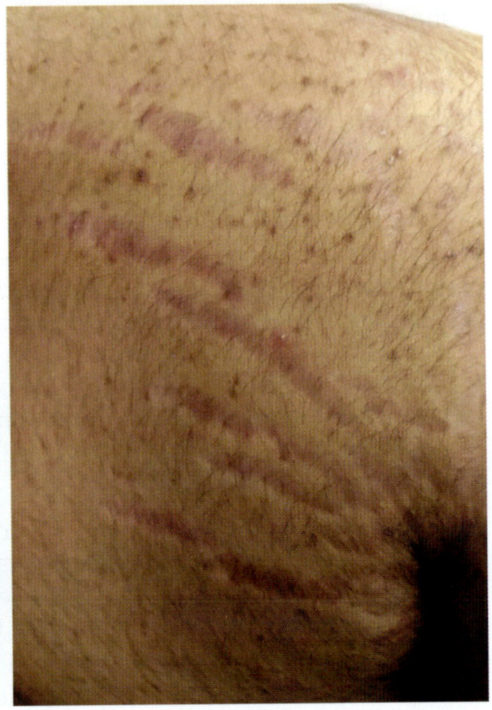

Fig. 9.8: Purple striae in Cushing's syndrome

healing, hypertension, diabetes, proximal myopathy, osteoporosis, growth retardation (in children), depression, menstrual irregularities, and increased susceptibility to infections (e.g., tuberculosis).

Addison's disease (primary adrenal insufficiency and hypocortisolism)

- *Clinical features:* Anorexia, loss of weight, extreme fatigability, weakness, pigmentation of skin (over knuckles, creases of palm, elbows, knees, areola, recent scars) and mucous membrane (oral cavity), hypotension with postural drop, abdominal pain, sparse axillary and pubic hair, and amenorrhoea.

Q. Give some idea about diseases like pheochromocytoma and diabetes insipidus.

- ***Pheochromocytoma:*** A pheochromocytoma is a neuroendocrine tumour of adrenal medulla, which secretes high amount of catecholamines (catecholamines are adrenaline, nor-adrenaline and dopamine). The patient usually presents with episodes of sympathetic drive with symptoms like headache, palpitations, pallor, sweating, apprehension, nervousness, anxiety and fear of death. Hypertension may be paroxysmal or persistent; due to sudden rise of BP along with fluctuating BP, patients may present with acute LVF, AMI or stroke. The patients may have associated hyperglycaemia. The 24-hour urinary vanillylmandelic acid (VMA) is high in pheochromocytoma.
- ***Diabetes insipidus:*** It is the persistent excretion of large amount of hypotonic (specific gravity < 1010 and osmolality < 300 mOsm/kg) but otherwise normal urine (i.e.,

hypotonic polyuria) due to deficiency of vasopressin or ADH; the patient feels intense thirst. Remember, uncontrolled diabetes mellitus gives rise to hypertonic polyuria. **NB:** Normal osmolality of blood and urine is respectively 280–300 mOsmol/kg and 400–750 mOsmol/kg.

Q. Can you give a short account of gynaecomastia?

When the male breast looks like that of a female, it is known as gynaecomastia; even the nipple and areola give rise to a feminine appearance. The common causes are:

- Physiological: Newborn, adolescence (Fig. 9.9), old age
- Klinefelter's syndrome
- Hepatocellular failure, especially from alcoholic cirrhosis
- Hypogonadism
- Leprosy, bronchogenic carcinoma
- Drug-induced e.g., spironolactone, cimetidine, digitalis, etc.

Gynaecomastia gives rise to a severe psychological problem to the patient. So, early detection of its aetiology as well as management is essential.

Q. What are the 'endocrine emergencies' commonly encountered in a hospital?

The common endocrine emergencies are:

1. Hypoglycaemia
2. Diabetic ketoacidosis
3. Thyroid storm or thyrotoxic crisis
4. Myxoedema coma
5. Pituitary apoplexy
6. Adrenal crisis or Addisonian crisis
7. Severe hypercalcaemia (from malignancy or primary hyperparathyroidism).

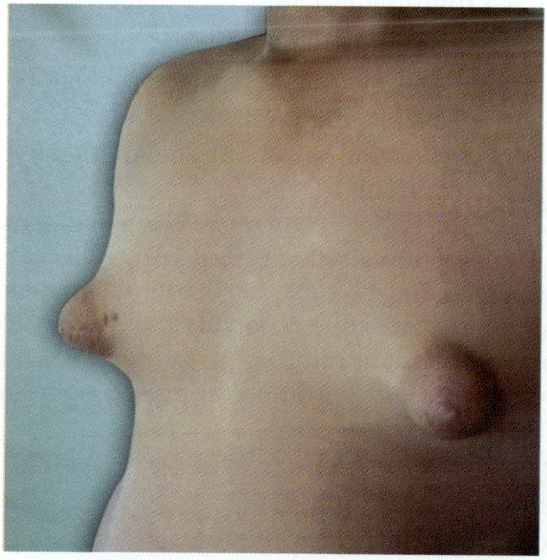

Fig. 9.9: Puberty gynaecomastia

Q. What is diabetes mellitus?

It is a clinical syndrome characterised by high blood sugar level (i.e., hyperglycaemia) and glycosuria (i.e., sugar present in urine) due to relative or absolute deficiency of insulin secretion and/or action, or insulin resistance that arises from genetic as well as environmental factors and thereby leads to disturbances in carbohydrate, protein, fat metabolism, and water and electrolyte homeostasis.

Usually diabetes mellitus is of two types like:
Type 1 (β-cell destruction, leading to absolute insulin deficiency)
Type 2 (insulin resistance ranging from deficiency to secretory defect).

Q. What are the diagnostic criteria of diabetes mellitus?

The WHO diagnostic criteria for diabetes mellitus:

- Symptoms of diabetes plus 'random' blood glucose concentration ≥ 200 mg/dL, or
- 'Fasting' plasma glucose ≥126 mg/dL, or
- '2 hours-postload' plasma glucose ≥200 mg/dL during an oral GTT (glucose tolerance test), or
- HbA_{1C} ≥6.5%

The diagnostic criteria for pre-diabetes and diabetes are:

- In these criteria, the categories of FPG (fasting plasma glucose) are:
  FPG <100 mg/dL = Normal fasting glucose
  FPG ≥100 mg/dL and <126 mg/dL = Impaired fasting glucose (IFG)
  FPG ≥126 mg/dL = Provisional diagnosis of diabetes (of more than one occasion)
- The corresponding categories when the oral GTT is used, are as follows:
  In these criteria, the categories of 2 hPG (2-h postload glucose) are:
  2 hPG <140 mg/dL = Normal glucose tolerance
  2 hPG ≥140 mg/dL and <200 mg/dL = Impaired glucose tolerance (IGT)
  2 hPG ≥200 mg/dL = Provisional diagnosis of diabetes (must be confirmed on a subsequent day)

NB: Patients with IGT (140–199 mg/dL), and/or IFG (100–125 mg/dL), or HbA_{1C} ≥5.7–6.4% are now regarded as **'pre-diabetes'**.

Blood glucose concentration in mg/dL should be divided by 18 to get the value in mmol/l, e.g. 140 mg/dL= 7.8 mmol/l.

Oral GTT is a test where the patient consumes 75 mg of glucose dissolved in 300 ml of water in 5 minutes, after an unrestricted carbohydrate diet taken 3 days prior to the test. A treated diabetic person may take his/her recommended meal instead of glucose. Then blood and urine samples are collected every half-hourly for at least 2 hours.

HbA_{1C} (or, glycosylated haemoglobin) provides an accurate and objective measurement of blood glucose concentration for preceding 6–8 weeks.

Q. How a diabetic patient presents? Why diabetes is so important a disease?

Mode of presentation of diabetes mellitus:

- *Asymptomatic:* Detected by chance on routine examination (e.g., pre-operative check up).

- *Typical triad of symptoms:* Polyuria, polydipsia and polyphagia (P_3 symptoms); usually patients come with H/o loss of weight (instead of polyphagia), which is unexplained and unintentional.
- *Common presentation:* Tiredness or fatigue, recurrent boils or abscess formation, delayed wound healing, non-resolving pneumonia, pruritus vulvae or balanitis, blurred vision due to refractory error, or resistant tuberculosis.
- *Presentations with complications:* Diabetic ketoacidosis, nephropathy, sudden blindness or myocardial infarction (silent).

Diabetes mellitus is an important disease because it a very common devastating illness which increases the morbidity and mortality to several times. The number of people affected by diabetes is rising at a rocket speed and as such it is now a global pandemic. It kills thc patient by the dual mode of microangiopathy as well as macroangiopathy. Moreover, the host resistance is also decreased by diabetes (like diabetes, immunosuppression is also common in lymphoma, leukaemias, multiple myeloma, corticosteroid therapy, post-radiotherapy, renal failure and AIDS). Even a minor surgery in a diabetic patient may prove fatal. Therefore, the 'need of the hour' is to understand its aetiology and to develop preventive strategies, which are the keys to improve the health of the public and thereby to reduce the burden on the health care system.

During history taking, it is the duty of a student to take the history of diabetes (and hypertension too) in each and every patient.

Q. What is the outline of management of diabetes?

The success of treatment of diabetes depends on patient's patience and proper understanding. The mainstay of treatment is:

- Diabetic diet (healthy eating).
- Lifestyle modification (weight control, exercises like brisk walking, swimming, cycling for at least 30 minutes/day).
- *Drugs:* Oral hypoglycaemic agents (sulphonylureas, biguanides, meglitinides, thiazolidinediones, dipeptidyl peptidase-4 inhibitors, glucagon-like peptide 1 analogue, α-glucosidase inhibitors) and insulin.

(Simultaneous treatment of complications like hypertension, obesity, dyslipidaemia, coronary heart disease, UTI, etc. should be taken into account).

Q. What are the complications of diabetes?

The life-history of diabetics is full of complications involving different organs/systems. The complications are:

Acute

- Hypoglycaemia
- Diabetic ketoacidosis (DKA)
- Hyperosmolar non-ketotic coma (HONK)
- Infections (due to low immunity e.g., urinary tract infection, tuberculosis, pneumonia)
- Acute circulatory failure
- Lactic acidosis (rare).

Late (or, chronic complications)

- Circulatory abnormalities (microangiopathy and macroangiopathy)
- Retinopathy (loss of vision, cataract, rubeosis iridis)
- Nephropathy (proteinuria, nephrotic syndrome, CRF, ESRD)
- Neuropathy (peripheral and autonomic neuropathy, diabetic amyotrophy)
- Gastrointestinal disorders (gastric atony, chronic pancreatitis)
- Dermatological complications (recurrent pruritus vulvae/balano-posthitis, diabetic dermopathy—Fig. 9.10)
- Recurrent infections (tuberculosis, herpes zoster, fungal infections—Fig. 9.11)
- Diabetic foot (non-healing ulcer, gangrene)
- *Others:* Emphysematous cholecystitis, malignant otitis externa, rhinocerebral mucormycosis, hypertriglyceridaemia, cardiomyopathy, musculoskeletal involvement ('Prayer sign'—Fig. 9.12).

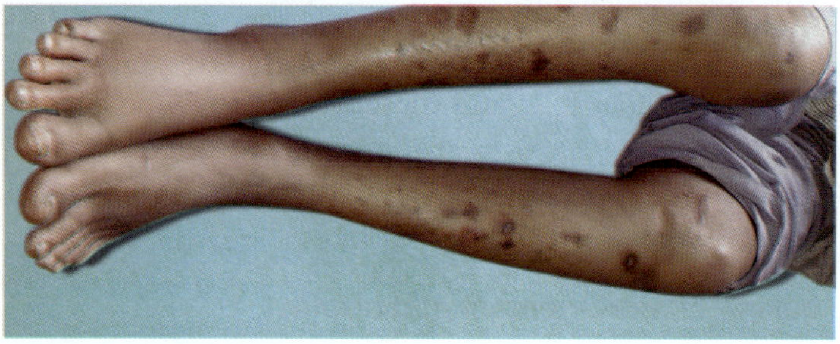

Fig. 9.10: Diabetic dermopathy (shin spots)—small rounded brown plaque which are hyperpigmented and scaly, and located over anterior tibial surface

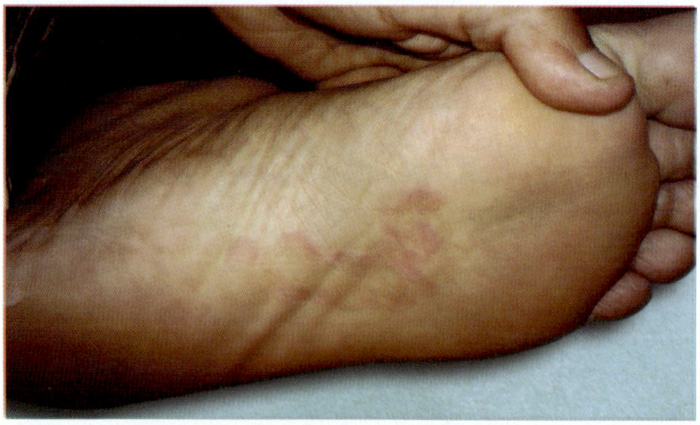

Fig. 9.11: Tinea pedis—ringworm (fungal) infection in sole of foot

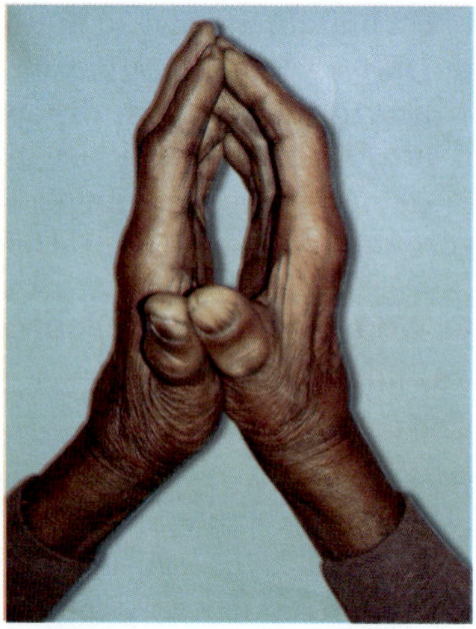

Fig. 9.12: Prayer sign—diabetic arthropathy affecting hands when the patient cannot appose the hands properly as in prayer

Q. How to differentiate hypoglycaemic coma from hyperglycaemic coma?

Coma in diabetes is due to hypoglycaemia, hyperglycaemia (DKA), HONK, CVA, renal failure or hepatic coma. In hypoglycaemic coma, blood sugar is usually <55 mg/dL. It is essential to differentiate hypoglycaemia from hyperglycaemia at the earliest. The differentiating points are:

Features	*Hypoglycaemic coma*	*Hyperglycaemic coma (i.e., diabetic ketoacidosis)*
1. History	Missing a meal, overdose of insulin or hypoglycaemic drugs, vigorous exercise	Missed insulin or hypoglycaemic drugs and/or infection/fever
2. Symptoms/signs	• Sweating, palpitation, hunger, tremor, dizziness, confusion	• Polyuria, thirst, vomiting, pain abdomen
	• Skin and tongue are moist	• Dry skin and tongue
	• Pulse: Normal or tachycardia	• Pulse: Weak
	• BP: Normal or high	• BP: Low
	• Breathing: Normal or shallow	• Breathing: Air hunger/Kussmaul's breathing
	• Jerks: Often brisk	• Jerks: Diminishes or absent
	• Plantar response: Bilaterally extensor	• Plantar response: Flexor
	• Smell: No smell of acetone	• Smell: Smell of acetone
3. Blood	Low sugar, pH normal	High sugar, pH low
4. Urine	Ketone bodies absent	Ketone bodies and sugar: Both are present

Q. What is diabetic microangiopathy and macroangiopathy?

The angiopathy in diabetes is of two types:

- *Microangiopathy (small vessel disease):* Retinopathy, nephropathy and neuropathy (altogether known as 'triopathy') are due to microangiopathy.
- *Macroangiopathy (large vessel disease):*
  - Coronary artery disease (angina pectoris, silent myocardial infarction, cardiomyopathy).
  - Cerebrovascular disease (cerebrovascular accidents or CVA).
  - Peripheral vascular disease [intermittent claudication, gangrene, impotence (on a vascular basis), diabetic foot].
  - Systemic hypertension.

Q. Metabolic syndrome (syndrome X): A short note.

The criteria (cluster of metabolic risk factors) minutely changes from country to country, association to association but the subsets remain same, and they are:

- Hypertension
- Hyperglycemia (fasting)
- Hypertriglyceridaemia
- Reduced high-density lipoprotein cholesterol (HDL-C)
- Abdominal obesity (increased waist circumference).

WHO criteria of metabolic syndrome require 'insulin resistance' to fulfil the criteria. **Insulin resistance** is clinically suspected at the bedside by the presence of acanthosis nigricans, skin tags (acrochordons), central obesity, lipodystrophy and features of polycystic ovarian disease (PCOD).

Decoding Abbreviations

GTT	Glucose tolerance test
IFG	Impaired fasting glucose
IGT	Impaired glucose tolerance
WHO	World Health Organisation.

Chapter 10

Haemopoietic (Lymphoreticular) System

Q. Discuss the common symptoms (chief complaints and H/o present illness) of haematological disorders.

Symptomatology	*Possible haematological disorder/s*
• Pallor/anaemia (weakness, palpitations, breathlessness, ankle oedema, dizziness)	Aplastic anaemia, lymphoma, leukaemias
• Enlargement of lymph nodes anywhere in body	Lymphoma, acute and chronic leukaemias
• Dragging pain in left upper abdomen	Massive splenomegaly e.g., chronic myeloid leukaemia, thalassaemia
• Epistaxis, gum bleeding, menorrhagia	Immune thrombocytopenic purpura (ITP), aplastic anaemia, acute leukaemias
• Haemarthrosis (collection of blood in the joint) or prolonged bleeding	Coagulation disorders e.g., haemophilia
• Haemorrhagic spots in skin or mucous membrane	Thrombocytopenia from ITP, leukaemias, aplastic anaemia, or vessel wall abnormalities (Henoch-Schönlein purpura/HSP)
• Skin rash	SLE with haematological aberration, lymphoma
• Fever	Leukaemias, lymphoma, infection with immuno-suppression
• Bone pain	Multiple myeloma, acute leukaemias
• Joint pain	Leukaemias, HSP
• Paraesthesia	Vitamin B_{12} deficiency
• Jaundice	Haemolytic anaemia
• Loss of body weight	Haematological malignancies (lymphoma, leukaemias)

Q. How to proceed to examine the haemopoietic (lymphoreticular/reticulo-endothelial) system?

The telegraphic outline of schematic examination is:

1. Anaemia (remember, jaundice may be looked for haemolytic anaemia).
2. Haemorrhagic manifestations into skin or mucous membrane (petechiae, purpura, ecchymosis, etc.)

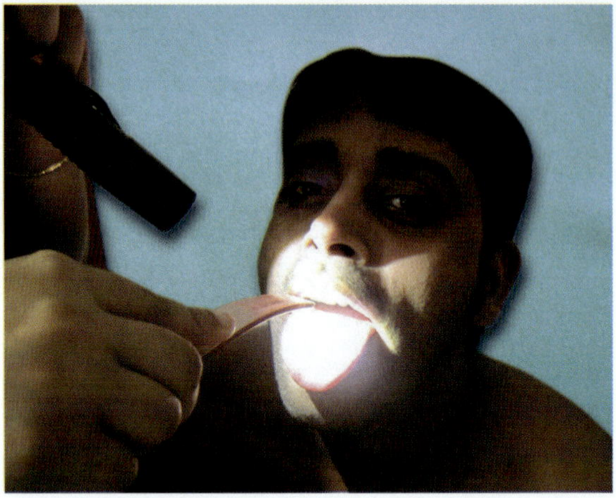

Fig. 10.1: The oral cavity is being examined with the help of spatula (tongue depressor) and torch

3. Oral cavity (gum bleeding, Waldeyer's ring in lymphoma, or any ulcer) (Fig. 10.1).
4. Lymph nodes all over the body (generalised lypmhadenopathy in lymphoma) (Fig. 10.2).
5. Liver and spleen (e.g., hepatomegaly in lymphoma, splenomegaly in thalassaemia, and absence of hepatosplenomegaly in aplastic anaemia or sickle cell anaemia).
6. Sternal tenderness.
7. Ophthalmoscopy (fundus of eye should be examined for retinal haemorrhage, papilloedema, etc).

*Read anaemia and lymphadenopathy from the section on 'General examination', and examination of liver and spleen from 'GI and hepatobiliary system'.

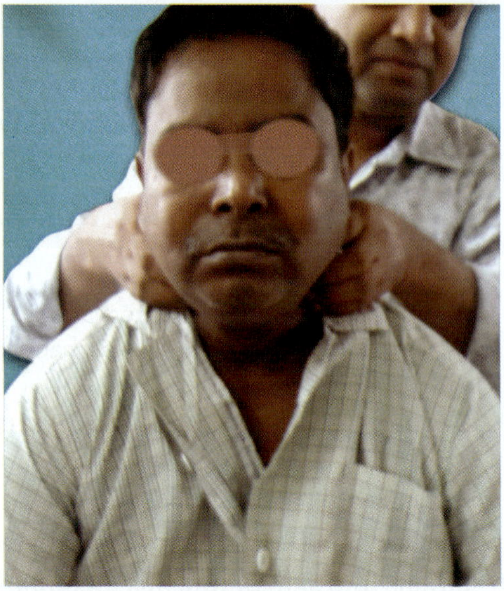

Fig. 10.2: Method of examination of neck glands from behind

Q. Clinically, what are the haemorrhagic spots (Fig. 10.3)?

Loosely, these haemorrhagic spots are known as 'purpuric spots'. They denote extravasation of blood into skin and mucous membrane, which *never blanches on application of pressure (applied by a pinhead or a glass slide)*. They are:

- Petechiae: 1–2 mm (tiny, pinhead)
- Purpura: 3–5 mm (a bit larger haemorrhagic spots)
- Ecchymosis or bruise: >5 mm large, confluent purpuric lesions
- Haematoma: Large haemorrhages in the skin with surface elevation.

Q. Can you classify purpuric spots or haemorrhagic spots?

They are classified as below:

- Thrombocytopenic (quantitative defects)—ITP, drug-induced (quinine, heparin, penicillins), aplastic anaemia, infections, SLE, SBE, acute leukaemias.
- Non-thrombocytopenic
  - Vessel wall abnormalities—HSP, infections (e.g., meningococcus), senile purpura, Cushing's syndrome, scurvy, uraemia, vasculitis.
  - Platelet functional defects (qualitative defects)—thrombasthenia or Glanzmann's disease.

NB: ITP (idiopathic/immune thrombocytopenic purpura) is an autoimmune disorder which leads to immune-mediated destruction of platelets. It is common in females and has two forms, acute and chronic.

Q. How to elicit 'sternal tenderness' (Fig. 10.4)?

Press the upper part of the body of sternum with the ball of the thumb for 2–3 seconds. If sternal tenderness is present, the patient winces with pain or shows facial grimace. Sternal tenderness is a vital clinical sign at the bedside, and is due to proliferation and hypercellularity of bone marrow, which is present in conditions like:

- Acute leukaemias (acute myeloid leukaemia/AML and acute lymphoblastic leukaemia/ALL)

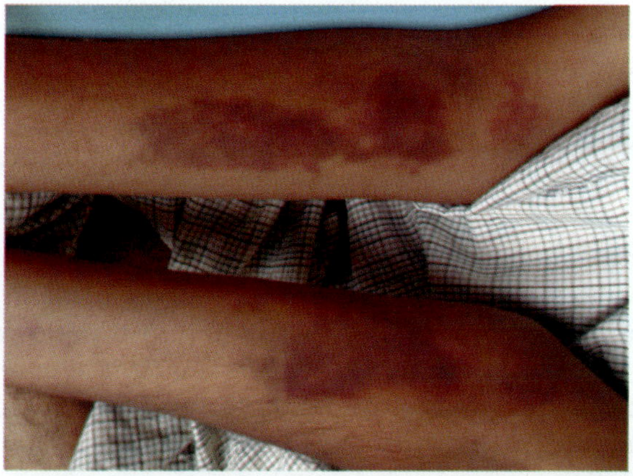

Fig. 10.3: Haemorrhagic spots—ecchymoses are seen in both forearms; few petechiae and purpura are also there

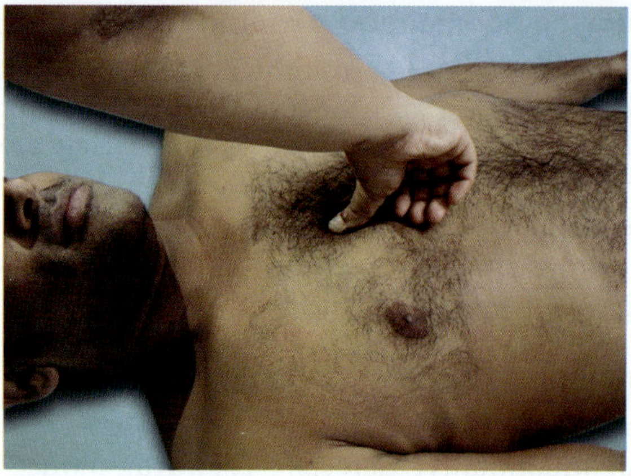

Fig. 10.4: Elicitation of sternal tenderness by pressing the upper part of the body of sternum by clinician's ball of the thumb

- Chronic myeloid leukaemia (CML)
- Severe anaemia due to any cause (except aplastic anaemia)
- Secondary metastasis in bones and multiple myeloma
- Rarely in osteomalacia and osteoporosis.

Q. What is aplastic/hypoplastic anaemia?

Hypocellular bone marrow with pancytopenia (simultaneous presence of anaemia + leucopenia + thrombocytopenia) is aplastic anaemia. It is diagnosed by:

- *Presence of precipitating factor:* Drugs (e.g., chloramphenicol), chemicals, radiation, congenital.
- *Features of anaemia:* Easy tiredness, vertigo, black-out, exertional dyspnoea, palpitations.
- *Features of leucopenia:* Fever with chill and rigor, sore throat (i.e., pain in the throat), features of depressed immunity (i.e., enhanced chance of infection).
- *Features of thrombocytopenia:* Bleeding manifestations into skin and mucous membrane like petechiae, purpura, ecchymosis; epistaxis and gum bleeding.

NB: Pancytopenia may be due to: Bone marrow failure, aplastic anaemia, bone marrow infiltration (e.g., carcinoma, multiple myeloma, acute leukaemias), ineffective haematopoiesis (e.g., megaloblastic anaemia) and peripheral destruction (e.g., hypersplenism).

Spleen is never enlarged in aplastic anaemia.

Q. What is megaloblastic anaemia?

Here, the red blood cells (RBC) count is low and the RBCs are larger in size. This is a macrocytic anaemia, and is commonly due to vitamin B_{12} and folic acid deficiency. Pernicious anaemia is a variety of megaloblastic anaemia where there is atrophy of gastric mucosa which leads to loss of parietal cells and thereby leading to deficiency of intrinsic factor resulting into disturbance in absorption of vitamin B_{12}.

Remember, iron deficiency anaemia is a microcytic anaemia.

Read *details of anaemia* from the section on 'General examination'.

Q. What is leukaemia? Classify leukaemias.

It is a progressive malignant disease of the haematopoietic stem cells where there is rapid overproduction of *abnormal or immature WBCs or leucocytes* in the bone marrow or peripheral blood.

Traditionally, leukaemias are classified into four main subsets:

- *Acute:*
  - Acute myeloid leukaemia (AML)
  - Acute lymphoblastic leukaemia (ALL)
- *Chronic*
  - Chronic myeloid leukaemia (CML)
  - Chronic lymphocytic leukaemia (CLL).

Most common variety of leukaemia is CLL. Loosely, leukaemias are called 'blood cancer' but common examples of *haematological malignancies* in a true sense are leukaemias, lymphoma and multiple myeloma.

Q. What are clinical manifestations in leukaemias?

- ***Acute:*** Symptoms result from bone marrow failure, or from organ infiltration with leukemic cells, or both. It is a sudden onset illness along with high fever, intermittent infections, anaemia, anorexia, weakness, loss of weight, haemorrhagic manifestations (Fig. 10.5) (e.g., gum bleeding, petechiae, purpura, etc.), gum hypertrophy (Fig. 10.6), hepatosplenomegaly, lymphadenopathy (more in ALL in comparison to AML) and presence of sternal tenderness. Children and young adults are affected mainly. The disease course is stormy and of short duration, if not diagnosed and treated early.
- ***Chronic:*** CML patients present in 30–80 years of age. They may be asymptomatic, or complains of dragging pain in left hypochondrium (as a result of massive

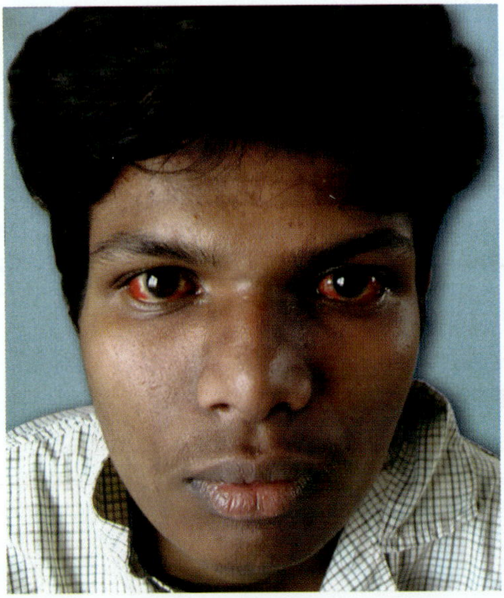

Fig. 10.5: Subconjunctival haemorrhage in acute leukaemia

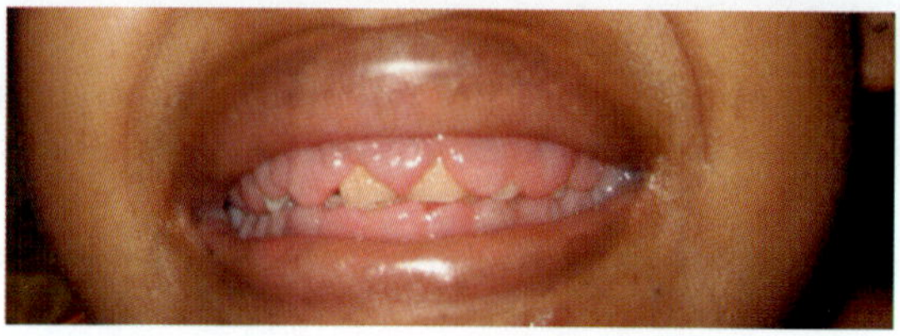

Fig. 10.6: Gum hypertrophy in acute myeloid leukaemia

splenomegaly), or presents with non-specific symptoms like loss of appetite, tiredness, loss of weight, anaemia and infections; sternal tenderness is present. There is presence of *Philadelphia chromosome* in blood, which is nothing but shortening of long arms of chromosome 22 due to balanced reciprocal translocation of genetic material with chromosome 9.

In CLL (peak age 65 years), the onset is insidious like CML where anaemia develops slowly. The patient presents with painless, firm and discrete lymphadenopathy (generalised); sternal tenderness is absent but moderate splenomegaly is present.

Q. What are myeloproliferative disorders?

In myeloproliferative disorders, there is uncontrolled clonal proliferation of one or more of the cell lines in the bone marrow, and are classified as:

- Chronic myeloid leukaemia (proliferation of WBC)
- Polycythemia vera (proliferation of RBC)
- Essential thrombocythemia (proliferation of thrombocytes)
- Myelofibrosis (excessive scar tissue forms in the bone marrow which impairs its ability to produce normal blood cells).

Q. What is thalassaemia?

It is an autosomal recessive disorder of haemoglobin production, where there is partial or total failure to synthesise a specific type of globin chain. Thalassaemia is of two types:

- *α-thalassaemia:* Reduction or absence of α-chain synthesis
- *β-thalassaemia:* Reduction or absence of β-chain synthesis (commonest variety).

Haemolytic anaemia is divided into hereditary and acquired (falciparum malaria, SLE, drugs like primaquine, eclampsia, lymphoma) types. Other than thalassaemia, other hereditary haemolytic anaemias are sickle cell anaemia, hereditary spherocytosis, haemoglobin E disease and G6PD deficiency.

Q. How thalassaemia patients present in a hospital?

The characteristic presentation of thalassaemia patients are:

- Young patient with positive family history (both the parents are thalassaemia minor or carrier).
- Anaemia (moderate to severe).
- Jaundice (mild).
- Stunted growth.

- Recurrent infections (commonly in the respiratory tract).
- Typical mongoloid facies (read 'Facies' in 'General examination').
- Splenomegaly (huge) and hepatomegaly (mild to moderate).
- May give past H/o repeated blood transfusions in different hospitals.

Q. Outline of treatment in thalassaemia.

A thalassaemia patient requires lifelong treatment and it is:

- *No oral or parenteral iron therapy to correct anaemia.*
- Transfusion therapy (repeated)—with a target Hb concentration of 9.5–10 g/dL. Previous target of therapy with hypertransfusion (Hb kept >10 g/dL) and supertransfusion (Hb kept >12 g/dL) is not popular nowadays.
- Iron chelation with desferrioxamine, if indicated.
- Folic acid 5 mg/day continued lifelong to replace the increased demand due to ineffective erythropoiesis. Antibiotics, as and when necessary, to treat infections.
- Splenectomy (in requirement of excessive blood transfusions, mechanical problems and features of hypersplenism) which is preceded by pneumococcal, *H. influenzae* and meningococcal vaccine.
- Definitive therapy: Allogenic bone marrow transplantation.
- Gene therapy with genetic counselling.

NB: Thalassaemia minor only requires folic acid (5 mg/day) therapy with genetic counselling.

Q. Normal haemoglobin pattern in an adult.

Normal haemoglobin	*Pattern/type*	*Structure*
Adult	• HbA (97%) • HbA_2 (1.5–3.5%) • HbF (<2%)	• $\alpha_2\beta_2$ • $\alpha_2\delta_2$ • $\alpha_2\gamma_2$

NB: At term, HBF (fetal haemoglobin) accounts for 70–90% of total haemoglobin. As charted in the table above, adults have <2% of HbF. In thalassaemia major, HbF increases enormously (thus, *haemoglobin electrophoresis which detects HbF >2% of total Hb confirms the diagnosis of thalassaemia*); in thalassaemia minor, HbA_2 is increased and helps in detection of thalassaemia carrier (e.g., blood test done during pre-marriage counselling).

Q. What is lymphoma?

They are heterogenous group of malignant diseases of lymphoreticular origin. The patient of lymphoma presents with fever, loss of weight, anorexia associated with generalised lymphadenopathy. The major types of lymphoma are Hodgkin's disease (HD) and non-Hodgkin's lymphoma (NHL). They are classified in the following subdivisions:

Hodgkin's disease (WHO pathological classification), which is a minor modification of previous Rye classification:

- Nodular lymphocyte-predominant HD
- Classical HD
  - Nodular sclerosis HD (commonest)
  - Mixed cellularity HD
  - Lymphocyte-rich HD
  - Lymphocyte-depleted HD (rare).

Non-Hodgkin's lymphoma

- Rappaport's classification:
  - Nodular (low grade and prognostically better)
  - Diffuse (high grade and prognostically worse)
- International Working Formulation:
  - High grade
  - Intermediate grade
  - Low grade.

NB: Clinical staging of lymphoma is done by **Ann Arbor staging classification** (especially HD; clinical staging is not very helpful in NHL as it disseminates frequently haematogenously throughout the body at the time of diagnosis).

Final diagnosis of lymphoma comes from lymph node biopsy (Fig. 10.7).

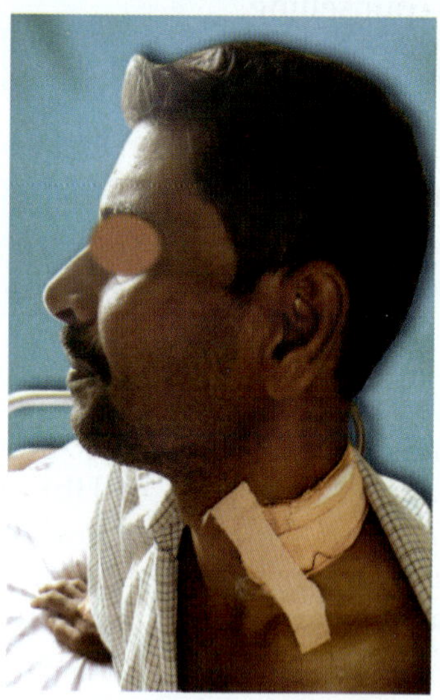

Fig. 10.7: Patient of lymphoma undergone lymph node biopsy from neck

Q. Basic differentiation of HD and NHL.

Features	*Hodgkin's disease*	*Non-Hodgkin's lymphoma*
• Age	Bimodal (15–35 yrs and >50 yrs). Less common (30%)	Any age. More common (70%)
• Lymph node involvement	Unifocal origin; 90% nodal, 10% extranodal; well localised at diagnosis	Multicentric origin; 60% nodal, 40% extranodal; widespread at diagnosis

• Anaemia	Late	Early
• B-symptoms*	Early and prominent	Late and non-prominent
• Lymph node character	Rubbery elastic feel, no matting	Variegated or firm feel, matted rarely
• Pel-Ebstein fever	May be present	Absent
• Pruritus	Common	Less common
• Involvement of:		
a. Waldeyer's ring and epitrochlear nodes	Less common	Common
b. Splenomegaly	More common	Common
c. GI tract and CNS involvement	Not common	Common
• Reed-Sternberg cell in histology of lymph nodes	Present (hallmark of diagnosis)	Absent
• Prognosis (outcome)	Cure rate is high	Cure rate is low

***B-symptoms:** Fever >38°C, drenching night sweats and 10% loss of body weight in previous 6 months. Characteristics of lymphadenopathy in HD and NHL are described in the section of 'Lymph nodes' in 'General examination'.

Q. How patient of multiple myeloma presents?

It is the neoplastic proliferation of plasma cells which infiltrate different tissues in the body along with the bone marrow. The patient is classically a male person in between 60 and 70 years of age, and presents with:

- Back pain (bone pain at the back is the commonest presentation)
- Weakness, wasting, pyrexia
- Syncope, vertigo, breathlessness as a result of severe anaemia
- Renal failure
- Recurrent respiratory tract infections
- Hyperviscosity syndrome (as a result of aggregation of IgM paraproteins, and is manifested by headache, bleeding gum, Raynaud's phenomenon, paraesthesia, CCF, fluctuating consciousness).

NB: An aged patient with back pain and pallor make the clinician suspicious of multiple myeloma. Diagnosis is done by the presence of any two of the following investigations like:

1. Monoclonal immunoglobulin, or light chains in blood or urine (done by protein electrophoresis)
2. Bone marrow infiltration with malignant plasma cells (by bone marrow biopsy)
3. Osteolytic bone lesions seen in skull, ribs or vertebrae (by radiology).

Q. What are 'bleeding disorders'?

Bleeding disorders are due to:

- ***Platelet disorders*** (quantitative diminution and/or qualitative defects in platelets): There is H/o gum bleeding (Fig. 10.8), epistaxis or bleeding from vagina along with presence of petechiae, purpura or ecchymosis. Bleeding occurs spontaneously or

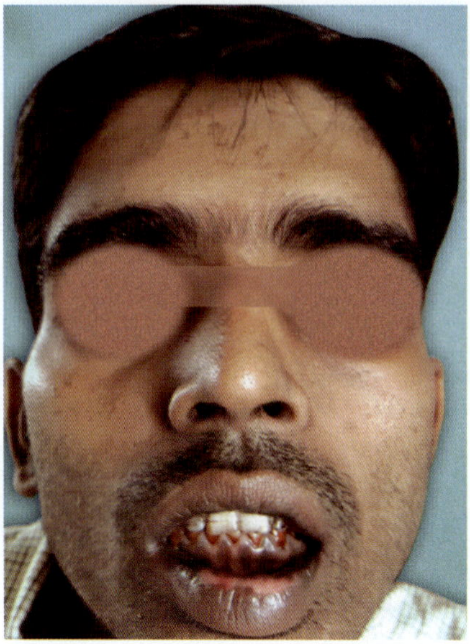

Fig. 10.8: Gum bleeding in thrombocytopenia (staining of teeth by blood is seen)

immediately after trauma and local pressure can stop bleeding. Bleeding time (BT) is prolonged but coagulation time (CT) remains normal, while platelet count may be diminished (in quantitative diminution).

- ***Coagulation disorders*** e.g., haemophilia or Christmas disease. Only affects males while females are the carriers. These are X-linked diseases with oblique transmission (uncle and nephew may be the sufferers). Bleeding occurs in viscera, muscles, retroperitoneum and joints; bleeding from nose, mouth, urinary tract may occur. Bleeding starts hours after trauma but notorious for persistence; local pressure can not stop bleeding. BT is normal while CT is prolonged with normal platelet count. Factor VIII or IX assay can confirm the diagnosis.
- ***Vessel wall abnormalities:*** Commonly seen in old age. This abnormality is common in HSP, infections (e.g., meningococcus), senile purpura, Cushing's syndrome or prolonged corticosteroid therapy, uraemia and vasculitis. Petechiae, purpura, and bleeding immediately after trauma is common; local pressure can stop bleeding. The BT is prolonged with normal CT and normal platelet count.

  Conditions like septicaemia or uraemia affect all the three abnormalities described above.

Q. Mention the major hazards of blood transfusion.

The hazards of blood transfusion are:

1. Febrile or pyrogen reaction with rigors
2. Allergic reactions
3. Haemolytic reactions
4. Thrombophlebitis
5. Circulatory overload (e.g., may be dangerous in a patient with heart failure)

6. Transmission of infections (e.g., hepatitis B and C, HIV, malaria)
7. Air embolism
8. Complications of massive transfusion (e.g., hypothermia, citrate intoxication)
9. Immunological sensitisation (e.g., Rh-isoimmunisation)
10. Transfusion-associated graft-versus-host disease (GvHD).

Q. Different blood components and products.

Recently, there is a trend that whole blood is rarely used for transfusions, rather transfusions are done by the of blood components. Blood components are prepared from single donations and they are:

1. *Blood components:* Red cell concentrate, granulocyte concentrate, platelet concentrate, fresh frozen plasma (FFP), cryoprecipitate (e.g., concentrate of factor VIII or vW factor).
2. *Blood products:* Albumin, coagulation factor concentrates and immunoglobulins are made from plasma.

Q. Describe about food rich in iron, folic acid and vitamin B_{12}.

- *Iron:* Liver, meat, poultry, seafood and fish; cereals, green leafy vegetables (e.g., spinach), nuts, peas, legumes and dried fruits (e.g., apricots). It is important to remember that cow's milk and breast milk are deficient in iron. Daily requirement in males: 0.5–1 mg/day, and in menstruating women: 1–3 mg/day.
- *Folic acid:* Fruits, green leafy vegetables and animal protein (e.g., liver, kidney, yeast). Daily requirement is 200 µg.
- *Vitamin B_{12}:* Meat, egg, kidney, liver, heart and dairy products; vegetables are deficient in vitamin B_{12} (*true vegetarian suffer from its deficiency*). Daily requirement is 1–2 µg.

NB: The so-called haematinics (nutrients required for the formation of blood cells) are iron, folic acid, and B_{12}.

Decoding Abbreviations

BT	Bleeding time
CT	Clotting or coagulation time
Hb	Haemoglobin
HD	Hodgkin's disease
NHL	Non-Hodgkin's lymphoma
SBE	Subacute bacterial endocarditis
SLE	Systemic lupus erythematosus
HSP	Henoch-Schönlein purpura
G6PD	Glucose-6-phosphate dehydrogenase.

Chapter 11

Musculoskeletal (Locomotor) System

Q. What is meant by musculoskeletal (MSK) system?

It is also known as *locomotor system* which provides support, stability and movement of the body. It is an organ system which is made up of bones (forming skeleton), muscles, cartilages, joints, ligaments, tendons and different other connective tissues.

Q. What are the common symptomatology in MSK disorders?

A. *Chief complaints:* Pain in joints (arthralgia), or pain and swelling in joints (arthritis) with onset and duration, axial (spine) or appendicular (peripheral) joints involved; large or small joints, single or multiple joints affected; fleeting (rheumatic arthritis), additive (rheumatoid arthritis) or intermittent (gout) joint involvement; whether associated with morning stiffness, muscle weakness, joint deformity, loss of appetite or loss of weight, fever, conjunctivitis, skin rash, oral or genital ulcer, dry mouth, alopecia, or lymphadenopathy.

B. *Past history:* Trauma, tuberculosis, dengue or chikungunya, bleeding diathesis (e.g., haemophilia), dysentery or UTI, sexual exposure, sore throat, miscarriage.

C. *Family history:* Tuberculosis, bleeding diathesis (e.g., haemophilia), ankylosing spondylitis, gout.

D. *Personal history:* Regarding dietary history, a patient of gout should be asked whether he is taking red meat, alcohol or seafood.

E. *Occupational history:* Should be taken into account (e.g., prolonged table work may initiate back pain).

F. *Obstetric history:* H/o foetal loss is common in anticardiolipin antibody syndrome.

Q. Mention a few terminologies to be decoded in MSK system.

- *Rheumatologist:* An internist or pediatrician with a special interest in rheumatology who treats musculoskeletal diseases i.e., disorders of the joints, muscles and ligaments, and systemic autoimmune disorders, commonly referred to as rheumatic diseases.
- *Arthralgia:* Subjective presence of joint pain only (no inflammation, no swelling).
- *Arthritis* (inflammation of the joint i.e., pain plus swelling of the joint)

- Monoarthritis: Affection of single joint
- Oligoarthritis or pauciarthritis: Affection of 2–4 joints
- Polyarthritis: Involvement of ≥5 joints.

- *Soft tissue rheumatism or periarthritis:* Involvement of joint capsule and periarticular structures like ligament, tendon, bursa, fascia, muscle, etc. (i.e., non-articular in origin); common examples are fibromyalgia, frozen shoulder, tennis elbow, carpal tunnel syndrome.
- *Enthesitis:* Inflammation of enthesis (i.e., the site of ligament, tendon, or articular capsule insertion into periosteum and bone), which is common in ankylosing spondylitis.

Q. How to examine a patient of MSK disorder?

The joints are examined simply by—'look, feel and move'.

- *Inspection:*
  - Number of joint or joints involved
  - Attitude of the limb, swelling, deformity
  - Signs of inflmmation over joints
  - Muscle wasting, skin changes
- *Palpation:*
  - Corroboration of the findings of inspection
  - Temperature, tenderness and swelling of the joints
  - Muscle power testing
- *Movements (passive and active both):*
  - Pain on movement; any grating sensation?
  - Restricted movement or increased mobility (e.g., hypermobile joint)
  - Any muscular spasm?
- *Measurements:*
  - Any shortening of limb
  - Thoracic and lumbar ankylosis (e.g., in ankylosing spondylitis)
  - Measure joint movement by goniometer
- Examination of spine (e.g., tenderness, kyphosis, scoliosis, lordosis)
- Examination of gait
- Systemic examination—fever, anaemia, hepatosplenomegaly, pleurisy, pericarditis, lymphadenopathy, etc.

Q. What are causes of mono-, oligo- and polyarthritis in clinical practice?

They are as follows:

- *Monoarthritis:* Septic arthritis (*Staphylococcus aureus*, *Neisseria gonorrhoeae*, Salmonella, etc.), crystal arthropathy (gout, pseudogout), tuberculous arthritis, osteoarthritis, trauma, SpA, haemarthrosis (from trauma or haemophilia), monoarticular flare of polyarticular disease, Charcot joint.
- *Oligoarthritis:* SpA, psoriatic arthropathy, gout, osteoarthritis, juvenile idiopathic arthritis (JIA), septic arthritis, oligoarticular flare of polyarticular disease.
- *Polyarthritis:* Rheumatoid arthritis, viral arthritis (e.g., Parvovirus B19, hepatitis B and C, chikungunya, rubella, HIV), SLE, psoriasis, chronic gout, JIA, ReA, rheumatic

arthritis (from acute rheumatic fever), generalised osteoarthritis, hypertrophic osteoarthropathy (e.g., from bronchogenic carcinoma), sarcoidosis, haemochromatosis (an iron storage disorder with tissue damage), SBE, Lyme disease (a tick-bite disease caused by bacterium *Borrelia burgdorferi*).

Q. What are common causes of arthralgia (pain in joints)?

Viral and bacterial/inflammatory (RA, SpA, SLE, systemic sclerosis or scleroderma)/ degenerative (osteoarthritis) joint disorders, gout, trauma (e.g., road traffic accidents), chronic pain disorders (e.g., fibromyalgia), hypermobile joints (Marfan's syndrome—Fig. 11.1) are common causes in clinical practice.

Q. What are common causes of myalgia (pain in muscles)?

Pyrexia (viral or bacterial infections), hypothyroidism, vitamin D deficiency, fibromyalgia, drug-induced (e.g., statins, triptans), polymyalgia rheumatica, myositis, dermatomyositis, muscle tear or haematoma, rhabdomyolysis (breakdown of damaged skeletal muscle) are very common causes.

Q. What are the common age and sex of arthritis?

Age and sex of a patient immensely help in clinical diagnosis in rheumatology like:

- *Age:*
  - Children: Haemophilia, JIA
  - Young: Gonococcal arthritis, trauma
  - Adults: SpA, ReA, SLE, RA (middle age), gout, psoriasis
  - Old age: Osteoarthritis.
- *Sex:* Majority of inflammatory arthritis are commoner in females except ankylosing sapondylitis, gout and ReA which are common in males.

Q. How diseases are differentiated by musculoskeletal pain?

Pain is the universal feature of MSK system. MSK diseases can be differentiated by taking a careful history and making a meticulous clinical examination, which may be added by selective laboratory tests to reach a provisional diagnosis. The approach should be:

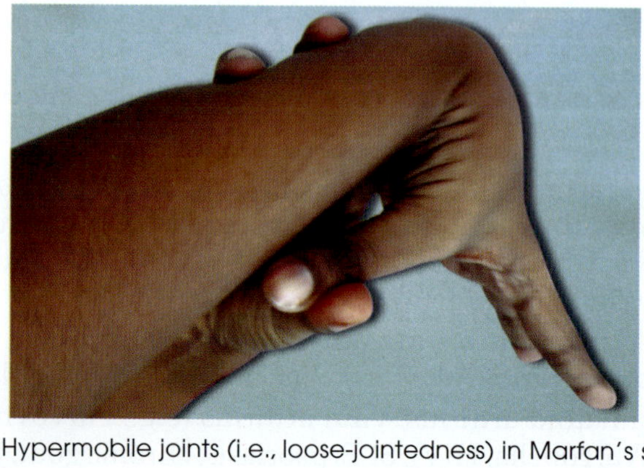

Fig. 11.1: Hypermobile joints (i.e., loose-jointedness) in Marfan's syndrome

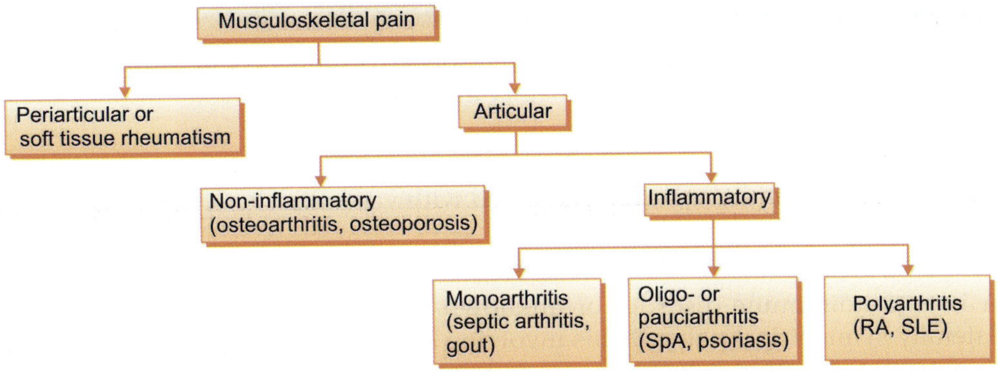

***Common terminologies:** RA—rheumatoid arthritis, SpA—spondyloarthropathy, SLE—systemic lupus erythematosus, ReA—reactive arthritis, MCP—metacarpophalangeal, MTP—metatarsophalangeal, PIP—proximal interphalangeal, DIP—distal interphalangeal, DMARD—disease-modifying anti-rheumatic drugs, NSAIDs—non-steroidal anti-inflammatory drugs, RF—rheumatoid factor, ANF—antinuclear factor, CRP—c-reactive protein.

Q. How to differentiate inflammatory from non-inflammatory arthritis?

At the bedside, it is differentiated by:

Features	*Inflammatory arthritis*	*Non-inflammatory arthritis*
• Early 'morning stiffness'	> 30 minutes	Absent
• On taking rest	Pain aggravates	Pain reduces
• On gentle use of joints	Symptomatic improvement	No such improvement
• Spontaneous flares (up-and-down course)	Common	Uncommon
• Constitutional symptoms like low-grade fever, night sweats, fatigue, loss of appetite and loss of weight	Present	Absent
• High ESR or CRP	Present	Absent

Q. What is 'Rheumatoid factor (RF)'?

Rheumatoid factors are antibodies [usually immunoglobulin (Ig) M or IgM] developed against Fc portion of IgG. RF is commonly found in different autoimmune disorders and chronic infections. RF is positive in approximately 70% cases of RA.

Q. What are seropositive and seronegative diseases?

Rheumatic diseases are divided according to presence or absence of RF:

- *Seropositive (i.e., RF positive):* Sjögren's syndrome, RA (70%), Felty's syndrome, SLE, systemic sclerosis, polymyositis and dermatomyositis, vasculitis.
- *Seronegative (i.e., RF negative):* SpA, gout, osteoarthritis, RA (30%), JIA (majority), rheumatic arthritis, Still's disease.

NB: RF may be positive in non-rheumatological diseases like fibrosing alveolitis, chronic hepatitis, syphilis, tuberculosis, leprosy, malignancy, and in normal population (5–20% females > 65 years).

Q. Prototype arthritis in rheumatology to be acquainted with.

1. *Rheumatoid arthritis (RA):* Inflammatory arthritis (seropositive or seronegative)
2. *Spondyloarthropathy (SpA):* Inflammatory arthritis (seronegative)
3. *Gout:* Crystal arthropathy
4. *Osteoarthritis:* Degenerative joint disease
5. Different autoimmune arthritis associated with vasculitis

Q. How a rheumatoid arthritis (RA) patient presents?

RA is an autoimmune disorder of unknown aetiology characterized by chronic, bilaterally symmetrical polyarthritis involving small and large joints with persistent synovitis, which ultimately gives rise to joint erosion, destruction and deformity resulting in gross disability of the patient (Fig. 11.2). Different extra-articular manifestations of RA are fever, weight loss, anaemia, pyoderma gangrenosum, pleural effusion, fibrosing alveolitis, pericarditis, conduction defects, episcleritis (Fig. 11.3), carpal tunnel syndrome, or amyloidosis.

MCP and PIP joints of hands are commonly involved (DIP joints are usually spared) and lumbosacral spines are not involved in RA.

Q. What is seronegative spondyloarthropathy (SpA)?

These are group of inflammatory arthritis which are characterised by inflammatory low back pain in addition to peripheral arthritis. They are diagnosed by the presence of:

- Asymmetrical oligoarthritis (lower limb >upper limb)
- Association with HLA-B27 allele

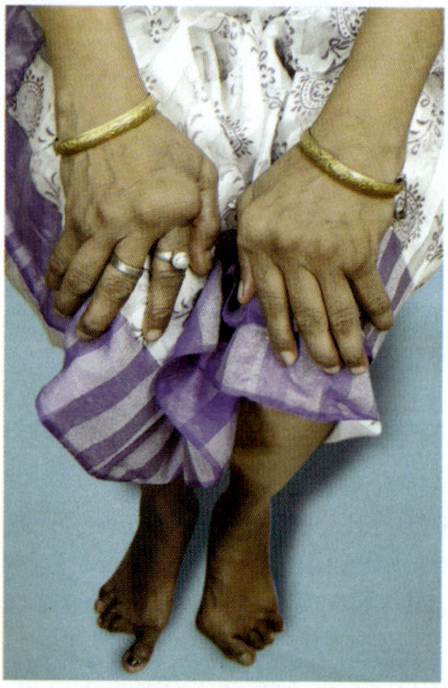

Fig. 11.2: Deformities in hand and feet in long-continued rheumatoid arthritis

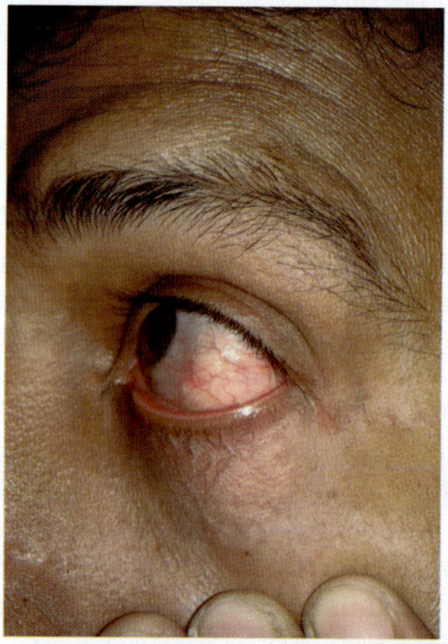

Fig. 11.3: Episcleritis in left eye in rheumatoid arthritis

- Sacroiliitis and/or inflammatory spondylitis
- Enthesitis
- Anterior uveitis (Fig. 11.4)
- The rheumatoid factor (RF) is persistently negative.

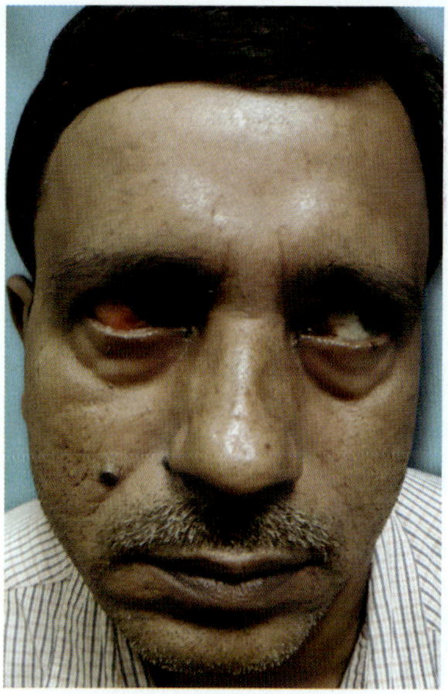

Fig. 11.4: Uveitis in right eye in spondyloarthropathy (i.e., ankylosing spondylitis)

SpA includes these five disorders:

1. ***Ankylosing spondylitis*** (M:F = 3:1, peak incidence in 2nd or 3rd decade with recurrent episodes of back pain which is marked in the morning; this inflammatory arthritis commonly affects the sacroiliac joint and spine (*axial involvement*), and ultimately progresses to bony fusion of the spine with marked stiffness in the body along with severe pain; there may be alternating buttock pain along with different *peripheral joint involvement*. Rest increases but exercise improves pain. There may be extra-articular manifestations like plantar fasciitis, Achilles tendonitis or aortic incompetence).
2. ***Reactive arthritis*** (previously known as Reiter's syndrome—Fig. 11.5): The classical triad of urethritis, conjunctivitis and arthritis following gastrointestinal (Salmonella, Shigella, Campylobacter or Yersinia-induced) or genitourinary (non-gonococcal urethritis or sexually acquired infection with Chlamydia) infection usually results in ReA. This inflammatory arthritis typically affects young men (or women), 1–3 weeks after an episode of bloody diarrhoea or sexual exposure with involvement of large joints of lower limbs. Circinate balanitis, keratoderma blennorrhagica (Fig. 11.6) and nail dystrophy are extra-articular manifestations.
3. ***Psoriatic arthropathy:*** The patients have psoriasis with different types of joint involvement like oligoarthritis, polyarthritis, involvement of DIP joints (Fig. 11.7), spondylitis (back pain) or mutilation of joints with deformity (arthritis mutilans).
4. ***Arthritis associated with inflammatory bowel diseases*** i.e., ulcerative colitis and Crohn's disease (known as enteropathic arthritis).
5. **Undifferentiated SpA.**

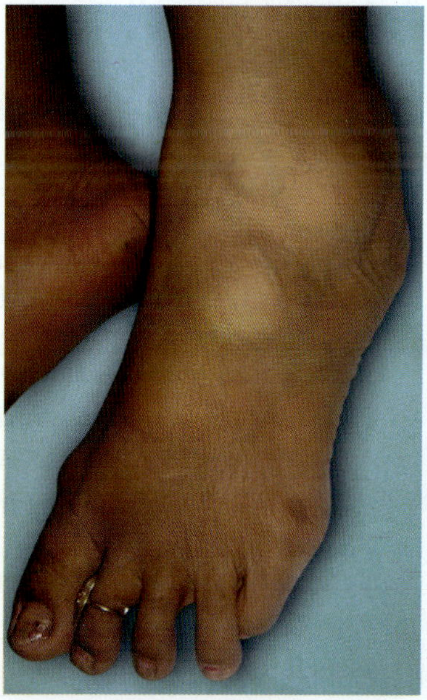

Fig. 11.5: Synovitis of the left ankle and tarsal joint in reactive arthritis

NB: According to a few rheumatologists, the sixth group is juvenile-onset SpA.

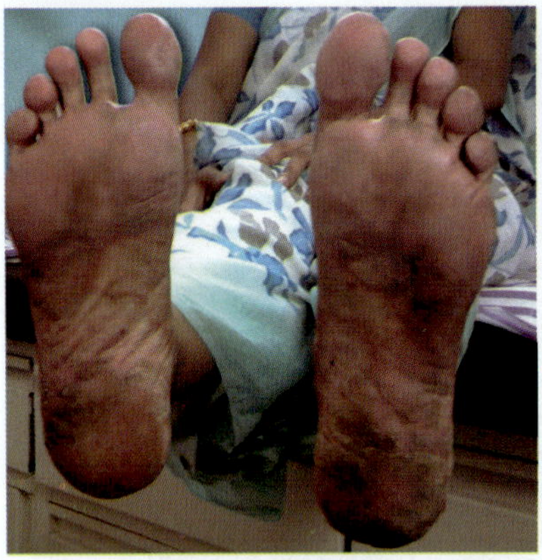

Fig. 11.6: Keratoderma blennorrhagica (painless red and raised pustules and plaques mimicking psoriasis) in soles in reactive arthritis (previous Reiter's syndrome)

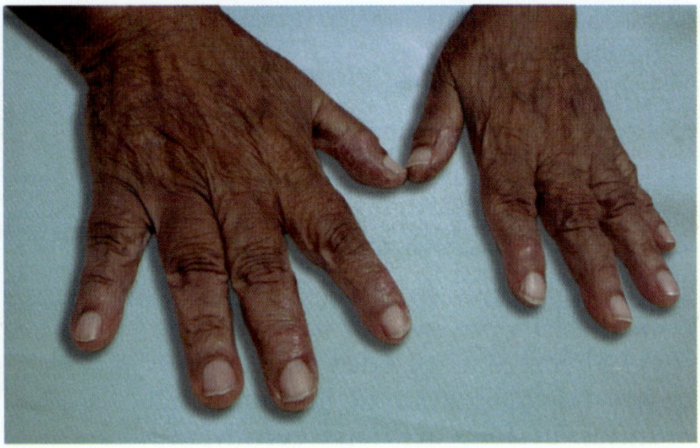

Fig. 11.7: Psoriasis with DIP joints involvement

Q. What is fleeting or migratory arthritis?

In *fleeting* arthritis when one joint is being affected, the inflammation of previous joint is subsided. But in *additive* arthritis, one fresh joint is involved over and above other involved joints (e.g., RA, ReA). Common causes of fleeting arthritis are:

1. Rheumatic arthritis i.e., from acute rheumatic fever (commonest).
2. Viral arthritis
3. SLE
4. Arthritis from inflammatory bowel disease (IBD), septicaemia, serum sickness.

Q. What is meant by collagen vascular disease (CVD) and connective tissue disorders (CTD)?

Though these two terms are pronounced in same breath, there is a minute difference like:

- CVDs are heterogenous group of autoimmune diseases characterised by presence of autoantibodies like SLE, RA, systemic sclerosis, polymyositis and dermatomyositis, mixed connective tissue disease (MCTD). Here collagen and blood vessels are affected and the disease is autoimmune in nature.
- CTD (affects the collagen tissues of the body):
  - *Autoimmune:* Same as CVDs
  - *Heritable:* Marfan's syndrome, Ehlers-Danlos syndrome, osteogenesis imperfecta.

Q. Synopsis of a few disorders/phenomenon.

- ***Felty's syndrome:*** A seropositive RA which is common in aged females and is associated with anaemia, neutropenia, thrombocytopenia and splenomegaly.
- ***Caplan's syndrome:*** It is seen in coal miners who is having RA with pneumoconiosis of the lung.

- ***Systemic lupus erythematosus (SLE):*** It is an inflammatory, autoimmune, multisystem disorder with arthralgia and skin rash as the most common clinical presentation. It virtually affects most of the systems in the body while renal and cerebral involvement pose serious problems. SLE is common in women of 20–40 years age group. Malar rash (butterfly rash in face—Fig. 11.8), discoid rash, photosensitivity, oral ulcers (commonly painless palatal ulcer—Fig. 11.9), arthritis/arthralgia, serositis (e.g., pleurisy or pericarditis), neurological (e.g., psychosis), renal (e.g., proteinuria), and haematological (e.g., leucopenia or thrombocytopenia) manifestations are common. The patient may present with 'pyrexia of unknown origin (PUO)'. The morbidity (refers to the distressed and unhealthy state of the individual) and mortality (the state of being subject to death) is high in SLE.

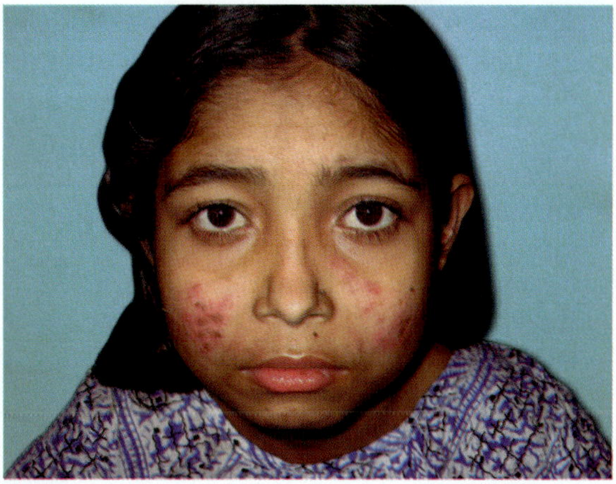

Fig. 11.8: Classical photosensitive butterfly rash over face with erythema and telangiectasia in SLE

- ***Gout*** (Fig. 11.10): It is a crystal-induced arthritis where monosodium urate (MSU) crystals are deposited in joints, tendons, bursa, etc. Gout is always associated with hyperuricaemia but all hyperuricamic patients do not suffer from gout. Acute gout usually affects the 1st MTP joint of the foot, especially after an alcoholic debauch (any joint may be affected) which is tremendously painful; if acute gout is not treated properly, the patient develops into chronic gout which may give rise to tophi formation (MSU crystal deposition in tendon, ligament or soft tissues) or renal involvement.
- ***Sjögren's syndrome:*** It is another autoimmune disease which affects the entire body. The patient presents with dry eyes (xerophthalmia), dry mouth (xerostomia),

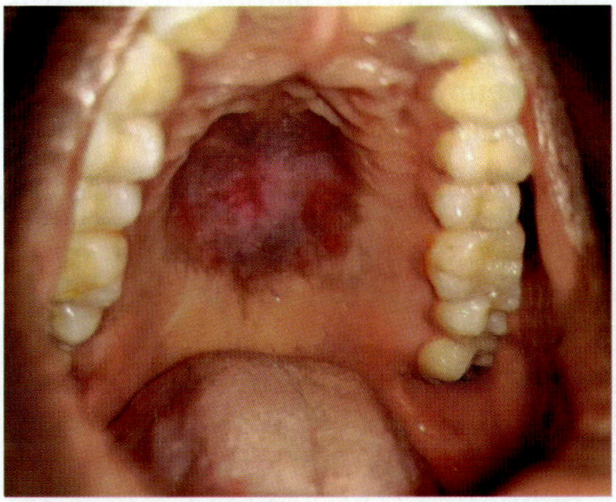

Fig. 11.9: Large palatal ulcer in SLE, which is usually painless

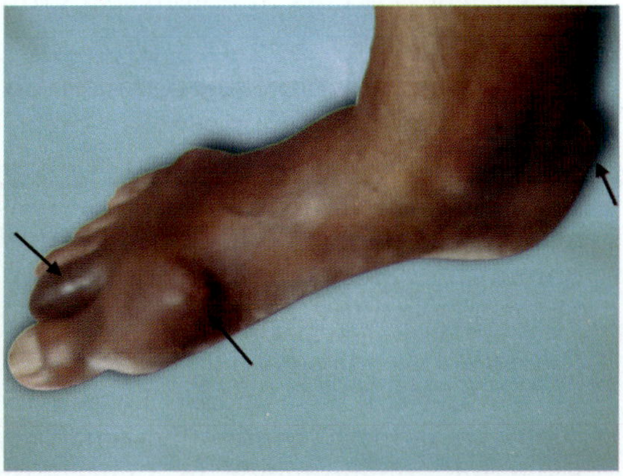

Fig. 11.10: Gout—arrows from left to right point blackening of toe, affection of 1st metatarsophalangeal joint and Achilles tendonitis respectively due to deposition of tophi

myalgia, arthralgia and fatigue. Older women are commonly affected. Bilateral parotid swelling may be a presenting feature. There is an increased chance of development of lymphoma.

- ***Osteoarthritis:*** It is the commonest form of arthritis in clinical practice and is usually regarded as a degenerative process due to ageing. Now it is thought that some amount of inflammation is also present in its pathology which affects the cartilage, subchondral bone, meniscus, ligaments, synovium and capsule of the joint. It may affect any weight-bearing joint but in India, knee joint is commonly affected while hip joint involvement is seen in western world. DIP joints of hands are commonly involved (Fig. 11.11). As there is no definite treatment of this disease, it is the commonest cause of disability in the older population.

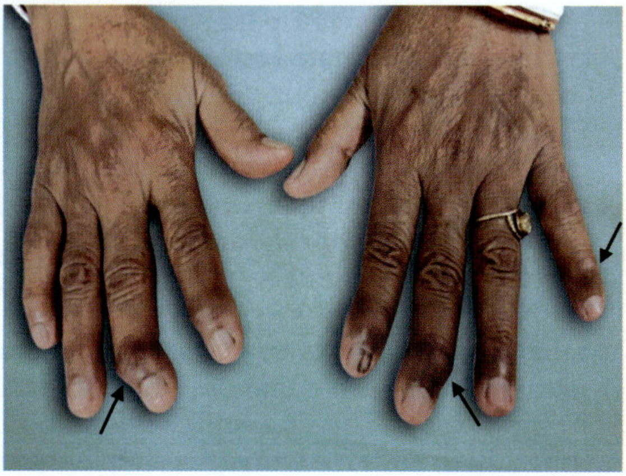

Fig. 11.11: Heberden's nodes are seen in distal interphalangeal (DIP) joints in osteoarthritis; some sort of deformity has developed

- ***Osteoporosis:*** It is defined as low bone density, which results in a micro-architectural deterioration of bone tissue and leads to increased bone fragility with enhanced risk of fracture. Common risk factors are female sex, post-menopausal women, prolonged immobilisation, CRF, diabetes, drugs (e.g., heparin), increasing age and smoking. Osteoporosis is being treated by calcium, vitamin D, bisphosphonates and recombinant human parathyroid hormone.
- ***Osteomalacia:*** It is the defective mineralization of newly formed bone matrix due to vitamin D deficiency in an adult; the patients may have bone pain (bone tenderness too) and muscle weakness. When this defective mineralization (as a result of vitamin D deficiency) occurs in epiphyseal growth plate in children before puberty, it is known as rickets.
- ***Fibromyalgia:*** It is one of the common soft tissue rheumatism. The disease is common in females who complain of widespread body pain, ongoing tiredness and tender points detectable on application of pressure on their muscles. The disease is often associated with irritable bowel syndrome (IBS), migraine, dysmenorrhoea, tension headache, etc. The diagnosis is clinical and is commonly due to disturbed or unrefreshing sleep. The disease is due to 'abnormal pain perception' by the patient. The response to treatment is unsatisfactory.
- ***Raynaud's phenomenon*** (Fig. 11.12): It is a vasospastic disorder, manifested clinically by 'triphasic colour response' i.e., sequential development of pallor, cyanosis and rubor (i.e., redness), commonly seen in fingers and toes. Exposure to cold precipitates Raynaud's phenomenon in a susceptible individual. The common causes are scleroderma, SLE, thoracic inlet syndrome, hyperviscosity syndrome (e.g., multiple myeloma), and ergot or β-blocker-induced. It is being treated by different vasodilators.

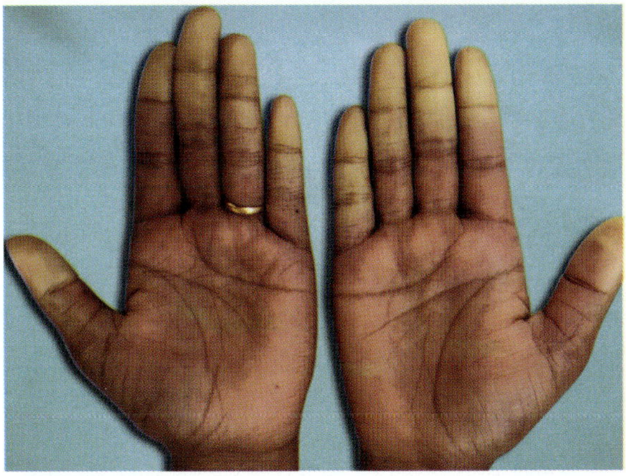

Fig. 11.12 Raynaud's phenomenon—it is characterised by 'tiphasic colour response' with sequential development of blanching, cyanosis and redness of fingers and toes; blanching reaction is pronounced in this patient of systemic lupus erythematosus (SLE)

Q. What are the common blood tests done in rheumatology?

Common blood tests done in rheumatology are TC and DC (total count and differential count), ESR, CRP, RF, anti-CCP (antibody to cyclic citrullinated peptide; found in RA), ANA (antinuclear antibody; found in SLE), ANCA (anti-neutrophil cytoplasmic antibody; found in Wegener's granulomatosis), ASO titre (antistreptolysin O, found in acute rheumatic arthritis), anti-ds DNA (antibody to double stranded DNA; common in SLE) and HLA-B27 (positive in spondyloarthropathies). Moreover, serum uric acid, calcium and phosphate level, alkaline phosphatase and 25-OH vitamin D level help in diagnosis.

Q. What are NSAIDs, DMARDs and biologics?

- *NSAIDs (non-steroidal anti-inflammatory drugs):* These are the common pain relievers. They are divided into COX-1 and COX-2 inhibitors (COX is cyclooxygenase enzyme). Cox-2 inhibitors (i.e., coxibs) are safer than cox-1 inhibitors so far as gastric and renal toxicities are concerned. The examples of cox-1 inhibitors are ibuprofen, diclofenac, indomethacin, etc.
- *DMARDs (disease-modifying anti-rheumatic drugs):* The common drugs are methotrexate, hydroxychloroquine, sulphasalazine, leflunomide, etc. They are used in persistent inflammatory synovitis present in different autoimmune diseases.
- *Biologics:* These are revolutionary drugs to treat autoimmune diseases when traditional DMARDs fail. The common drugs used are TNF-α blockers (etanercept, infliximab, adalimumab), abatacept (selective T-cell co-stimulation modulator), rituximab (anti-CD 20) and tocilizumab (interleukin-6 inhibitor). These drugs are used parenterally and are more expensive than DMARDs. Recently, an oral biologic [janus kinase (JAK) inhibitor] has been introduced for treatment of RA i.e., tofacitinib.

Decoding Abbreviations

MCTD	Mixed connective tissue disease
HLA	Human leucocyte antigen.

Index

Reader's Notes

Reader's Notes